Transgender and Gender Nonconforming Health and Aging

Cecilia Hardacker • Kelly Ducheny
Magda Houlberg
Editors

Transgender and Gender Nonconforming Health and Aging

Springer

Editors
Cecilia Hardacker
Howard Brown Health Centre
Chicago, IL
USA

Kelly Ducheny
Howard Brown Health Center
Chicago, IL
USA

Magda Houlberg
Rush University College of Nursing
Howard Brown Health Centre
Chicago, IL
USA

ISBN 978-3-319-95030-3 ISBN 978-3-319-95031-0 (eBook)
https://doi.org/10.1007/978-3-319-95031-0

Library of Congress Control Number: 2018959627

This Springer imprint is published by the registered company Springer Nature Switzerland AG
The registered company address is: Gewerbestrasse 11, 6330 Cham, Switzerland

To all the fierce TGNC people we have lost, too soon and too many.

To those resilient TGNC pioneers who endeavor to live respected, authentic, and fulfilled lives and who provide resources and support for generations that follow.

To all TGNC people who choose to live privately or cannot live publicly for any reason.

To all the TGNC communities that advocate for, support, and elevate their members.

To the reader whose desire to deepen the affirmative care provided to the TGNC community will surely help improve the quality of their lives.

Foreword

This book was created to offer providers and health-care teams better knowledge and insight needed to provide affirmative, respectful, and personalized care to transgender and gender non-conforming (TGNC) older adults. Specialized skills and awareness are required to partner with TGNC older adults to best support their holistic health, given the unique needs of this remarkably diverse and growing population. The ability to provide such affirmative and informed care is a national imperative and a matter of life and death.

The editors worked hard to bring together a wide range of contributing authors with diverse identities to speak to the provision of holistic, community-driven care for older TGNC people from multidisciplinary perspectives. The authors come from a range of gender identities, races, sexual orientations, ages, lived experiences, and socioeconomic (SES), geographic, and professional backgrounds. For the culminating chapter of the book entitled *VOICES*, TGNC older adults were invited to share their stories and speak directly to the provider and care team readers, offering their personal perspectives on the care they have received and the guidance they would like to offer their caregivers. The insight they offer is broad and distinct, in their own words and stemming from their individual experiences.

We begin the book with the *Essentials* chapter that explores concepts that are critical to understanding the experience of TGNC people, useful terminology, and culturally sensitive skills for care provision. The *Essentials* chapter helps readers begin a process of personal introspection and knowledge acquisition to develop a framework for intentional, affirming communication with TGNC older adults. Reading the *Essentials* chapter before moving deeper into the book is strongly recommended, since it allows the reader to anchor knowledge learned in the later chapters upon *Essentials* frameworks.

The editors asked that the authors strive to integrate their experience and knowledge with the existing literature and research, offering best practices and insight for providing care to TGNC older adults. It is our hope that readers will take this information, apply it, and share it widely. It is also our hope that this book will inspire innovation and future models of care, progressively improving the affirmative, community-driven care provided to and with the TGNC older adult community. Readers are reminded that while this book offers potential patterns, treatment approaches, health-care needs, barriers, and resiliencies, TGNC older adults do not share a universal narrative or life experience, but instead should be treated as unique, vibrant individuals.

TGNC aging presents us with a spectrum of lived experiences. Some older adults socially and/or medically transition in older adulthood, while others enter older adulthood having transitioned earlier in life. No two journeys are the same. Years of experiencing discrimination presents a different struggle than delaying one's transition. Both deserve affirming care and attention, and we have made space in this anthology for as many stories from TGNC older adults as possible.

Throughout the book we asked authors to use the term "TGNC" to include all people whose gender identity does not align with their sex assigned at birth, including gender queer, gender fluid, non-binary, third gender, two spirit, gender fabulous, gender questioning, gender non-conforming, and transgender people. There are some exceptions where specific reported research made use of other terminology. "TGNC" was used to maintain consistency within the book, understanding that not everyone would use this term to describe themselves. We intend its use respectfully to include a wide variety of identities and lived experiences under its umbrella.

TGNC older adults have long sought affirming care from community health centers like Howard Brown Health and others, primarily in urban areas. The search for comprehensive care across the lifespan motivates TGNC people to pursue centers of excellence, sometimes traveling long distances and across the nation to urban centers, seeking evidence-based, gender affirming care. Howard Brown is deeply committed to providing affirmative, respectful, and personalized care to the TGNC community. We are honored by the choice of many TGNC people to receive their care at our health center and feel an urgent sense of responsibility and obligation to share what we have learned to create a wider range of competent healthcare options for the community.

Howard Brown envisions a future where the health and wellness of TGNC people is affirmed with health care as a human right, where progressive social policy and enlightened societal norms uplift the lives of TGNC people and their families, and where affordable, accessible, and culturally competent care from non-judgmental healthcare professionals is available and provided to all who seek it. This book is part of our contribution to furthering that vision.

Contents

Contributors

Stacy Agosto, LCSW Behavioral Health Services, Howard Brown Health Center, Chicago, IL, USA

Zyer Beatty, M.Ed Department of Counseling and Human Development Services, University of Georgia, Atlanta, GA, USA

Mark Brennan-Ing, PhD Brookdale Center for Healthy Aging, Hunter College, The City University of New York, New York, NY, USA

Rory Meyers College of Nursing, New York University, New York, NY, USA

Sand Chang, PhD Department of Health Promotion and Behavior, University of Georgia, Atlanta, GA, USA

Jules Chyten-Brennan, DO Montefiore Medical Center, Bronx, NY, USA

Claire Niemet, MPH Parkinson's Disease and Movement Disorders Program, Rush University Medical Center, Chicago, IL, USA

Loree Cook-Daniels, MS FORGE, Inc., Milwaukee, WI, USA

Kelly Ducheny, PsyD Behavioral Health Services, Howard Brown Health Center, Chicago, IL, USA

Cecilia T. Hardacker, MSN, RN, CNL Howard Brown Health Center, Chicago, IL, USA

Ruben A. Hopwood, MDiv, PhD The Danielsen Institute, Boston University, Medical Department, Fenway Health, Boston, MA, USA

Magda Houlberg, MD, AAHIVS, CMO Medical Services, Howard Brown Health Center, Chicago, IL, USA

Jacqueline Boyd, BS, CEO The Care Plan, Chicago, IL, USA

Katt Ross, LSW Social Services, Howard Brown Health Center, Chicago, IL, USA

Kelly Rice, MPH Social Services, Howard Brown Health Center, Chicago, IL, USA

Alix Komar, MD, FACOG Weiss Hospital, Chicago, IL, USA

Adam M. Messinger, PhD Justice Studies Department, Northeastern Illinois University, Chicago, IL, USA

Tatyana Moaton, MBA-HRM Human Resources, Howard Brown Health Center, Chicago, IL, USA

Channyn Parker Youth Development, Howard Brown Health-Broadway Youth Center, Chicago, IL, USA

Kristen E. Porter, PhD, Mac, Lac Zen Executive LLC, Boston, MA, USA

Kristin Reitz, LCSW Behavioral Health Services, Howard Brown Health Center, Chicago, IL, USA

Jennifer Roark, PhD, MSW Department of Sociology, Social Work, and Anthropology, Utah State University, Logan, UT, USA

Vanessa Sheridan, BA Center on Halsted, Chicago, IL, USA

Anneliese A. Singh, PhD Department of Counseling and Human Development Services, University of Georgia, Atlanta, GA, USA

Greg Storms, MA Center on Halsted, Chicago, IL, USA

K. Tajhi Claybren, A.M Behavioral Health Services, Howard Brown Health-Broadway Youth Center, Chicago, IL, USA

Hector Torres, PsyD Center on Halsted, Chicago, IL, USA

Natalia Truszczynski, MPH Department of Health Promotion and Behavior, University of Georgia, Atlanta, GA, USA

Lindsay White, MPH Department of Health Promotion and Behavior, University of Georgia, Atlanta, GA, USA

The Essentials: Foundational Knowledge to Support Affirmative Care for Transgender and Gender Nonconforming (TGNC) Older Adults

1

Kelly Ducheny, Cecilia T. Hardacker, K. Tajhi Claybren, and Channyn Parker

1.1 Introduction

Long before the word "transgender" was introduced into our vocabulary, there existed a constellation of individuals who have always been a foundational part of what is known today as the lesbian, gay, bisexual, transgender, and queer (LGBTQ) community. This unique set of soldiers, both known and unknown, spanning oceans and time, have been erased and unwritten throughout history by the patriarchal pen. Transgender and gender nonconforming (TGNC) people have long stood at the forefront of battles for liberation and equality. With this book, we pay homage to and salute our community's most valuable resource, our TGNC elders.

In the last 15 years, there has been an explosion of research [3], literature, media, and publication about TGNC identities, TGNC people, and the new frontier of affirmative health care [41, 72]. TGNC voices and identities have reached mainstream society and professional networks in new ways, with TGNC voices amplified and role models visible. Much of the exposure has highlighted TGNC people as an "emerging" population, with deep focus on youth who are exploring TGNC

K. Ducheny (✉)
Behavioral Health Services, Howard Brown Health Center, Chicago, IL, USA
e-mail: kellyd@howardbrown.org

C. T. Hardacker
Howard Brown Health Center, Chicago, IL, USA
e-mail: ceciliah@howardbrown.org

K. Tajhi Claybren
Behavioral Health Services, Howard Brown Health-Broadway Youth Center, Chicago, IL, USA
e-mail: kTajhiC@howardbrown.org

C. Parker
Youth Development, Howard Brown Health-Broadway Youth Center, Chicago, IL, USA
e-mail: channynp@howardbrown.org

M. Houlberg et al. (eds.), *Transgender and Gender Nonconforming Health and Aging*, https://doi.org/10.1007/978-3-319-95031-0_1

identities [63] and TGNC adults in their 20s or 30s. Much less attention has been focused on TGNC older adults' unique life experiences, resiliency, and challenges.

Less attention has been focused on TGNC older adults because of ageist invisibility and the rarity of a TGNC person surviving into older adulthood. It is frequently stated by members of the TGNC community that TGNC people have an average lifespan of 30–35 years [62], although no demographic evidence can be cited. TGNC community members are accorded elder status in their 30s and 40s. To emerge into their 50s, 60s, or 70s as older adults, TGNC people must have survived hate, violence, and attempted murder, suicide and depression, limited access to education, housing, and employment, systematic oppression, a profound lack of health care, and constant risk of exposure and expulsion in a transphobic world [71]. Survival of TGNC older adults is a testament to their resilience, creativity, determination, resourcefulness, and perseverance [32].

TGNC people make up 0.53% of the US population, of those a greater number are transwomen (0.28%) compared to transmen (0.16%) or gender nonconforming people (0.08%) [20]. Other research estimates the percentage of TGNC people as low as 0.3% in North Dakota and as high as 0.8% in Hawaii with only 0.5% of the total over the age of 65 [26]. Data collection is limited by survey question inconsistency and lack of viewing gender on a continuum [34] or gender spectrum that includes queer and non-binary identities.

With an increase in culturally adept, affirmative health care, and a broadening awareness and acceptance in mainstream society, more TGNC people will have the opportunity to grow into older adulthood. Increasing the number of TGNC older adults and improving their quality of life will evolve the essence and depth of TGNC communities, preserving knowledge and connection, and intergenerational networks and support, interrupting the erasure and silencing of the TGNC community. TGNC communities themselves are learning how to age and what it means to be an older adult, since many TGNC people have never seen living into older adulthood as a possibility. While most care systems are unprepared to provide affirmative, respectful health care to TGNC elders [41], the need is extremely high given TGNC people's low access to affirmative care for decades of their lives and their understandable hesitance to approach health care, given previous, consistent experiences in transphobic and damaging care systems [36].

An understanding of the compelling need for affirmative care is necessary but not sufficient for the provision of affirming, adept, and effective care for TGNC people. In addition to an understanding of need, health-care professionals must develop knowledge, skills, and attitudes that support affirmative service provision [36]. Such knowledge, skills, and attitudes are created in progressive layers, with a foundational infrastructure of cultural sensitivity providing a frame upon which more specialized intervention skills are built across time. This chapter is designed to offer the foundational knowledge a reader will need to understand and apply information found in the following chapters. The following chapters in this book are written at an intermediate or advanced level and presume that the reader has intentionally digested and learned the essential information presented below.

To understand and apply the content of this book, health-care professionals must take initiative to gather, digest, and incorporate learning that isn't taught in most training programs or available in most care settings [36]. Without this learning, even well-intentioned care professionals will do damage, interrupt affirmative care, and fail to establish trust with TGNC older adults that is pivotal to their engagement and participation in health care [3, 36]. While this learning can be personally challenging, it will deepen the care you can provide for TGNC people and for all people you serve by extension. The information in this chapter is an introduction; it is not exhaustive, but it is a critical starting point. Thank you for taking the next steps to deepen your understanding about TGNC people and improve the care you can offer to the TGNC older adult community.

1.2 Learning the Basics

This section will offer basic constructs and terminology that are pivotal when working with TGNC older adults. The goal is to provide the reader with foundational understanding of gender identity, gender expression, and sexual orientation and offer valuable insight into TGNC people's lives that is essential to providing care to TGNC older adults.

1.2.1 Gender Identity and Gender Expression

When born, children are assigned a sex of either male (M) or female (F) based on observed reproductive anatomy. Children who are born with a penis receive a male *gender marker* of "M"; children born with a vagina receive a female gender marker of "F" [3]. That gender marker is listed on the child's birth certificate. Children who are *intersexed* (born with ambiguous physical characteristics of both sexes) are assigned either a male or female sex and then may undergo unnecessary surgery to align body parts with the assigned sex [36, 47]. The government, society, health-care and school systems, and the child's parents have traditionally assumed that all children with a *female sex assigned at birth* will grow up to be women and all children with a *male sex assigned at birth* will grow up to be men. It has been assumed that people are *cisgender*, in other words, that people's sex assigned at birth was automatically identical to their *gender identity* – which is their personal felt experience of gender, of being male, female, a combination of male and female, or a unique blend of those genders [3]. It was also assumed that gender was *binary* [3] and that there are only two ways to experience gender either as a girl/woman or as a boy/man.

These assumptions have been proven wrong. Research has demonstrated that a significant number of people are *transgender or gender nonconforming (TGNC)* [20], an umbrella term to describe people whose sex assigned at birth is not aligned with their gender identity [3]. In addition, research has shown that people experience a wide range of gender identities, with gender identity being a spectrum [33, 52] rather than a binary option of either boy/man or girl/woman [3, 5, 41]. How a person externally expresses their gender identity is called their *gender expression* [3]. Each person has a unique way of expressing their gender identity which can include, but is not limited to, how people dress, their hair length/style, wearing jewelry or make up, chosen names and pronouns, self-portraits, gender markers on identification and birth certificate, the way a person moves, acts or speaks, and other aspects of physical presentation. A person's gender expression can evolve and change across time. A person's gender identity can never be predicted based on outward appearance [3]. Some TGNC people may select not to express their true gender identity due to comfort level, issues of safety, or ongoing identity evolution and development. Regardless of outward expression, a person's gender identity should always be honored and respected.

1.2.2 Sexual Orientation and Gender Identity

The "LGBT" acronym implies that lesbian, gay, bisexual, and transgender people are the same, grouped for affinity and identity [36]. This is not accurate. *Sexual orientation* refers to a person's openness to or desire for emotionally, romantically, and sexually intimate relationships with different types of other people [2, 3]. A person's sexual orientation can be lesbian, gay, bisexual, heterosexual, queer, pansexual, or asexual [3]. Gender identity, in turn, refers to an individual's internal felt sense of gender [3]. TGNC people can have any sexual orientation. This can be confusing because, in the past, sexual orientation was identified based on each person's sex assigned at birth. Given our evolving knowledge of gender, best practice is to use each person's gender identity (not sex assigned at birth) to describe sexual orientation. For example, a *transgender man* (assigned female sex at birth, male gender identity) who is only attracted to men would be gay, while a *transgender woman* (assigned male sex at birth, female gender identity) who is only attracted to men would be heterosexual. To best support TGNC people, allow them to share important information pertaining to sexual partners and sexual behaviors as TGNC communities include all sexual orientations.

1.2.3 Transition

Transition is the process of aligning a TGNC person's gender expression with their self-identified gender identity [3]. The process of transitioning can include medical, social, and legal changes that support a TGNC person to actualize and share their gender identity. Medical transition can include hormone therapy, surgery, and a range of medical procedures that physically alter the body to align it more closely with a person's gender identity [16]. Social transitioning can include sharing a TGNC identity with family, friends, and people in community, asking others to use gender pronouns or a chosen name that align with gender identity, and dressing/

grooming in ways that align with gender identity [49]. Legal transition can include changing a person's legal name or gender marker and revising the gender marker or name on legal documents (social security card, birth certificate, passport, insurance card, state ID or driver's license, credit cards, life insurance policies, etc.) [25]. It is critical to understand that there is no right way to transition; there is no correct sequence or combination of choices [73]. Transition choices may change across time as gender identity evolves [73]. If someone chooses to pursue certain forms of transitioning and/or does not medically, socially, or legally transition, their gender identity still has great integrity and value; they are no less TGNC than someone who chooses a more traditional pathway. Each person's transition, whether visible to other people or not, is deeply personal and individualized to the needs and desires of that person.

1.2.4 Disclosure

Disclosing a TGNC identity, or *coming out*, can be intimately connected to a person's access to support and resources, sense of agency, and issues of safety and control [3]. Before sharing their identity with others, TGNC people go through a process of self-awareness and discovery, first understanding their own gender identity and then deciding whether and when to disclose to others. This includes family, friends, loved ones, colleagues, and care providers. A person can develop self-awareness of a TGNC identity at any age; some TGNC older adults may have known since childhood, while others discover it in the later stages of their life after parents have passed and they are free to explore their own identity [3, 41]. The age at which someone identifies that they may be TGNC should not impact the validity and value of that identity.

Coming out is never "finished," with TGNC people having to make daily decisions about what to share throughout their lives [74]. If and how someone decides to disclose their identity is a personal choice; others should never impose that choice or thoughtlessly share information about someone's gender identity without permission. If and how a TGNC person decides to disclose their identity can change across their lifespan [7]. Choices may change or evolve as a person's control over living conditions and care provision change, as resources and support shift, as their identity evolves, and as circumstances that could increase the danger of rejection, violence, loss of employment, injury, or discrimination develop. Some people choose not to disclose that they are TGNC and instead make efforts to *pass* or to be consistently perceived to be cisgender by others [30]. For TGNC people who select to live a *stealth* life [3], their ability to pass and not be *clocked* (identified as TGNC) is paramount. The more a TGNC person's gender expression and behavior align with cultural expectations of either masculinity or femininity, the increased possibility the TGNC person will pass and will not be *outed* or identified as TGNC by others. Worries about being clocked and outed by others can create intense social anxiety and worry, making public interaction self-conscious and vulnerable [30]. Some TGNC people may only seek to pass in specific situations or locations to increase safety and comfort, since falling out of narrow cultural expectations of gender and being clocked as TGNC can result in violence, discrimination, and even death, depending on who does the clocking. However, not every TGNC person is interested in passing [3]. Some TGNC people are not concerned with passing because their gender identity and/or gender expression fall outside of cultural expectations of masculine and feminine identities, such as a *non-binary gender* identity or a *gender nonconforming* identity (identities that do not exclusively align with either masculine or feminine) [3, 41]. For them, passing may not be of interest; instead they may pursue a more robust understanding of gender identity and expression that allows for and honors gender nonconformity and gender expansiveness. Other TGNC people may realize that based on physical, financial, or health reasons, the ability to pass is not an option. The ability to pass should not be pressed, prioritized, or diminished by others. Instead, TGNC people's experiences and choices should be valued, with a focus on helping the TGNC person actualize their gender presentation goals.

1.2.5 Resilience

Despite the many adversities that TGNC people navigate to access basic human rights such as education, employment, housing, social services, and affirming health care, TGNC people demonstrate deep resilience, creativity, and resourcefulness [64]. Resilience is an essential component of the livelihood of TGNC people and a strength of TGNC communities [3, 55, 70]. TGNC people make passionate and valuable contributions to their surrounding communities and around the world. For many TGNC people, their resilience is rooted in their community connection and chosen families [48] rather than *biological families* (family you were born into). Some TGNC people develop a *chosen family* that is a group of individuals who select one another to serve significant roles in each other's lives, resembling a "family structure" even though individuals are not biologically or legally related. Chosen families can be essential when a TGNC person is rejected or unable to access support or resources from their biological family or mainstream society. Chosen family members have few legal rights and are often unrecognized by hospitals for visitation and medical decision-making and by legal systems (i.e., wills, deeds, shared homes, intended inheritance), unless legal documentation is specifically created to establish those rights [4]. The resilience of TGNC people can be awe-inspiring, with TGNC people creating networks of supports, economic opportunities, services, celebrations, and resources that are outside of official economic systems and mainstream society and that are shared by word-of-mouth and community networking [4]. Due to the structural oppression that TGNC communities experience, many TGNC people, particularly those with multiple marginalized intersecting identities, find their livelihood and overall well-being connected to work and earning opportunities outside of official economic systems that are based on street economies and sex work ([38], [75], [66]).

1.2.6 Gender-Affirming Communication

When communicating with TGNC people, there are several components of gender-affirming communication that are critical to practice and apply. These include name preference, gender pronouns, and how TGNC anatomy is understood and discussed. TGNC people may prefer to use a name that is not the same as the name on their legal documents, such as state ID, social security card, or insurance card (*legal name*) [25]. *Preferred names* are chosen by TGNC people to represent their identity and personality; names may change across time as identity evolves or may remain steady. For various reasons, not everyone is able to legally change their name. Some TGNC people choose to and are able to legally change their name. Upon completing a *name change process*, the legal name of the person is no longer the name given to them at birth but is the name they selected for themselves. Regardless of whether a TGNC person has completed a legal name change, their preferred name should always be respected and used. When first meeting any person, ask the name that person would like you to use while working with them. It is important to use a person's preferred name regardless of whether that person is there to hear it [36]. Consistent use of preferred names with health teams and colleagues reinforces the person's choice, communicates respect, and offers the team practice at using the correct name even when it might be counterintuitive by a person's appearance (i.e., a person with long hair and makeup with a preferred name of Peter). As TGNC people align legal documentation with their gender identity, they may change the gender marker on their state ID, social security card, passport, or birth certificate. Similar to state-based name change requirements, different states have different requirements to change the gender marker on any of these documents [25]. Having documentation that aligns with a TGNC person's gender identity further supports efforts to socially, legally, and medically transition.

Another critical component to respectful communication is the use of *gender pronouns* (he, him, his; she, her, hers; they, them, theirs; ze, zir, zirs) chosen by the TGNC person [22]. Gender pronouns should never be assumed based on appearance. Instead, every person should be asked what gender pronouns they use. Just like the range of gender identities and expressions, there are a range of gender pronouns outside of she/her/hers and he/him/his. Some people with non-binary or gender nonconforming identities use they/them/theirs to refer to themselves [3]. While using "they" as a singular pronoun (Amilie said they would meet us in their office) may feel initially awkward, it is a common usage in TGNC communities and in professions and care systems that serve TGNC people that should be learned and integrated into daily practice [3]. If a mistake is made and a TGNC person is *misgendered* (spoken to or about using the wrong pronouns) [56], best practice is to acknowledge the error, genuinely apologize for the mistake, and then take action to avoid repeating the error. Mistakes are inevitable, but an authentic apology and an intentional process that holds the system and healthcare team accountable for improvements communicate value and build true trust with the TGNC community [36].

1.2.7 Bathrooms

Bathroom use is a complex, persistent issue for TGNC people. Binary bathroom designations (women's room and men's room) can place a TGNC person in uncomfortable and potentially dangerous situations. Forced choice bathrooms require TGNC people to publicly declare an identity that may or may not match who they are or how they present. Forced choice bathrooms also require TGNC people to anticipate and manage the potentially aggressive, frightening, or demeaning reaction of others using the bathrooms they choose [35]. To avoid this choice and these situations, many TGNC people avoid using public bathrooms, even to the detriment of their health [35]. Best practice is to offer *gender-neutral* single stall bathrooms that can be used by anyone with any gender identity in privacy. A men's room or women's room can be converted to a gender-neutral bathroom, and when that does not occur, TGNC people should be able to use the bathroom that aligns with their gender identity without questioning from others.

The section above offers a range of concepts and vocabulary. Like all aspects of society and communication, word choice and language used by the TGNC and health-care communities will continue to evolve. Language and vocabulary in this area change at a fast rate, requiring regular refreshment and awareness [3]. While language used by the TGNC community can change quickly, it is important to listen to and reflect the preferred terminology of TGNC older adults as they discuss their lives and identities. While some TGNC older adults will incorporate the newest vernacular, some may prefer to use language that existed at defining times of their lives, even if language in community and the profession has changed. It is critical to respect TGNC older adults' language choices while still introducing new terms and concepts that deepen their awareness of options and self-determination. The American Psychological Association [3] offers an excellent resource to explore these concepts in greater depth that includes an informative glossary of terms.

1.3 Cultural Context and Generational Cohort

In understanding TGNC older adults, it is critical to examine the lives they have led and the social, historical, and cultural contexts they have experienced. At this point in time, TGNC older adults were born in the early 1960s and before. Though many TGNC older adults will not self-identify as gender nonconforming or non-binary, some will identify as transsexual [19], a term that is used less frequently in contemporary culture. TGNC older adults lived their younger years in stigmatizing and dangerous environments, and they have endured medical practices that pathologized transgender identities [50, 68, 69]. The approach to care for TGNC people has evolved deeply since they came of age.

Historically in the United States, TGNC people have had few resources available to them. Affirming health care has been limited in the United States until recently and was more established in European countries and in Thailand [21] between 1940 and 1990. To be openly TGNC during these decades in the United

States was fraught with peril. In the 1940s, during the Second World War, approximately 15,000 gay men and transgender people were exterminated in German concentration camps [14]. In the 1950s, there was no cultural, legal, or medical safe space for TGNC people who were often committed to psychiatric institutions for reparative therapy or forced to live lives in isolation or seclusion [18]. Even in the 1960s, a time widely recognized as the beginning of civil rights for gays and lesbians, TGNC people were largely excluded despite their active involvement in the early movement [18]. TGNC people have borne decades of lack of care and absolute danger to their lives.

Care for TGNC individuals in the 1960s focused solely on psychiatric care for gender identity disorder [43]. Medical care for TGNC people, as we understand it today, with affirming treatment with hormones, behavioral health, and surgical options, was not available. Additionally, treatment in the 1960s through the 1990s was isolating and rigid, requiring that TGNC people adhere to a narrow, specific, and binary narrative or the limited care available to them was blocked [3]. Currently in the United States, older adults are seeing a dramatic shift in care options and visibility. In the last 15–20 years, with much of the growth and activity in the last 5 years, older TGNC adults have growing access to care that they have not been able to experience for most of their lives. Changes in access to services covered by insurance, specifically Medicare, have made available long-denied services [15].

When working with TGNC older adults, it is imperative to consider each individual and their life experience as the foundation of their care. Consider TGNC older adults' age of self-awareness of their own identity as TGNC and how that played out in their lives. Be mindful of their age of coming out to others, if they are out, and the generational assumptions of their younger years [3]. The experience of coming out at 18 years old in 1960 will be very different from coming out at 70 years old in 2015. For each individual, there will be a unique personal narrative, important for the provider to appreciate and respect.

1.4 TGNC Health Disparities

As previously mentioned, the current and emerging generations of TGNC older adults came of age between the 1960s and 1980s when homosexuality was illegal and criminalized, and a TGNC identity was pathologized by the medical community and mainstream society [24]. The onset of the HIV/AIDS epidemic in the 1980s created further barriers to societal acceptance, positive health outcomes, and equal access to physical and mental health services for many TGNC people [34]. The discrimination and victimization TGNC older adults experienced in their formative adult years created layers of trauma, caution, and well-founded mistrust of health-care systems and mainstream society, reified by continued experiences of poor care, discrimination, and mistreatment [36]. This trauma can result in caution disclosing gender identity or personal details to health-care providers, worries about the loss of existing services should their TGNC identity be discovered, and a distrust of health service staff and systems by TGNC older adults [36].

Little information is available on the number of TGNC older adults and the health disparities they experience. Several factors appear to contribute to this gap of information including, but not limited to, the low number of TGNC people living to older ages, TGNC community concern about how collected information would be used by researchers and health systems [39], the invisibility of TGNC people in current research [3], inability to collect gender identity demographic data in electronic health records, low national priority and lack of research funding, and the need for some TGNC older adults to de-transition when moved into unsupportive care facilities [40]. Given a potentially higher mortality rate, fewer TGNC people may survive to older ages compared to the general population, creating complex challenges in finding TGNC older adult populations and studying their lives and health. Given the long history of non-affirmative and harmful health care and the past use of data to pathologize TGNC identities, the TGNC community is appropriately cautious about engaging in research [37, 54]. In addition, most research ignores gender identity as a demographic variable, making the TGNC community invisible [34]. Available research on the health disparities and specific needs of TGNC older adults has historically been limited, frequently considered a taboo subject of governmental and academically funded research. Data on gender identity is not routinely collected by the US Census Bureau [12], the greater medical community, or through federally funded demographic research. Prior to 2015, there was no national directive to collect sexual orientation and gender identity (SOGI) data in research or through patient information [41]. In addition, TGNC older adults may choose to or be forced to "de-transition" (deny their TGNC gender identity and shift gender presentation back to sex assigned at birth) when shifting into assisted living systems or nursing homes [40].

Since 2015, as part of Meaningful Use Guidelines Stage 3 [13], electronic health record (EHR) systems across the United States have been adding capacity to collect sexual orientation and gender identity data. This critical information collection allows TGNC communities to be visible in significant ways [12]. Without data collection, health inequities that exist for these vulnerable populations had minimal opportunity to be discovered and therefore were not addressed. Now that these groups, especially TGNC communities, can be addressed in a meaningful way in terms of research, the impact on specific subgroups can be illuminated and studied [13].

In the past, research and data collection regarding the health needs of TGNC people has largely focused on transition-related care and HIV/AIDS health disparities [9]. The limited amount of research completed on these topics has been conducted with small and often ineffective convenience samples or samples obtained in nonsystematic ways [44]. As the number of TGNC older adults increase, there is a critical need to better understand the specific health needs of this growing, and oftentimes vulnerable, population. TGNC older adults will not only have health conditions that are customarily associated with aging, including hypertension, diabetes, heart disease, and degenerative memory disorders, but could also face uncertain health conditions that are not yet fully understood. These uncertainties include the long-term effects of the use of hormones and silicone injections, long-term surgical complications, older adult HIV disease management, and the overall mental and social health of aging TGNC individuals.

TGNC people are habitually subjected to various forms of discrimination including social stress, violence, prejudice, workplace hostility, and institutional and systematic barriers to care [41]. The impact of social stress, including violence, transphobia, and stigma, is significantly felt by TGNC people, and even more so by aging persons within this population. This social stress can result in depressive symptoms, suicidal ideation, interpersonal trauma exposure, substance abuse disorders, and anxiety [67]. TGNC people are also disproportionately victimized through physical and verbal abuse, sexual assault, property damage, and denial of access to health-care services. One study found that 40% of transgender individuals reported being denied health care or were provided inferior care based on their gender identity [42]. Additionally, another study of over 27,000 TGNC people published in 2016 found that 46% of respondents reported verbal harassment; 24% were physically threatened; 58% reported being mistreated by law enforcement officials; 19% were not hired for a job, fired, or not promoted; 54% experienced intimate partner violence; and 47% were sexually assaulted. These incidence rates are frequently found to be higher among TGNC populations compared to cisgender peers [41].

The workforce can be a particularly challenging environment for TGNC people. There are significant links between workplace hostility and suffering psychological distress [8]. Nearly 50% of transgender individuals report workplace discrimination based on their gender identity [46]. This discrimination can take the form of hostility, isolation, lack of collaboration, lower pay, and lack of advancement opportunities. The ability to advocate for one's self can also be significantly altered by past and current victimization and discrimination based on gender identity [11]. Realized and perceived discrimination within the workplace can also affect a TGNC person's ability to maintain long-term employment, sustain a positive career advancement trajectory, and attain occupational gratification and aspirations [10, 51]. In turn, it adversely affects an individual's lifetime earning potential, ability to financially plan for retirement, maintain health insurance, and achieve an overall sense of financial security [17]. TGNC people may enter the workforce later than cisgender peers, may have been held at entry level positions for longer periods of time, and are more likely to have been involved in street economies that provide less reliable income and financial safety. TGNC older adults find themselves moving into their older age having earned consistently less than their cisgender peers [46] and rarely having had the opportunity to plan or save for retirement or for a time in their lives when they are no longer able to work. This financial insecurity impacts the individual's ability to access health care [27] and can increase feelings of depression, hopelessness, and fear. According to the 2013 Aging with Pride: National Health, Aging, Sexuality and Gender Study, 50% of all transgender adults aged 50 or older live at or below 200% of the federal poverty level, compared to only 30% of their LGB counterparts, and 25% of transgender adults experience financial barriers to health services compared to only 6.4% of non-transgender individuals [28].

Within many institutions and social service operations, supportive resources available to older adults are not systematically inclusive of TGNC people's life experiences and needs. Many social programs and services within senior centers, long-term care facilities, and in-home health services operate under the assumption that all individuals served are heterosexual [44] and cisgender. Institutional providers of these services and programs must utilize culturally competent care delivery systems, respectful and affirming language, informed intake procedures, and inclusive operating procedures. The absence of these practices may cause TGNC individuals to be excluded, shamed, misunderstood, and forgotten.

Access to gender-affirming services remains a significant problem within the health-care system. TGNC individuals are found to have lower rates of insurance coverage, reduced social support, lack a primary care provider, delay seeking medical care, and experience harassment within health-care settings [41]. These factors can lead to higher rates of mental stress/illness, emergency room visits, and hospitalizations [58]. A significant institutional deterrent to positive health outcomes for TGNC older adults is the inequities that exist within the private and public insurance systems. While it has been found that TGNC people with private insurance are subjected to less discrimination within health-care settings, there are still exclusions for TGNC affirmative care within many private insurance plans [42]. The exclusions make it difficult or impossible for consumers to receive gender affirmative surgery and hormone prescriptions. While Medicare has formally removed such exclusions [57], other changes within the Medicare system and a lack of providers willing to accept Medicare payment rates for gender affirmation surgery may make it difficult to access a full continuum of affordable health care through public assistance plans. Exclusion policies for Medicaid and private insurance plans vary state by state, making the continued advocacy for TGNC patients' rights to accessible and affirmative health-care coverage essential.

Beyond the difficulties and trauma of navigating health and societal systems, TGNC people frequently experience family rejection, stress, and oppression [3]. In lieu of unsupportive biological family relationships, many TGNC people create support systems through a chosen family. A chosen family provides a TGNC older adult with a personal safety net of friends, neighbors, and loved ones who provide meaningful support to each other over time. A chosen family is a community- and individual-level coping mechanism that aids in mitigating stress and establishing meaningful, affirming relationships that can replace nonsupportive biological family members [31]. One study has shown that some aging TGNC people with close relationships to their biological families can actually show more depressive symptoms than those that do not maintain these relationships [43], although some TGNC people experience supportive, caring relationships with their biological families. For TGNC older adults who remain connected to their families of origin, it can be stressful to wonder whether relationships will remain strong across time to rely upon family members when support and advocacy are needed to ensure the TGNC older adult receives affirmative care and respect through older adulthood and death.

1.5 Affirmative Care

Central to serving aging TGNC people is the provision of gender-affirming care, defined as "care that is sensitive, responsive, and affirming to trans patients' gender identities and/or expressions" and "health care that holistically attends to transgender people's physical, mental, and social health needs and well-being while respectfully affirming their gender identity" [61]. Research has consistently shown that TGNC people are more likely to experience positive life and health outcomes when they receive social support and affirmative care [3, 65]. Affirmative, patient-centered care must recognize and support each individual; there is no "one-size-fits-all" approach [61]. In practice, this means that all health care providers will need to not only educate themselves but also their care teams to provide this life-saving and life-affirming care. To begin, providers should immerse themselves in the available literature and develop a skill set that they can share with their teams. Development of day-to-day practices, including appropriate use of terminology and recognition of chosen name and pronouns, elimination of stigma, use of evidence-based protocols, and a consistent commitment to personal introspection, are all essential to creating a safe and welcoming space for TGNC people [3].

A foundational component of affirmative care is the recognition that TGNC identities can be healthy and self-affirming and are not inherently pathological [16]. While a person's identity is healthy, chronic exposure to societal stigma and discrimination can result in persistent distress associated with discordance between a person's gender identity and body or sex assigned at birth [3, 9, 16], defined as gender dysphoria in the *Diagnostic and Statistical Manual of Mental Disorders, Fifth Edition* (DSM-5) [1]. Not every TGNC person experiences gender dysphoria, but supporting those who do is a critical health-care need. The World Professional Association for Transgender Health (WPATH) has a comprehensive resource available that describes standards of care for TGNC individuals [16]. The Center of Excellence for Transgender Health at the University of California San Francisco (UCSF) has similar guidelines for the "Primary and Gender-Affirming Care of Transgender and Gender Non-binary People" [23], and multiple progressive LGBT community health centers across the country utilize these care protocols [59].

It is critically important that TGNC people have agency in all aspects of their health and wellness. As with many people who are aging, TGNC older adults may experience loss of power and agency, especially as others involve themselves in their care. An adult child or caregiver may invalidate a TGNC person's identity by not using correct pronouns or telling the provider that it doesn't matter, referring to their transfeminine parent as "my dad" or "him," giving the provider permission to do the same. Providers will demonstrate advocacy for their patient by adhering to the patient's chosen name and pronoun in spite of what family and outside systems may suggest, and will ultimately be of more benefit to the patient.

Self-determination of the TGNC person regarding their identity, choices in care, and plans for transition is the heart of patient-centered, affirmative care. Health-care providers must place the TGNC older adult in the guiding role and, working in concert, offer affirming pathways of care [60]. During the 1990s, Howard Brown Health, an LGBT-centric federally qualified health center in Chicago, along with Callen-Lorde Community Health Center in New York City, began developing an informed consent model for hormone use that excluded the need for psychotherapy, a mental health letter, and "proof" of having a "real" TGNC identity [59]. Community and patient feedback, in addition to clinical data, led to the adoption of this model of care. This pioneering approach eliminated required lengthy mental health evaluations and the requirement that an individual prove real-life experience (RLE) (living as their intended gender for a year) prior to acquiring a prescription for hormones. The informed consent model, simply stated, provides that if the patient is of age of consent, has no unmanaged medical conditions, and has the capacity to consent, they will be able to gain a prescription of hormones, many times in their first appointment [25].

The role of the health care provider in providing affirmative care for TGNC older adults is multifaceted and, most importantly, demands interdisciplinary communication [25]. Support for older TGNC people will require the provider and the care team to provide more patient navigation and support than usual, coordinating communications between other health specialists and making best efforts to carve affirmative pathways to needed services. In affirmative interdisciplinary care, the role of the care team expands to link patients to other affirmative care systems and, when possible, to protect TGNC people from or prepare them to interact with systems that are unsupportive or damaging [25]. For instance, a health care provider may call ahead after referring a patient to a hospital for mammography, to advise the clinic on providing respectful care to a transgender man who has breasts. In addition, health care providers often write letters for TGNC people to change their gender markers on a driver's license and state identification documents; requirements to change gender markers vary from state to state, but these all-important letters are required to navigate these government offices [76].

In all encounters with TGNC people, there may be an understandable issue of distrust on the part of the patient. The establishment of a successful relationship begins the moment a provider and health care team meet a new patient. A best practice to utilize in the first patient encounter is for the provider to introduce themselves with their name and pronoun, ask for the same from the patient, and, throughout the interview, always ask permission to discuss sensitive topics and explain the intent of questions. In cases when a physical exam is needed, be sure to ask for shared language to describe body parts as the patient may use different terminology. Allow for time to discuss any procedure, even allowing for the procedure to be done another day if the prospect of an exam causes a patient distress [45]. Be mindful to screen and treat body parts the patient has as it pertains to the purpose of the visit [23]. It may be that an older transwoman may need a screening for prostate cancer and an older transman may need a hysterectomy. Inspection of genitalia is not indicated when a patient is visiting for a physical injury or illness that does not involve those body parts.

Multiple challenges exist within institutional spaces that create barriers to care. For example, most EHRs do not support the ability to use a name other than the name used for billing in documentation and offer inadequate support in creating affirmative documentation for referrals [76]. In terms of documentation, it is important to use a patient's preferred name and pronouns regardless of who reads it, unless it is unsafe for the patient or if the patient has requested that different pronouns be used in the medical records [13].

To actualize affirmative care, an interdisciplinary method must be employed to support TGNC patients. An interdisciplinary collaborative care (ICC) team is defined as a team that "aspires to a more profound level of collaboration (than a multidisciplinary team), in which constituents of different backgrounds combining their knowledge mutually complete different levels of planned care" [6]. This collaboration moves beyond traditional institutions of health care [25]. Consider a team supporting a person transitioning as an older adult – this team may include a primary care provider, behavioral health provider, spiritual adviser, and legal advocate, with referrals to electrolysis, and case management or social service to aid with housing, nursing home entry, or hospice care. This coordinated symphony of care is needed for the unique challenges older TGNC people experience.

Many care systems do not have mechanisms in place to support ICC teams, which can involve unbillable collaborative time; however, such collaboration and interdisciplinary communication is pivotal in supporting TGNC people [25]. When working to build affirmative care pathways, team members who are more familiar with TGNC resources and affirmative care will facilitate the learning of colleagues and will maximize their colleagues' effectiveness working with TGNC patients. A provider new to TGNC care will find this framework an invaluable support. If leading this team building process, it is important to do this in a manner that solidifies the team rather than disrupts it and, ultimately, amplifies and supports the voice of the TGNC person to involve them in active participation as a care team member. Some TGNC individuals who have not had their voices heard or respected in previous health-care experiences, or who have learned from their community to expect disrespectful and damaging treatment, may present to the care team as less willing to tolerate delay or more assertive about their health-care choices than other patients. This behavior can sometimes be interpreted by care systems as insistent, entitled, or even resistant. Care teams are encouraged to reframe their understanding of this behavior, recognizing that this behavior has enabled TGNC people to protect themselves in often uninformed and damaging care systems, supporting them in their fight to ensure body integrity and access medically necessary care. It is fueled by resilience and has supported the survival of TGNC elders. Providers are encouraged to work with the patient as the center of the care team and make every attempt to support TGNC people in establishing agency and authentic equal participation in care decisions [36].

As a provider and advocate to aging TGNC patients, it is critical that organizations move to establish safe, welcoming, and knowledgeable health care spaces. Moving this work forward will require exerting the power and privilege inherent in the role of provider and health care team to create safe and affirmative care systems and laws, with every step toward affirmation building improved health outcomes.

1.6 Ongoing Learning and Closing Thoughts

When providing care for TGNC older adults, it is important that health-care providers and all care team members are aware of the depth and limitations of their current knowledge and skill base and continuously work to deepen them to support TGNC people [25, 55]. A lack of knowledge or skill, or unexamined beliefs about gender identity and gender expression on the part of a provider, can impact a TGNC person's willingness to trust them and their care team's ability to offer affirmative care [28]. The topics and guidance covered in this book are not exhaustive but offer some necessary tools to offer affirmative care to TGNC patients. As such, it is imperative that health-care providers and care teams continue to educate themselves through training, mentorship, and authentic digestion of TGNC patient and community feedback. It is not the responsibility of the patient to inform health-care providers of best practices for offering affirmative care. TGNC patients can and will share important details specific to their individualized care. However, it is the health-care professional's responsibility to deepen their education and the knowledge and skills of their team and to consistently improve the system in which they provide care [25].

While the development of knowledge and skills are critical to the provision of affirmative care, so is the introspection required to understand one's unexamined beliefs about gender identity and expression. Societal learning has embedded transphobic beliefs, judgments, stereotypes, and assumptions about gender identity and gender presentation in all people and systems [53]. Unexamined beliefs of this nature will be obvious in language and behavior; even if they are actualized in subtle ways, these beliefs will impact the care of the patient and their trust in the care team [29]. As providers and care teams work to educate themselves, it is important to devote time to the examination of beliefs, judgments, stereotypes, and assumptions as they relate to patients, to the necessity and perceived value of care, and to the possibility of best health for TGNC older adults. This examination may be exciting and simultaneously uncomfortable as care team members work to learn more, evolve understanding, and take critical steps to provide consistent and progressively stronger affirmative care. We truly thank each person for reading this book and for the affirmative care that will be provided to TGNC communities as a result.

References

1. American Psychiatric Association. Diagnostic and statistical manual of mental disorders. 5th ed. Washington, DC: American Psychiatric Association; 2013.
2. American Psychological Association. Guidelines for psychological practice with lesbian, gay, and bisexual clients. Am Psychol. 2012;67(1):10–42. https://doi.org/10.1037/a0024659.
3. American Psychological Association. Guidelines for psychological practice with transgender and gender nonconforming people. Am Psychol. 2015;70(9):832–64. https://doi.org/10.1037/a0039906.
4. American Society on Aging, MetLife. "Still Out, Still Aging": the MetLife study of lesbian, gay, bisexual and transgender baby boomers. 2013. Retrieved from: https://www.metlife.com/assets/cao/mmi/publications/studies/2010/mmi-still-out-still-aging.pdf.

5. Benjamin H. The transexual phenomenon. New York: The Julian Press, Inc; 1966.
6. Bernard-Bonnin AC, Stachenko S, Bonin D, Charette C, Rousseau E. Self-management teaching programs and morbidity of pediatric asthma: a meta-analysis. J Allergy Clin Immunol. 1995;95(1):34–41.
7. Bockting W, Coleman E. Developmental stages of the transgender coming out process: toward an integrated identity. In: Ettner R, Monstrey S, Eyler AE, editors. Principles of transgender medicine and surgery. New York: Haworth Press Inc; 2007. p. 185–208.
8. Bockting WO, Miner MH, Swinburne Romine RE, Hamilton A, Coleman E. Stigma, mental health, and resilience in an online sample of the US transgender population. Am J Public Health. 2013;103(5):943–51.
9. Bockting W, Coleman E, Deutsch MB, Guillamon A, Meyer I, Meyer W, Reisner S, Sevelius J, Ettner R. Adult development and quality of life of transgender and gender nonconforming people. Current Opin Endocrinol Diabetes Obes. 2016;23(2):188–97. https://doi.org/10.1097/MED.0000000000000232.
10. Brewster ME, Velez BL, Mennicke A, Tebbe E. Voices from beyond: a thematic content analysis of transgender employees' workplace experiences. Psychol Sex Orientat Gend Divers. 2014;1:159–69. https://doi.org/10.1037/sgd0000030
11. Budge SL, Tebbe EN, Howard KAS. The work experiences of transgender individuals: negotiating and transition and career decision-making processes. J Couns Psychol. 2010;57:377. https://doi.org/10.1037/a0020472. Advance online publication
12. Cahill S, Makadon H. Sexual orientation and gender identity data collection in clinical settings and in electronic health records: a key to ending LGBT health disparities. LGBT Health. 2014a;1(1):34–41.
13. Cahill S, Makadon HJ. Sexual orientation and gender identity data collection update: U.S. Government takes steps to promote sexual orientation and gender identity data collection through meaningful use guidelines. LGBT Health. 2014b;1(3):157–60.
14. Cant B. 'Anyone who thinks of homosexual love is our enemy': remembering the experiences of lesbian, gay, bisexual and transgender people during the Nazi terror. Divers Health Care. 2012;9(4):239–41.
15. Civic Impulse. (2017). H.R. 3590 — 111th congress: patient protection and affordable care act. Retrieved from https://www.govtrack.us/congress/bills/111/hr3590.
16. Coleman E, Bockting W, Botzer M, Cohen-Kettenis P, DeCuypere G, Feldman J, et al. Standards of care for the health of transsexual, transgender, and gender-nonconforming people, version 7. Int J Transgend. 2012;13(4):165–232.
17. Cook-Daniels L. Trans aging. In: Kimmel D, Rose T, David S, editors. Lesbian, gay, bisexual and transgender aging: research and clinical perspectives. New York: Columbia University Press; 2006. p. 20–35.
18. Cook-Daniels L. Living memory GLBT history timeline: current elders would have been this old when these events happened…. J GLBT Fam Stud. 2008;4(4):485–97.
19. Cook-Daniels L. Understanding transgender elders. In: Handbook of LGBT elders. Cham: Springer; 2016. p. 285–308.
20. Crissman HP, Berger MB, Graham LF, Dalton VK. Transgender demographics: a household probability sample of US adults, 2014. Am J Public Health. 2017;107(2):213–5.
21. Chokrungvaranont P, Tiewtranon P. Sex reassignment surgery in Thailand. Med Assoc Thai. 2004;87(11):1402–8.
22. Darr B, Kibbey T. Pronouns and thoughts on neutrality: gender concerns in modern grammar. Pursuit-The Journal of Undergraduate Research at the University of Tennessee. 2016;7(1):10.
23. Deutsch MB, editor. Guidelines for the primary and gender-affirming care of transgender and gender nonbinary people. San Francisco: University of California; 2016.
24. Drescher, J. Out of DSM: Depathologizing homosexuality. Behav Sci (Open Access Journal of Psychology and Cognition) (2015). doi: https://doi.org/10.3390/bs5040565 5, 565. Retrieved from https://www.ncbi.nlm.nih.gov/pmc/articles/PMC4695779/.
25. Ducheny, K., Hendricks, M.L., Keo-Meier, C.L. (2017). TGNC-affirmative interdisciplinary collaborative care, In A.A. Singh L.M. Dickey (Eds.), Affirmative counseling and psychological

practice with transgender and gender nonconforming clients (pp. 69–93). Washington, DC: American Psychological Association.
26. Flores AR, Brown TN, Herman J. Race and ethnicity of adults who identify as transgender in the United States. UCLA School of Law: Williams Institute; 2016.
27. Frazer MS, Howe EE. Transgender health and economic insecurity: a report from the 2015 LGBT health and human services needs assessment survey. New York: Empire State Pride Agenda; 2015. www.prideagenda.org/lgbtdata
28. Fredriksen-Goldsen KI, Cook-Daniels L, Kim HJ, Erosheva EA, Emlet CA, Hoy-Ellis CP, Muraco A. Physical and mental health of transgender older adults: an at-risk and underserved population. The Gerontologist. 2014;54(3):488–500. https://doi.org/10.1093/geront/gnt021.
29. Fredriksen-Goldsen KI, Kim HJ. The science of conducting research with LGBT older adults – An introduction to aging with pride: National Health, Aging, and Sexuality/Gender Study (NHAS). The Gerontologist. 2017;57(supl_1):S1–S14.
30. Fütty JT. Challenges posed by transgender-passing within ambiguities and interrelations. Grad J Soc Sci. 2010;7(2):57–75.
31. Gates T. Chosen families. In: Carlson J, Dermer S, editors. The sage encyclopedia of marriage, family, and couples counseling, vol. 1. Thousand Oaks: SAGE Publications, Inc; 2017. p. 240–2. https://doi.org/10.4135/9781483369532.n74.
32. Grant JM, Mottet LA, Tanis J, Harrison J, Herman JL, Keisling M. Injustice at every turn: a report of the National Transgender Discrimination Survey. Washington, DC: National Center for Transgender Equality and National Gay and Lesbian Task Force; 2011.
33. Harrison J, Grant J, Sherman JL. A gender not listed here: genderqueers, gender rebels and otherwise in the National Transgender Discrimination Study. LGBT Policy Journal at the Harvard Kennedy School. 2012;2:13–24.
34. Herbst J, Jacobs E, Finlayson T, McKleroy V, Neumann M, Crepaz N. Estimating HIV prevalence and risk behaviors of transgender persons in the United States: a systematic review. AIDS Behav. 2008;12(1):1–17.
35. Herman JL. Gendered restrooms and minority stress: the public regulation of gender and its impact on transgender people's lives. J Public Manag Soc Policy. 2013;19(1):65–80.
36. Association of American Medical Colleges Implementing curricular and institutional climate changes to improve health care for individuals who are LGBT, gender nonconforming, or born with DSD, a resource for medical educators. Association of American Medical Colleges. 2014. Downloaded July 18, 2018 from https://www.aamc.org/download/414172/data/lgbt.pdf
37. Hwanng SJ, Lin A. The health of lesbian, gay, bisexual, transgender, queer, and questioning people. In: Trinh-Shervrin C, Islam N, Rey M, editors. Asian American communities and health: content, research, policy, and action. San Francisco: Jossey-Bass; 2009. p. 226–82.
38. Hwanng SJ, Nuttbrock L. Sex workers, fem queens, and cross-dressers: differential marginalizations and HIV vulnerabilities among three ethnocultural male-to-female transgender communities in New York City. Sex Res Soc Policy. 2007;4:36–59. https://doi.org/10.1525/srsp.2007.4.4.36.
39. Institute of Medicine. The health of lesbian, gay, bisexual, and transgender people: building a foundation for a better understanding. Washington, DC: National Academy of Sciences; 2011.
40. Ippolito J, Witten TM. Aging. In: Erickson-Schroth L, editor. Trans bodies, trans selves: a resource for the transgender community. New York: Oxford University Press; 2014. p. 476–97.
41. James SE, Herman JL, Rankin S, Keisling M, Mottet L, Anafi M. The report of the 2015 U.S. Transgender Survey. Washington, DC: National Center for Transgender Equality; 2016.
42. Kattari SK, Hasche L. Differences across age groups in transgender and gender nonconforming people's experiences of health care discrimination, harassment, and victimization. J Aging Health. 2016;28(2):285–306.
43. Kimmel D, Rose T, Orel N, Greene B. Historical context for research on lesbian, gay, bisexual, and transgender aging. In: Kimmel DC, Rose T, David S, editors. Lesbian, gay, bisexual, and transgender aging: research and clinical perspectives. New York: Columbia University Press; 2006. p. 1–19.

44. Kimmel D. Lesbian, gay, bisexual, and transgender aging concerns. Clin Gerontol. 2014;37:49–63.
45. Klein DA, Malcolm NM, Berry-Bibee EN, Paradise SL, Coulter JS, Keglovitz Baker K, et al. Quality primary care and family planning services for LGBT clients: a comprehensive review of clinical guidelines. LGBT Health. 2018;5(3):153–170
46. Lee J. Lost in transition: the challenges of remedying transgender employment discrimination under title VII. Harv JL & Gender. 2012;35:423.
47. MacLaughlin DT, Donahoe PK. Sex determination and differentiation. N Engl J Med. 2004;350:367–78. http://dx.doi.org/10/1056/NEJMra022783
48. Metlife Mature Market Institute®2 & The Lesbian and Gay Aging Issues Network of the American Society on Aging. Out and aging: the MetLife study of lesbian and gay baby boomers. J GLBT Fam Stud. 2010;6(1):40–57. https://doi.org/10.1080/15504280903472949.
49. Miller LR, Grollman EA. The social costs of gender nonconformity for transgender adults: implications for discrimination and health. Sociol Forum. 2015, September;30(3):809–31.
50. Mizock L, Lewis TK. Trauma in transgender populations: risk, resilience, and clinical care. J Emot Abus. 2008;8(3):335–54.
51. Mizock L, Meuser KT. Employment, mental health, internalized stima and coping with transphobia among transgender individuals. Psychol Sex Orientat Gend Divers. 2014;1:146–58. http://dx.doi.org/10/1037/sgd0000029
52. Monroe S. Beyond male and female: poststructuralism and the spectrum of gender. Int J Transgend. 2005;8(1):3–22. https://doi.org/10.1300/J485v08n01_02
53. Nadal KL, Rivera DP, Corpus JH, Sue DW. Sexual orientation and transgender microaggressions. In: Microaggressions and marginality: manifestation, dynamics, and impact. 2010. p. 217–240.
54. Namaste VK. Invisible lives: the erasure of transsexual and transgendered people. Chicago: University of Chicago; 2000.
55. Porter KE, Brennan-Ing M, Chang SC, Dickey LM, Singh AA, Bower K, Witten TM. Providing competent and affirming services for transgender and gender nonconforming older adults. Clin Gerontol. 2016;39(5):366–88.
56. Poteat T, German D, Kerrigan D. Managing uncertainty: a grounded theory of stigma in transgender health care encounters. Soc Sci Med. 2013;84:22–9.
57. Proctor K, Haffer SC, Ewald E, Hodge C, James CV. Identifying the transgender population in the Medicare program. Transgender Health. 2016;1(1):250–65.
58. Progovac AM, Le Cook B, Mullin B, McDowell A, Sanchez MJ, Wang Y, Creedon TB, Schuster MA. Identifying gender minority patients' health and health care needs in administrative claims data. Health Affairs. 2018;37(3):413–20.
59. Radix AE. Medical transition for transgender individuals. In: Eckstrand KL, Ehrenfeld JM, editors. Lesbian, gay, bisexual, and transgender healthcare. New York: Springer International Publishing; 2016. p. 351–62.
60. Reisner SL, Bradford J, Hopwood R, Gonzalez A, Makadon H, Todisco D, et al. Comprehensive transgender healthcare: the gender affirming clinical and public health model of Fenway Health. J Urban Health. 2015;92(3):584–92.
61. Reisner SL, Radix A, Deutsch MB. Integrated and gender-affirming transgender clinical care and research. J Acquir Immune Defic Syndr (1999). 2016;*72*(Suppl 3):S235.
62. Richards J. Op-ed: It's time for trans lives to truly matter to us all. February 18, 2015. The Advocate, downloaded May 5, 2018 at https://www.advocate.com/commentary/2015/02/18/op-ed-its-time-trans-lives-truly-matter-us-all.
63. Shields JP, Cohen R, Glassman JR, Whitaker K, Franks H, Bertolini I. Estimating population size and demographic characteristics of lesbian, gay, bisexual, and transgender youth in middle school. J Adolesc Health. 2013;52(2):248–50.
64. Singh AA, Hays DG, Watson LS. Strength in the face of adversity: resilience strategies of transgender individuals. J Couns Dev. 2011;89(1). https://doi.org/10.1002/j.1556-6678.2011.tb00057.x

65. Singh A, Dickey LM, editors. Perspectives on sexual orientation and diversity. Affirmative counseling and psychological practice with transgender and gender nonconforming clients. Washington, DC: American Psychological Association; 2017.
66. Stanley EA. Fugitive flesh: gender self-determination, queer abolition, and trans resistence. In: Stanley EA, Smith N, editors. Captive genders: trans embodiment and the prison industrial complex. Oakland, CA: AK Press; 2011. p. 1–11.
67. Valentine SE, Shipherd JC. A systematic review of social stress and mental health among transgender and gender non-conforming people in the United States. Clin Psychol Rev. 2018; https://doi.org/10.1037/14957-000.
68. White JT, Gendron TL. LGBT elders in nursing homes, long-term care facilities, and residential communities. In: *Handbook of LGBT elders*. Cham: Springer; 2016. p. 417–37.
69. Williams ME, Freeman PA. Transgender health: implications for aging and caregiving. J Gay Lesbian Soc Serv. 2007;18(3–4):93–108.
70. Witten TM. It's not all darkness: robustness, resilience, and successful transgender aging. LGBT Health. 2014;1(1):24–33.
71. Witten TM, Carpenter B. Invisibility squared: the challenges of living as a transgender older adult. 2015. Downloaded July 18, 2018 at https://psychologybenefits.org/2015/03/09/invisibility-squared-thechallenges-of-living-as-a-transgender-older-adult/.
72. Wylie K, Knudson G, Khan SI, Bonierbale M, Watanyusakul S, Baral S. Serving transgender people: clinical care considerations and service delivery models in transgender health. Lancet. 2016;388(10042):401–11.
73. Diamond LM, Pardo ST, Butterworth MR. Transgender experience and identity. In: Schwartz S, Luyckx K, Vignoles V, editors. Handbook of identity theory and research. New York: Springer; 2011. p. 629–47.
74. Eliason MJ, Schope R. Shifting sands or solid foundation? Lesbian, gay, bisexual, and transgender identity formation. In: Meyer IH, Northridge ME, editors. The health of sexual minorities. Boston: Springer; 2007. p. 3–26.
75. Grant JM, Mottet LA, Tanis J, Harrison J, Herman JL, Keisling M. Injustice at every turn: a report of the national transgender discrimination survey. Washington: National Center for Transgender Equality and National Gay and Lesbian Task Force; 2011.
76. Keo-Meier C, Ducheny K, Hendricks M. Identity and support letters. In: Kauth MR, Shipherd JC, editors. Adult transgender care: an interdisciplinary approach for training mental health professionals. New York: Routledge; 2017. p. 194–207.

Endocrinology, Hormone Replacement Therapy (HRT), and Aging

2

Magda Houlberg

The function of gender roles within society continues to evolve along with the norms and attitudes regarding gender expression and identity. For many individuals, how they were raised, what they could and could not do, and positions in society based on gender roles continue to evolve and change as well. When considering biomedical interventions for gender-affirming care, the effectiveness of the treatment versus the risks and managing expectations regarding reasonable response to treatment should be considered. Many binary definitions which were required for access to hormone replacement therapy (HRT) now have been deconstructed from a medical perspective [30]. This chapter addresses practice recommendations for the assessment and treatment of transgender and gender nonconforming (TGNC) older adults who are seeking to access gender-affirming HRT and shared clinical decision-making with patients.

There are excellent clinical general practice guidelines available for HRT, including the World Professional Association for Transgender Health (WPATH) Standards of Care (SOC) ([12]), University of California San Francisco (UCSF) Center of Excellence (CoE) for Transgender Health Guidelines for the Primary and Gender-Affirming Care of Transgender and Gender Non-binary People [14], and the Endocrine Society Clinical Practice Guidelines [25]. These guidelines do not focus specifically on older adults but do mention some considerations in regard to a clinical approach that takes into account issues of comorbidities and diseases of aging that are impacted by HRT.

Gender-affirming medical and surgical interventions are designed to improve people's quality of life and account for diversity in gender identity and expression, including non-binary identities. It is recommended to utilize a biopsychosocial approach that examines the impact of life course events, experiences, and

M. Houlberg (✉)
Medical Services, Howard Brown Health Center, Chicago, IL, USA
e-mail: magdah@howardbrown.org

M. Houlberg et al. (eds.), *Transgender and Gender Nonconforming Health and Aging*,
https://doi.org/10.1007/978-3-319-95031-0_2

interventions such as HRT on the dimensions of successful aging such as physical and mental health, social engagement, and well-being. When considering biomedical interventions for gender-affirming care for older adults, the benefit of the treatment versus the risks and managing expectations regarding reasonable response to treatment should be considered.

This biopsychosocial approach complements current aging paradigms that include intersecting domains of successful aging, productive aging, and civic engagement later in life [16]. These paradigms are based on fixed assumptions of heterosexuality and the male/female gender binary. Yet, norms and attitudes regarding gender expression and gender roles are not static, either at the individual or societal level, and can evolve over the course of a lifetime. Mid-life is a critical period for transgender adults as they anticipate challenges of aging [31]. The exploration of gender identity for individuals may occur any time in the life cycle. It is well-known in transgender communities that many baby boomers only began to seriously contemplate gender transitions in their later years [16].

Data is sparse in estimating the total population of people who identify as TGNC. The Williams Institute analyzed data from population-based surveys and estimated that 0.6% of adults (1.4 million people) identify as transgender, and an estimated 217,050 of those individuals are 65 and older [20]. The 2015 US Transgender Survey, the largest transgender survey to date, had 27,715 respondents, and while 43% of those that elected to start HRT were between 25 and 44 years old, 13% of those individuals began HRT after 45 years old [27].

2.1 Physiologic Theories of Aging

It is not yet understood why all living things age. If biomedical aging is defined as the loss of organism homeostasis, hormones are influenced by and drive aspects of the aging process and are also influenced by that process. Hormones are the biomedical messengers of the body and signal and regulate cells, tissues, and organ system. One of the theories regarding the biologic underpinnings of the aging process is that the endocrine system changes during the normal aging process.

In the endocrine theory of aging [28], it suggests that the synthesis and secretion of many hormones change. Additionally, the expression of cell receptors in tissues changes both in number and signaling capacity. Circadian cycles of hormone secretion can become irregular. Maintaining homeostasis may change as these hormone levels impact organ tissues. The hormonal effects on aging or the effect of endogenous administration of sex hormones such as estrogen, progesterone, and testosterone or the impact of androgenic blocking on aging on a cellular or organ system level are not yet fully understood. Exogenous hormone treatment has been most extensively studied with patients where the sex at birth aligns with their gender identity and is androgenic replacement of endogenous hormone secretion that has reduced with aging, or circumstances where hormone-sensitive cancers are treated with hormone-modulating medications.

2.2 Patient Assessment

Each of the clinical guidelines, the WPATH [12], the UCSF [14], and the Endocrine Society guidelines [25], has clear frameworks for how to conduct patient assessments for HRT. Patient assessment candidacy for HRT can be accomplished by a variety of medical providers, including medical providers that are trained in family medicine, internal medicine, geriatrics, obstetrics and gynecology, endocrinology, and other fields. In most clinical protocols, patient candidacy for gender-affirming hormone therapy requires the clinical provider to identify persistent and documented gender dysphoria/gender incongruence; and in addition, the patient must be able to make a fully informed decision and consent for treatment, and any mental health concerns should be well controlled [12, 17].

As treatment models of care for TGNC patients continue to modernize and progress, the process by which a TGNC individual has access to HRT continues to evolve. The implementation and use of the informed consent model has become increasingly prevalent by medical providers who treat TGNC patients and clients. Past clinical models required the TGNC person to obtain the diagnosis of gender dysphoria, undergo ongoing psychotherapy, and pass a "real-life experience test" which consistened of living full-time in their identified gender for 6-24 months. These steps would need to be completed prior to the therapist recommending medical interventions such as hormone treatment or surgery, and a "gender dysphoria" diagnosis, as described within the DSM-5, would be required before HRT or surgical options could be explored with medical care teams. The current informed consent model (a) promotes a departure from the use of the diagnosis of gender dysphoria as a prerequisite for accessing transition services and (b) attempts to impact the way that transgender individuals experience and access healthcare by removing the psychotherapy/gatekeeping requirement. Within this model of care, the role of the practitioner is to provide TGNC patients with information about risks, side effects, benefits, and possible consequences of undergoing gender confirmation care and to obtain informed consent from the patient [41].

The informed consent model allows the patient to make an educated decision regarding the options available to them for HRT and, if desired, potential surgical procedures [45]. When utilizing the informed consent model, the rate of regret is very low [13]. Additionally, for patients seeking to continue HRT or have been treated with HRT for many years, this informed consent process removes lengthy barriers to accessing HRT where interruptions in treatment may present health issues.

Criteria for the clinical assessment of candidacy for HRT is focused on hormone initiation and assessment of patients who are treatment naïve. In older adults, the candidacy for HRT may already be well established, and clinical providers may be asked to continue HRT in circumstances where the patient has already been treated with HRT for many years. Candidacy for HRT in older adults who may be initiating HRT for the first time is focused on analysis of comorbidities and diseases of aging and identification of a treatment strategy informed by patient choice.

For the purpose of informed consent, the provider needs to develop an understanding of the individual's relative risks of treatment and should also fully understand the risks of withholding hormone treatment for gender affirmation.

Categorization and individualized estimates of the risk require clinical expertise in treatment of older adults and a detailed understanding of the progression of normal aging. The medical management of HRT is well within the scope of primary care and often is the least complex part of the individual's clinical care. Denial, rejection, or refusal to treat patients with HRT can have a deleterious effect on the patient that may outweigh the risks of provision of treatment. Shared decision-making is critical to care provision and should be the mainstay of any clinician's approach to care.

2.3 Establishing Goals of Treatment

Assessment of patients' expectations from accessing HRT is a key part of shared decision-making and can be customized to allow for clinicians to identify any misconceptions, assess the patient's general level of knowledge about the process, and also provide a space for people with non-binary identities where the goals of treatment may not be at either end of a traditional gender spectrum [36]. For this reason and to be intentionally inclusive, further discussion of patient goals for HRT will be described with feminizing and masculinizing effects as the primary aim. (Only in specific cases when research refers to individuals as *transgender man*, *transgender woman*, *transman*, or *transwoman* will this terminology be utilized.) Identifying what the patient hopes for when accessing hormones can be especially helpful in customizing and adjusting the treatment strategy. Additionally, identifying any areas of patient concern regarding non-desired effects of treatment can help to manage expectations regarding the progressive timeline of physical changes. This allows the clinician to identify expectations and helps to customize the discussion of risks and benefits of treatment. Inquiry includes how long has treatment been contemplated and if there has been a previous treatment course for gender affirmation. Identification of the patient's goals for accessing HRT can also help inform follow-up assessment visits and helps the clinician to identify unrealistic expectations.

2.4 Insurance and Financial Costs of Care

For masculinizing or feminizing HRT, the costs of care are modest in comparison with other common treatments and medications for older adults. Medicare and managed Medicare, the most common health insurance for older adults and people with disabilities, cover medically necessary transition-related medical and preventative care [5] regardless of the gender marker listed on the identification card [34]. For many older adults who receive Medicare coverage, the supplemental insurance may have different coverage policies. There may still be significant barriers and confusion about the definition of medical necessity and the use of hormones that are incongruent with the gender marker. Patients should seek insurance specialty support if encountering these barriers.

2.5 Approach to Patients with Multiple Chronic Conditions

Before initiating HRT, patients should have a complete health history that includes documentation of current or past medical conditions, cancer screening and history, past and present medications, and family history including family longevity, surgical history, social history, and mental health history. Questions regarding reproductive intent are usually not applicable. For older adults who are advanced in age and/or have complex medical histories, treatment can certainly introduce some aspects of risk, but the risk can be managed and rarely poses an absolute contraindication to initiation of HRT [17].

Additionally, it is important to utilize estimates of life expectancy to understand that the risk of HRT may not be additive, i.e., the patient may have a functional status and conditions that are more likely to contribute to morbidity and mortality and so the risk of hormone administration is minor in comparison. Given the high value that patients place on HRT and the potential for alleviation of suffering, the perceived value from the patient's perspective can be great. Diseases of aging and organ system disease considerations are addressed in this chapter and summarize current research and clinical recommendations across disciplines.

Older TGNC adults often face challenges and obstacles when initiating HRT at advanced ages. HRT initiation for older individuals may be less effective at achieving secondary sex characteristics and carry additional side effects or complications not seen in younger TGNC patients. Additionally, gender confirmation surgeries that are often provided in tandem with HRT bring increased risk for aging adults as well.

Later in life, initiation of HRT and gender-confirming surgeries can also have mental health and behavioral risks. One study [8] concluded that participants who initiated HRT at an earlier age may have subsequently experienced less lifelong burden of gender dysphoria and, therefore, had been less likely to turn to at-risk alcohol use to cope with gender-related distress. Aging TGNC individuals may also have further difficulties transitioning with their biological families, within established careers, and throughout long-term social support systems. Therefore, aging TGNC adults should be monitored and evaluated by their care teams for the development or increased prevalence of mental health distress or significant changes in risk behaviors.

2.6 Primary Prevention and Health Screening

Studies of preventative care in TGNC individuals are sparse. Predominant clinical protocols recommend an organ system inventory approach to prevention, so if the individual possesses the organ, they should be screened based on preventative care guidelines. These guidelines are readily extrapolated to TGNC populations. In some cases such as prostate screening, the recommendations have evolved, and the use of laboratory values such as PSA is influenced by HRT treatment [18]. Hormone-mediated cancer screening has followed national guidelines. If the patient has breasts, cervix, or prostate, primary prevention for cancer screening should be offered, and the patient should be counseled on the risks and benefits of screening and that the reliability may be influenced by HRT.

Tobacco presents a major risk factor for morbidity and mortality, along with social determinants of health for TGNC individuals. Smoking among lesbian, gay, and bisexual adults in the United States is much higher than among heterosexual/straight adults [4]. About one in five (20.5%) lesbian, gay, or bisexual adults smoke cigarettes compared with about one in seven (15.3%) heterosexual/straight adults [4]. Further, cigarette smoking is also higher among transgender adults (35.5%) than among cisgender adults [9] and as such leads to higher than expected prevalence of risk factors for diseases associated with or exacerbated by smoking (e.g., heart disease) [21].

As with all aging populations, greater sexual health counseling and STI prevention efforts need to be integrated into care and community messaging. As people age, their immune system function naturally declines, a process called immunosenescence, diminishing the body's innate ability to fight off infections. With the growth in the population of older adults, it has become increasingly important to emphasize maintaining good health status and preventing infections, including sexually transmitted infections (STIs) [40]. Despite the fact that STIs rank highly among patient concerns, providers of health services need to be educated that older adults continue to be sexually active, and discussing sex and healthy aging is important [33].

According to the National Social Life, Health, and Aging Project survey of more than 3000 people between the ages of 57 and 85, approximately 75% of people between 57 and 64 reported being sexually active. More than half of people between 65 and 74 reported being sexually active, and more than a quarter of those 75–85 reported being sexually active [33]. These data points report on sexual activity of all populations of aging individuals, including TGNC persons.

Half of all people currently living with HIV are aged 50 or older [11]. Older adults are acquiring HIV in the same ways as their younger counterparts. Many people are successfully aging with HIV because medication regimens are highly effective, easy to take, and side effects are minimal and easy to manage, yet it can be more difficult for older adults to manage HIV than younger adults. In the United States, there are currently 1.25 million people living with HIV, and as of 2015, 50% of these individuals were over the age of 50. By 2020, it is estimated that 70% of those living with HIV will be over age 50 [33]. Ongoing HIV prevention, testing, and partner services need to continue to be available to TGNC patients to ensure continued health for both HIV-positive and HIV-negative individuals.

Osteoporosis screening has special importance in TGNC older adults due to a confluence of risk factors. TGNC populations carry a higher burden of tobacco use, which is a major risk factor for osteoporosis, as is hypogonadal states such as menopause or surgical removal of testicles or ovaries and HIV infection. Cisgender male osteoporosis and hypogonadal-related osteoporosis increases with age yet remains lower than cisgender females of similar ages [23]. Studies with the greatest statistical power show increased rates of osteopenia in transgender women on HRT [39].

There is disagreement regarding the bone density reference ranges for cisgender male and female patients and TGNC people who have established cross-sex hormone therapy (CSHT), with some experts advocating for a combined standard reference range. Providers less familiar with post CSHT must carefully assess for changes in bone density.

There is insufficient evidence to estimate breast or reproductive cancer prevalence in the TGNC population. Gender-affirming hormones have not been shown to affect cancer risk [17, 29], but there is a clear need for more study on this topic.

2.7 Expected Changes with HRT

The initiation of HRT in TGNC individuals will have significant changes within the body. For older adults, these changes will be occurring at the same time as expected onset of conditions and diseases associated with aging, including, but not limited to, hypertension, diabetes, memory disorders, elevated cholesterol, and cardiovascular disease. Medical providers who serve TGNC patients must ensure the ongoing monitoring of these significant physiological changes along with expected conditions of aging.

2.8 Feminizing Hormone Treatment

The objective of feminizing hormone treatment is to decrease levels or decrease the effects of endogenous testosterone in the body while simultaneously adding physiologic doses of estrogen. Accepted protocols for prescribing and dosage of HRT can be found in multiple publicly available resource sites (Appendix A). Suppression of testosterone and its effects is usually achieved with androgen blockers, such as spironolactone and finasteride, or can be achieved by surgical removal of gonads. The reduction in testosterone alone will result in some degree of feminization. These changes are accompanied by the administration of parenteral or oral forms of estrogen. Permanent changes over time include breast growth, testicular atrophy, decreased sperm count, and decreased fertility, and these will remain if HRT is discontinued. Changes that are nonpermanent may revert over time if HRT is discontinued or interrupted, including changes in sex drive, morning erections, fat redistribution, decreases in muscular strength, softening of the skin and decreases of body hair, and reversal of male pattern baldness. Patients who have undergone removal of gonadal tissue and endogenous sources of sex hormones benefit from the presence of some sex hormone to maintain bone health and to avoid osteoporosis, which can be the result of hypogonadism where extremely low levels of sex hormone are present [23]. As previously mentioned, present clinical protocol for feminization treatment is the pairing of an antiandrogen such as spironolactone or finasteride and physiologic doses of estrogen. In the United States, this is the predominant approach; in other countries, other antiandrogen approaches may be used.

Beers Criteria are used to identify potentially inappropriate medication use in older adults and set guidelines for healthcare professionals to help improve the safety of prescribing medications for older adults [2]. These criteria are designed without consideration of masculinizing and feminizing treatment in TGNC populations and do not explore potential benefit or risks of HRT in this context. Using Beers Criteria, estrogens are identified as potentially inappropriate medications in patients 65 and older due to a demonstrated lack of cardiovascular protection or cognitive protection in research done with postmenopause cisgender women and due to carcinogenic potential, primarily in breast and endometrial tissue. Studies such as the 2002 Women's Health Initiative are not well-applied to TGNC aging populations, as the HRT utilized differs in formulation and involves progesterone forms not commonly utilized for gender-affirming HRT. In addition, the purpose and treatment outcomes and goals of treatment differ [43].

Feminizing treatment is accomplished through single-use medications or a combination of medications, often beginning with spironolactone in an off-label use. This medication is used as an antihypertensive potassium-sparing diuretic, and the mechanism of action is via mineralocorticoid (aldosterone) receptor antagonism. Spironolactone is a potent and direct antagonist of the androgen receptor, blocking androgens like testosterone from binding to and activating the receptor; as such, this can be integrated into their antihypertensive regimen in replacement of medications or in concert with them. No dose adjustment is necessary for hepatic impairment.

According to Beers Criteria, spironolactone should be avoided in patients 65 years and older with creatinine clearance <30 mL/minute due to risk of hyperkalemia [2]. Drug interactions for this medication are linked to enhancement of hypotensive effects of other medications, enhanced hypotensive effects in older adults based on propensity to orthostatic hypotension, enhancement of renal effects, and interactions that may increase potassium levels or decrease renal function. Many of these effects can be managed by close monitoring of therapy and dose adjustment. Absolute contraindications include hyperkalemia.

Another effective medication less frequently used in providing feminizing effects is finasteride. Finasteride competitively inhibits type II 5-alpha reductase, resulting in inhibition of the conversion of testosterone to dihydrotestosterone and marked suppression of serum dihydrotestosterone levels. It is manufactured for on- label use for benign prostatic hyperplasia and male pattern baldness, and off-label use for hirsutism and feminizing HRT. It is metabolized by the liver and so should be used with caution when hepatic impairment is present and is a minor substrate of CYP3A4. It does not, however, list significant drug-drug interactions with medications typically used in an aging population. Prostate cancer should be ruled out prior to initiation of the medication [35].

Finasteride reduces prostate-specific antigen (PSA) concentration by approximately 50% within 6 months of treatment, and to interpret serial PSAs, a new PSA baseline should be established ≥6 months after treatment initiation and PSA monitored periodically thereafter if prostate screening is desired. A confirmed PSA increase while on this medication, even if within normal limits, may be associated with an increased risk for prostate cancer and should be evaluated. The amount of total testosterone that is measured in serum after initiation of the medication is increased is generally quoted as a 10% increase, but the active form of serum dihydrotestosterone, the active form of testosterone, is reduced. Side effects of the medication can include hypotension that may be synergistic with other medications.

In addition to either androgen blocker spironolactone or finasteride, estrogens are typically introduced once testosterone effects are minimized. Estradiol or 17β-estradiol is a naturally occurring hormone that circulates endogenously within the human body. Estradiol plays an essential role in the development of secondary female sex characteristics, as well as in aging and several hormonally mediated disease states. Estrogen mediates its effects across the body through agonism of the estrogen receptor (ER). ERs are present in breasts, uterus, ovaries, skin, prostate, bone, fat, and brain tissue. Estradiol is available in a number of formulations, including oral, transdermal, and injectable. Estradiol is commercially produced to manage conditions associated with reduced estrogen production such as menopausal and perimenopausal symptoms as well as hypoestrogenism and TGNC HRT. It is sometimes used for the palliative treatment of some hormone-sensitive cancers like breast and prostate cancer.

Transdermal treatment with estrogen reduces the first-pass metabolism by the liver hepatic metabolism [6]. In studies in cisgender women, transdermal HRT may have less pronounced effects on hepatic protein synthesis, and this may mediate the thrombogenic risk [10]. Both oral and transdermal delivery systems have beneficial effects on high-density lipoprotein cholesterol to low-density lipoprotein cholesterol ratios [24]. The transdermal system has more favorable effects on triglycerides. Incidence of metabolic syndrome and weight gain appears to be slightly lower with a transdermal delivery system. In older adults, the use of transdermal or non-orally administered estrogen is recommended over oral [10]. Estrogen is metabolized by the liver, and there are a number of drug-drug interactions based on the CYP inhibitors and inducers that should be reviewed, and monitoring for these side effects is important. Patients who have been prescribed oral conjugated estrogens should be switched to transdermal or intramuscular administration of hormones. Recommended clinical protocols include frequent monitoring of estrogen and testosterone levels and monitoring for renal, liver, and hematologic effects more frequently (every 3 months) in long-term HRT [19, 25].

For feminizing treatment, the largest concern is some effects of venous thromboembolism (VTE). In studies with unconjugated estrogens from a population of transgender women in District of Columbia from chart audit from January 1, 2008, through March 31, 2016, 676 transgender women received oral estradiol-based cross-sex hormone replacement therapy (CSHT) for a total of 1286 years of hormone treatment and a mean of 1.9 years of CSHT per patient. Only one individual, or 0.15% of the population, sustained a VTE, for an incidence of 7.8 events per 10,000 person-years. There was a low incidence of VTE in this population of transgender women receiving oral estradiol [3].

A meta-analysis of research on HRT revealed that hormones utilized for masculinization may increase LDL-C and TG levels and decrease HDL-C level in individuals, whereas oral estrogens may increase TG levels in feminization [32], and the quality of the evidence was not high. In terms of outcomes of importance, there were few myocardial infarction, stroke, venous thromboembolism, and death events reported, but data is lacking.

Studies with the greatest statistical power show increased rates of osteopenia in transgender women on HRT [39]. Further research examined 100 transgender men and women after a mean of 10 years on HRT; 25% of transgender women experienced osteoporosis whereas transgender men did not [42]. Wierckx went on to suggest that this increase in bone mass could be due to either increased screening of transgender females, antiandrogen therapy itself, or prior administration of an antiandrogen for 1 year before the start of estrogen therapy.

Individuals receiving estrogen and antiandrogen treatment for feminization can expect decreases in sebum and acne, prostate size, sperm count and quality, lean mass, facial and body hair, male pattern baldness, systolic blood pressure, hemoglobin and hematocrit, testosterone, luteinizing hormone, and follicle-stimulating hormones. Increases in breast tissue, skin softness, fat mass, visceral fat, LDL cholesterol, triglycerides, and prolactin can be expected [14].

Cutaneous manifestations from feminizing estrogen therapy may include xerosis, brittle nails, and possible increased risk of melanoma and nonmelanoma skin cancers [38]. Estrogens rapidly and persistently reduce sebum production [26]. Indirectly, this can exacerbate dry skin (xerosis), including atopies, and older adults may experience increased pruritus and eczematous changes. Estrogens reduce and change pattern of body hair and can positively impact pattern hair loss but only partially reduces body hair growth so electrolysis and hair removal techniques may also be involved, particularly for removal of facial hair. Topical eflornithine can also be utilized to reduce but not eliminate unwanted hair growth.

Silicone injection as a method to achieve feminization was often the only method available and accessible to patients who are now in the TGNC aging cohort due to the barriers to accessing HRT in previous clinical protocols [45]. Skin complications from free silicone injection can include immediate reactions such as arterial occlusion, focal necrosis (related to venous occlusion), postinjection papules, discoloration of the skin, postinjection pain, redness, ecchymosis, bleeding, and swelling and hypersensitivity reactions. Longer-term effects can include pain, ecchymosis, pigmentation, inflammatory nodules, and pruritus. Longer-term potential complications include the formation of inflammatory nodules and silicone granulomata cellulitis with sterile abscesses [45]. Treatment for long-term complications can include a 4–6-week course of antibiotic therapy, inter-lesion injection of lesions, and resection of circumscribed lesions. NSAIDs can be used to reduce inflammation for refractory symptoms, and immunosuppressant medications have been attempted, but there is little outcome data on this approach. Anecdotally, free silicone injection as a body modification practice is not uncommon, but since there is little systematic data collection on this topic, the absolute risk of complications with this practice remains unknown [45].

There is insufficient evidence in the literature to estimate breast or reproductive cancer prevalence in the TGNC population. HRT utilized for gender-affirming treatment in this population has not been shown to affect cancer risk [42], but there is a clear need for well-designed robust studies to investigate further. Cancer screening should remain congruent with organs and established protocols regardless of hormone use [14].

There is little data on specific health disparities or effects in TGNC patients in regard to oral health. There is some research that suggests that estrogen deficiency is a risk factor for periodontal disease, and this is mostly in the context of hypogonadal states that are related to menopause or cancer treatment and surgical hypogonadism [37].

2.9 Masculinizing Hormone Treatment

The foundation for masculinizing treatment is the administration of exogenous testosterone to achieve virilization and secondary sex characteristics. As stated previously, accepted protocols for prescribing and dosage of HRT can be found in multiple publicly available resource sites (Appendix A). Cautions to treatment include the possibility of elevation of hematocrit, hyperviscosity, obstructive sleep apnea, and uncontrolled heart failure. Dosage forms are intramuscular, subcutaneous, and transdermal. Oral, sub-buccal, and internasal are not typically used in the United States. Concerns regarding long-term effects include breast cancer, cardiovascular disease, lipid profile changes, hepatic effects, polycythemia, and venous thromboembolism.

Testosterone may enhance the hypoglycemic effect of diabetes medications and may change the anticoagulant effect of warfarin, with the elderly at highest risk [7]. In general, this treatment can be administered regardless of the presence or absence of the uterus and ovaries, although there is some speculation that inducing an anovulatory state for a prolonged length of time would correlate to a greater risk of endometrial cancer. There is insufficient evidence to support this. Currently, studies have not demonstrated this risk [14].

Transgender men and gender nonconforming people also need to be carefully monitored as they age for endometrial cancer, polycystic changes, cardiovascular health, and musculoskeletal health. In a review of the effects of testosterone on surrogate risks of cardiovascular disease, testosterone administration affected some cardiovascular risk factors negatively, such as a decrease of high-density lipoprotein cholesterol, an increase of triglycerides, and inflammation factors, but notably, there was no induction of insulin resistance, which is a characteristic of hyperandrogenic conditions in women such as polycystic ovarian syndrome [22]. Medical management of testosterone will initially require frequent monitoring of labs, physical changes, and self-reported state of well-being. For some transgender men, initiating HRT in their later years and administering testosterone transdermally or by intramuscular injection can diminish dysphoria and depression [15].

As evidence accumulates for the benefits of supplemental testosterone in aging natal men, it has seen wider use in the aging population. Patients who have been receiving testosterone, particularly if they have undergone hysterectomy and oophorectomy, will require exogenous androgens to maintain bone health [23].

Transgender men and gender nonconforming people receiving testosterone therapy can expect to see decreases in HDL cholesterol, luteinizing hormone, follicle-stimulating hormones, estradiol, glandular tissue, and vaginal epithelium thickness. Increases can be expected in triglyceride count, hemoglobin and hematocrit, systolic blood pressure, hair density, fibrous connective tissue, clitoral size, lean mass, body weight, and grip strength. In a meta-analysis, hormones utilized for masculinization in TGNC individuals may increase LDL-C and TG levels and decrease HDL-C levels. In terms of outcomes of importance, there were few myocardial infarction, stroke, venous thromboembolism, and death events reported, but data is lacking [32].

Evaluation of dysplasia can be challenging on Pap tests from transgender and gender nonconforming patients on androgen therapy. Within the cohort of 11 patients taking testosterone, 43% of those evaluated had higher rates of unsatisfactory and abnormal Pap tests [1]. Pathologists should become familiar with the distinctive cytomorphological changes in the Pap tests from patients on androgen therapy [1]. In a literature review for cancer incidence in individuals on testosterone for masculinizing effects, an analysis of 228 articles reported 18 breast cancer cases, 5 ovarian cancer cases, 4 uterine/cervical cancer cases, and 1 vaginal cancer case [29]. There is insufficient evidence to estimate breast or reproductive cancer prevalence in the TGNC population. Gender-affirming hormones have not been shown to affect cancer risk in masculinizing treatment [29].

Conclusions For aging TGNC people, there are few absolute contraindications for hormone replacement therapy. Standards of care for HRT are readily available and can be easily integrated into complex geriatric patients' care provided that assessment of risks and benefits are thoroughly explored. Providers working in multiple disciplines can utilize these recommendations in addition to existing protocols to provide gender-affirming HRT for treatment-experienced or treatment-naive older TGNC adults. All conclusions have been formed with existing data and experience in primary care practice, yet further research studies are needed to provide an evidentiary basis for HRT care protocols for older TGNC adults.

Appendix A: Medication Prescribing and Dosage Resources

World Professional Association for Transgender Health (WPATH) Standards of Care (SOC) found at https://www.wpath.org/publications/soc

University of California San Francisco (UCSF) Center of Excellence (CoE) for Transgender Health Guidelines found at http://transhealth.ucsf.edu/trans?page=guidelines-home

Endocrine Society Clinical Practice Guidelines found at https://www.endocrine.org/guidelines-and-clinical-practice/clinical-practice-guidelines

References

1. Adkins BD, Barlow AB, Coogan AC, Desouki MM, Jack A, Schultenover SJ, Weiss VL. Characteristic findings of cervical Papanicolaou tests from transgender patients on androgen therapy: challenges in detecting dysplasia. Cytopathology. 2018;29:281. https://doi.org/10.1111/cyt.12525.
2. American Geriatrics Society. Updated beers criteria for potentially inappropriate medication use in older adults. J Am Geriatr Soc. 2015;63(11):2227–46. https://doi.org/10.1111/jgs.13702.
3. Arnold JD, Sarkodie EP, Coleman ME, Goldstein DA. Incidence of venous thromboembolism in transgender women receiving oral estradiol. J Sex Med. 2016;4(5):1241–6.
4. Babb SD, Gentzke AS, Jamal A, Phillips E, Homa DM, King BA, Neff LJ. Current cigarette smoking among adults — United States, 2016. Morb Mortal Wkly Rep. 2018;67:53–9. https://doi.org/10.15585/mmwr.mm6702a1.
5. Baker KE. The future of transgender coverage. N Engl J Med. 2017;376(19):1801–4.
6. Bergendal A, Kieler H, Sundström A, Linděn Hirschberg A, Kocoska-Maras L. Risk of venous thromboembolism associated with local and systemic use of hormone therapy in peri- and postmenopausal women and in relation to type and route of administration. Menopause. 2016;1:593. https://doi.org/10.1097/GME.0000000000000611.
7. Bjerrum L, Andersen M, Petersen G, Kragstrup J. Exposure to potential drug interactions in primary health care. Scand J Prim Health Care. 2003;21(3):153–8.
8. Bidwell, et al. Factors associated with gender-affirming surgery and age of hormone therapy initiation among transgender adults. Transgend Health. 2017;2(1):156–64. https://doi.org/10.1089/trgh.2017.0028.
9. Buchting FO, Emory KT, Scout, Kim Y, Fagan P, Vera LE, Emery S. Transgender use of cigarettes, cigars, and E-cigarettes in a national study. Am J Prev Med. 2017;53(1):e1–7. https://doi.org/10.1016/j.amepre.2016.11.022. Epub 2017 Jan 13
10. Canonico M, Plu-Bureau G, Lowe GD, Scarabin PY. Hormone replacement therapy and risk of venous thromboembolism in postmenopausal women: systematic review and meta-analysis. BMJ. 2008;336(7655):1227–31.
11. Centers for Disease Control and Prevention. Diagnoses of HIV infection among adults aged 50 years and older in the United States and dependent areas, 2010–2014. HIV Surveillance Supplemental Report 2016;21(2) http://wwwcdcgov/hiv/library/reports/surveillance/. Published May 2016. Accessed May 21, 2018.
12. Coleman E, Bockting W, Botzer M, Cohen-Kettenis P, DeCuypere G, Feldman J, et al. Standards of care for the health of transsexual, transgender, and gender-nonconforming people, version 7. Int J Transgend. 2012;13(4):165–232.
13. Deutsch MB. Use of the informed consent model in the provision of cross-sex hormone therapy: a survey of the practices of selected clinics. Int J Transgend. 2012;13(3):140–6.
14. Deutsch MB. Guidelines for the primary and gender-affirming care of transgender and gender nonbinary people. 2nd ed. San Francisco: Center of Excellence for Transgender Health, Department of Family and Community Medicine, University of California; 2016. Available at: www.transhealth.ucsf.edu/.
15. Ettner R. Care of the elderly transgender patient. Curr Opin Endocrinol Diabetes Obes. 2013;20(6):580–4. https://doi.org/10.1097/01.med.0000436183.34931.a5.
16. Fabbre VD. Gender transitions in later life: a queer perspective on successful aging. Gerontologist. 2015;55(1):144–53. https://doi.org/10.1093/geront/gnu079. Epub 2014 Aug 26
17. Feldman J. Medical and surgical management of the transgender patient: What the primary care clinician needs to know. In: World Professional Association for Transgender Health (WPATH), editor. Standards of care for the health of transsexual, transgender, and gender nonconforming people. 7th ed; 2009. p. 365–91.
18. Feldman J. Medical and surgical management of the transgender patient: what the primary care clinician needs to know. The Fenway Guide to Lesbian, Gay, Bisexual, and Transgender Health. 2nd ed. Philadelphia: American College of Physicians; 2015.

19. Feldman J, Safer J. Hormone therapy in adults: suggested revisions to the sixth version of the standards of care. Int J Transgend. 2009;11(3):146–82. https://doi.org/10.1080/15532730903383757.
20. Flores AR, Herman JL, Gates GJ, Brown TNT. How many adults identify as transgender in the United States? The Williams Institute. 2016. Published Web Location. http://williamsinstitute.law.ucla.edu/wp-content/uploads/How-Many-Adults-Identify-as-Transgenderin-the-United-States.pdf.
21. Gamarel KE, Mereish EH, Manning D, Iwamoto M, Operario D, Nemoto T. Minority stress, smoking patterns, and cessation attempts: findings from a community-sample of transgender women in the San Francisco Bay Area. Nicotine Tob Res. 2016;18(3):306–13. https://doi.org/10.1093/ntr/ntv066
22. Giltay EJ, Gooren LJ, Wierckx K. Cardiovascular disease in transsexual persons treated with cross-sex hormones: reversal of the traditional sex difference in cardiovascular disease pattern. Eur J Endocinol. 2014;170(6):809–19. https://doi.org/10.1530/EJE-14-0011. Epub 2014 Mar 10
23. Golds G, Houdek D, Arnason T. Male hypogonadism and osteoporosis: the effects, clinical consequences, and treatment of testosterone deficiency in bone health. Int J Endocrinol. 2017; https://doi.org/10.1155/2017/4602129. Epub 2017 Mar 16
24. Goodman MP. Are all estrogens created equal? A review of oral vs. transdermal therapy. J Womens Health (Larchmt). 2012;21(2):161–9. https://doi.org/10.1089/jwh.2011.2839.
25. Hembree WC, Cohen-Kettenis PT, Gooren L, Hannema SE, Meyer WJ, Murad MH, et al. Endocrine treatment of gender-dysphoric/gender-incongruent persons: an Endocrine Society clinical practice guideline. J Clin Endocrinol Metab. 2017;102(11):3869–903. https://doi.org/10.1210/jc.2017-01658.
26. Hermosura AT, Kabigting FD. Dermatologic care of the transgender patient. Dermatol Online J. 2016;22:10.
27. James SE, Herman JL, Rankin S, Keisling M, Mottet L, Anafi M. The report of the 2015 U.S. transgender survey. Washington, DC: National Center for Transgender Equality; 2016.
28. Jin K. Modern biological theories of aging. Aging and Disease. 2010;1(2):72–4.
29. Joint R, Chen ZE, Cameron S. Breast and reproductive cancers in the transgender population: a systematic review. BJOG (An International Journal of Obstetrics & Gynaecology). 2018; https://doi.org/10.1111/1471-0528.15258.
30. Jones BA, Brewin N, Richards C, Van Eijk M, Stephenson-Allen A, Arcelus J. Investigating the outcome of the initial assessment at a national transgender health service: Time to review the process? Int J Transgenderism. 2017;18(4):427–32.
31. Knochel KA. Are they prepared? A look at midlife transgender people and their anticipated adaptation to aging. Minneapolis: University of Minnesota; 2011.
32. Maraka S, Singh Ospina N, Rodriguez-Gutierrez R, Davidge-Pitts CJ, Nippoldt TB, Prokop LJ, Murad MH. Sex steroids and cardiovascular outcomes in transgender individuals: a systematic review and meta-analysis. J Clin Endocrinol Metabol. 2017;102(11):3914–23.
33. New York State Department of Health AIDS Institute (NYSDOH). Older adults and sexual health: a guide for aging services providers. 2017. https://aging.ny.gov/nysofa/Older%20Adults%20Sexual%20Health%20Guide%202017%20WEB%20version.pdf.
34. Proctor K, Haffer SC, Ewald E, Hodge C, James CV. Identifying the transgender population in the Medicare program. Transgender Health. 2016;1(1):250–65. https://doi.org/10.1089/trgh.2016.0031.
35. Rhoden EL, Morgentaler A. Testosterone replacement therapy in hypogonadal men at high risk for prostate cancer: results of 1 year of treatment in men with prostatic intraepithelial neoplasia. J Urol. 2003;170(6):2348–51.
36. Richards C, Bouman WP, Seal L, Barker MJ, Nieder TO, T'Sjoen G. Non-binary or genderqueer genders. Int Rev Psychiatry. 2016;28(1):95–102.
37. Russell S, More F. Addressing health disparities via coordination of care and interprofessional education: lesbian, gay, bisexual, and transgender health and oral health care. Dental Clinics. 2016;60(4):891–906.

38. Sabra JJ, Fang CX, Kundu RV. A knowledge-based assessment of dermatological care for transgender women. Transgender Health. 2018;3(1):71–3.
39. Safer JD, Weinand JD. Hormone therapy in transgender adults is safe with provider supervision; a review of hormone therapy sequelae for transgender individuals. J Clin Transl Endocrinol. 2015;2(2):55–60.
40. Schick V, Herbenick D, Reece M, Sanders SA, Dodge B, Middlestadt SE, Fortenberry JD. Sexual behaviors, condom use, and sexual health of Americans over 50: implications for sexual health promotion for older adults. J Sex Med. 2010;7(s5):315–29.
41. Schulz SL. The informed consent model of transgender care: an alternative to the diagnosis of gender dysphoria. First published Dec 13, 2017. Research Article. https://doi.org/10.1177/0022167817745217.
42. Wierckx K, Mueller S, Weyers S, Van Caenegem E, Roef G, Heylens G, et al. Long-term evaluation of cross-sex hormone treatment in transsexual persons. J Sex Med. 2012 Oct 1;9(10):2641–51.
43. Writing Group for the Women's Health Initiative Investigators. Risks and benefits of estrogen plus progestin in healthy postmenopausal women: principal results from the Women's Health Initiative randomized controlled trial. JAMA. 2002;288(3):321–33.
44. Wylie K, Knudson G, Khan SI, Bonierbale M, Watanyusakul S, Baral S. Serving transgender people: clinical care considerations and service delivery models in transgender health. Lancet. 2016;388(10042):401–11.
45. Zevin B, Deutsch MB. Center of Excellence for Transgender Health, Department of Family and Community Medicine, University of California San Francisco. In: Deutsch MB, editors. Guidelines for the primary and gender-affirming care of transgender and gender nonbinary people. 2nd ed. 2016. Available at www.transhealth.ucsf.edu/guidelines.

Transgender Physiology, Anatomy, and Aging: A Provider's Guide to Gender-Affirming Surgeries

3

Cecilia T. Hardacker, Jules Chyten-Brennan, and Alix Komar

3.1 Introduction

Multiple challenges exist for transgender and gender nonconforming (TGNC) and non-binary individuals as they age in relation to their physiology and anatomy. Many older TGNC people who desire gender-affirming surgery (GAS), who are attempting to have these medically necessary procedures, may find access difficult if not impossible. For TGNC individuals who have had GAS earlier in their lives, there may be long-term physical needs to address and multiple chronic health conditions as they age. For the purposes of this exploration, selected surgeries will be discussed in the context of TGNC individuals only and potential postoperative complications that may affect overall patient satisfaction and long-term outcomes. In this chapter, we will explore issues related to the physiology and anatomy of aging TGNC individuals and offer recommendations for providers to support their patients who desire GAS and those patients who have had GAS at some point in their life experience.

C. T. Hardacker (✉)
Howard Brown Health Center, Chicago, IL, USA
e-mail: ceciliah@howardbrown.org

J. Chyten-Brennan
Montefiore Medical Center, Bronx, NY, USA

A. Komar
Weiss Hospital, Chicago, IL, USA
e-mail: akomar@weisshospital.com

M. Houlberg et al. (eds.), *Transgender and Gender Nonconforming Health and Aging*,
https://doi.org/10.1007/978-3-319-95031-0_3

3.2 Access and Insurance

Transgender and gender nonconforming (TGNC) and non-binary people have begun to have greater access to multidisciplinary health care that seeks to affirm their physical and mental health and well-being. Behavioral Risk Factor Surveillance System (BRFSS) data from 2016 indicate there are an estimated number of 1.4 million people who identify as TGNC in the United States, and 217,050 of those are over the age of 65 [1]. Of these, only a portion of patients will desire and seek surgeries. In recent years, changes to health insurance law, primarily Section 1557 of the Affordable Care Act (ACA), interpreted to ban discrimination on the basis of gender identity, have increased availability of transition-related care to treat gender dysphoria [2]. Prior to 2010, gender dysphoria, defined as a strong misalignment of an individual's sense of self and their sex assigned at birth, was classified as a pre-existing condition [2]. Medically necessary transition-related care is described as a combination of hormone therapy and gender-affirming surgeries, and for patients experiencing gender dysphoria, mental health therapy is recommended on an individual basis [3]. For older TGNC individuals seeking this care, a 2014 ruling on Medicare's historical exclusion of coverage for transition-related care was deemed no longer justifiable, and the new coverage has expanded availability. In 2018, the Supreme Court is expected to rule on a case from Texas challenging this expanded protection [4]. Between 2002 and 2016, half of the US Fortune 500 companies have added gender transition care to their list of covered benefits, with some including gender-affirming surgeries [5]. In addition, in June of 2011, the Veterans Health Administration issued a directive to provide all transition-related care up to and after sex reassignment surgeries [7] showing a 40% increase of veterans seeking transition-related care in the first 2 years after issuance of the directive [7].

Even with this expanded coverage, older transgender individuals may face continued difficulty in attaining access to lifesaving surgeries. In May of 2015, Denee Mallon, a 75-year-old veteran of the Army, challenged the Medicare ban on paying for GAS, appealing to the Health and Human Services board; she won the right to have GAS paid through her Medicare benefits [8, 9]. In many cases, insurance options are limited and require lengthy navigation with representatives who are not welltrained or familiar with the surgical procedures and how to respectfully support TGNC or non-binary individuals. Older adults who have limited incomes and struggle with confusing health-care policies will more than likely experience impediments to GAS. Clinical settings that provide TGNC and non-binary patient navigation typically have dedicated staff, many times nurses, who work with the patient and insurance representatives to complete challenging approval processes.

3.3 Multiple Chronic Conditions

Few studies exist that explore the chronic disease burden of TGNC individuals. The 2015 United States Transgender Survey (USTS) and a 2016 study accessing Medicare claim records through the Centers for Medicare & Medicaid Services

(CMS) and Chronic Conditions Data Warehouse (CCW) provide two perspectives on chronic disease burden for aging transgender individuals.

The 2015 USTS connected with 27,715 respondents, 14% between 46 and 64, with an additional 2% over the age of 65, compared to 19% of the US population [10]. In terms of overall quality of life measures, respondents indicated they had difficulty with hearing, vision, walking, stairs, dressing, or bathing in similar rates as the general US population [10]. However, respondents reported having difficulty concentrating or remembering and making decisions because of a physical, mental, or emotional condition 6 times higher than their cisgender counterparts [10]. In addition, 3 times more respondents had difficulty doing errands alone, such as doctor's appointments or shopping, again, due to experiencing physical, mental, or emotional conditions. This psychological distress occurs at rates 4 times higher that of the general US population. Twenty percent of TGNC people over the age of 65 reported that they had lost their spouse or partner because of their transgender status, more often in trans-identified women [10]. Transgender, gender nonconforming and non-binary individuals over 65 are living with HIV at rates 5 times higher than the US population, with the highest burden in trans women of color (TWOC) [10]. Finally, 18% report using prescription medications for nonmedical reasons and a shocking 50% of TGNC people over 65 smoke tobacco [10]. In spite of these long-term health challenges, when asked about overall health, USTS respondents over 65 claimed very good (38%) or excellent (22%) health, in many cases based on familial support [10]. All of these conditions, though serious, are not insurmountable challenges to approval for GAS.

Recent access to extensive Medicare data has proven an illuminating resource to examine multiple chronic conditions (MCCs) in older transgender adults that receive benefits. Two separate groups of researchers worked to identify and describe older transgender individuals by examining data from 2013 in Centers for Medicare & Medicaid Services (CMS). In the 2016 study by Proctor et al., researchers followed an 8-step validation process reviewing multiple ICD-9 codes and diagnoses specific to transgender treatment, reviewing approximately one billion CMS fee-for-service claims, to ultimately analyze 4098 transgender Medicare beneficiaries [11]. The majority of cases reviewed identified as white (73.99%) from geographically diverse areas, the greatest number in California, 562, but with 13 states having 100 or more transgender beneficiaries [11]. Surprisingly, the majority of beneficiaries were below the age of 65, indicating qualification due to disability, rather than age, the primary vehicle for access to Medicare in the general population. Study data reveals specific chronic health issues for TGNC people as they age in comparison to their younger transgender cohort and, in another exploration of this data, their aging cisgender counterparts.

Health inequities for transgender individuals are well-documented here, revealing increased rates of smoking, substance use, HIV/AIDS, depression, and suicide [11], but research that examines multiple chronic conditions is scarce [12, 13]. The 2016 Proctor study of CMS data reviewed 20 chronic condition categories: acquired hypothyroidism, ischemic heart disease, COPD, PTSD, schizophrenia, diabetes, asthma, drug use disorders, obesity, personality disorders, rheumatoid arthritis/osteoarthritis, psychotic disorders, fibromyalgia, chronic pain and fatigue, anemia, tobacco use disorders, hypertension, hyperlipidemia, anxiety disorders, major depressive affective disorders, and depression [11]. In two typical aging health conditions, hypertension and hyperlipidemia, transgender individuals had >80% incidence compared to 50% in their younger transgender counterparts [11]. Over 50% of 65 and older transgender individuals are affected by anemia and depressive disorders, and >25% had one of these diagnoses related to anxiety, fibromyalgia, chronic pain or fatigue, rheumatoid arthritis/osteoarthritis, tobacco use, COPD, drug use disorders, asthma, ischemic heart disease, or acquired hypothyroidism [11].

Untreated hypertension, hyperlipidemia, asthma, COPD, anemia, and heart disease, in most cases, will delay or cause denial of surgery, but if medically managed, would not be cause to refuse authorization of gender-affirming surgeries. For many surgeons, tobacco use and excessive BMI are determining factors in surgery approval. For older adults in particular, tissue frailty becomes a crucial criterion that can eliminate any surgical option.

Research on older transgender individuals is limited, with most studies relying on a small participant number with rare exploration of multiple chronic conditions. In recent further analysis of CMS data by Dragon et al., eligible persons were selected by utilizing both ICD-10 codes and fee-for-service (FFS) beneficiaries who received transition-related care. Researchers utilized criteria based on ages of persons receiving benefits, showing persons younger than 65 had issues primarily related to disability compared to those 65 and older who had chronic disease burden as their central health issue. Conclusions indicate that transgender Medicare beneficiaries (TMB) have an 88.2% chronic disease burden (defined as more than one chronic condition) compared to 72.4% in their cisgender Medicare beneficiaries (CMB) counterparts. Specific comparisons where the health inequity is greater occur in overall mental health, pain, obesity, and some liver conditions [12] for both transgender persons over and under the age of 65. All categories show higher incidence of chronic disease processes, and most MCCs remain within a 10% increased range. Only chronic kidney disease, hyperlipidemia, and hypertension exceed a 10% increase and only depression more than doubles by comparison, a staggering 53.5% in TMB compared to 24.9% in their CMB counterparts [12].

For transgender persons seeking GAS, long-term health issues such as those identified, kidney disease, hyperlipidemia, and hypertension, are limiting factors for candidates for GAS only if these conditions are not well-managed and the patient is deemed "medically fit" [14]. As with most surgical procedures, stability of chronic conditions will be part of multiple factors that influence eligibility and readiness for top surgery, including breast augmentation or mastectomy, and bottom surgery, including vaginoplasty, phalloplasty, and metoidioplasty, discussed below.

For all providers with patients seeking GAS, being mindful of the appropriate use of the patient's name and pronouns as well as utilizing the same language they use to identify their bodies and body parts will build a foundation from which to build a trusting relationship and allow them to comfortably speak about themselves. As described in the essential chapter, these best practices will further support provider-patient communication, trust, and reduction of preoperative anxiety.

3.4 General Surgical Considerations

Surgery is inherently full of potential risks. Gender-related genitoplasty is no different in this regard. As a result, having a full discussion with the surgeon as well as the anesthesiologist prior to surgery and ensuring that all of the risks are well-understood is essential. Some of the potential risks during surgery may be modified (or the risk lowered) if the patient is well-prepared in advance. Research shows as a person enters older age, smoking, obesity, excessive alcohol use, illicit drug use, and any other unmanaged medical conditions may increase perioperative contraindications for surgery. While one's age cannot be altered, ensuring that the patient is up-to-date with all preventive health needs prior to consulting a surgeon will help lower the risks of surgery. Because complications can occur in any surgery, it is essential that the surgeon develops a trusting relationship with their patient and invest time to educate the patient to all the potential risks involved with each surgery.

3.5 Perioperative Risks

The perioperative risks that apply to almost any surgery fall into several categories: cardiac (heart), pulmonary (lung), venous thromboembolism (blood clots), hemorrhage (excessive bleeding), infection, injury to surrounding structures, poor wound healing, and need for a repeat procedure or return to the operating room.

3.5.1 Cardiac

The chance of complications related to the heart in the perioperative period is rare in young, healthy patients. However, the risk of major cardiac problems associated with surgery increases with certain factors: high-risk procedures, history of ischemic heart disease (heart attack, positive heart stress test, current chest pain, etc.), history of heart failure, history of cerebrovascular disease (stroke or mini-stroke), diabetes requiring treatment with insulin, and poor kidney function [15]. Major cardiac events include heart attack (myocardial infarction), fluid in the lungs (pulmonary edema), certain detrimental changes in the heart rhythm, and cardiac arrest. Even when a patient has one of the known risk factors, the chance of a major cardiac event around the time of surgery remains rare (Table 3.1).

Table 3.1 Rate of major cardiac event surrounding surgery [15]

No risk factors	0.5%
One risk factor	1.3%
Two risk factors	3.6%
Three or more risk factors	9.1%

3.5.2 Pulmonary

Similar to cardiac issues that may occur surrounding surgery, major pulmonary events related to surgery are also relatively infrequent. These potential risks include failure of the lung to expand fully, lung infection, inability to get enough oxygen, need to remain on a ventilator (breathing machine) for more than 48 hours, and worsening of underlying lung disease. Major complications related to the lungs are heavily related to the preoperative risk factors, as previously discussed (age, obesity, smoking, drug and alcohol use, and prior health conditions), in addition to surgery-specific risk factors that include surgical site and length of surgery [16].

3.5.3 Venous Thromboembolism

The American College of Chest Physicians has stratified patients undergoing surgery for the risk of blood clots surrounding the procedure. These groups are labeled very low risk, low risk, moderate risk, and high risk [17]. The group into which a patient is placed preoperatively is based on many factors including patient age, medical history, family history, and characteristics of the surgery. The risk of blood clots around the time of surgery can be high (10–80%); however, they are rarely fatal (0.1–0.8%) [18]. The potential serious consequences of a blood clot related to surgery are numerous and varied depending on the location of the clot. Some of the more severe possible outcomes are death, stroke, need to be on a ventilator, cardiac arrest, and loss of a limb. Most blood clots are so insignificant they are never diagnosed. There is not currently enough data in the literature to attribute a certain risk for blood clot associated with gender-related genitoplasty.

3.5.4 Hemorrhage

While not mutually exclusive to a blood clot, excessive bleeding may seem as though it is the opposite. In any surgery, control of surgical blood loss is paramount. The complicating factor is that while the general location and structure of blood vessels are similar among patients, no two humans are exactly the same. As a result of this anatomic variance, blood vessels can be inadvertently injured or must be disrupted to accomplish the surgery. Depending on the amount of hemorrhage during surgery, a blood transfusion may be required. This is necessary to maintain the function of the patient's vital organs and allow for healing. Surgeons and anesthesiologists do not transfuse blood products unless deemed medically necessary. The rates of infectious transmission related to red blood cell transfusion in the United States are low. The chance of getting a bacterial infection is 0.2 per million units of blood transfused [19]. Similarly low are the chances of transmitting a virus during transfusion of red blood cells: 0.2–0.7 per million unit risk for HIV [20] and less than 1 per million unit risk for hepatitis B and C [21]. Other risks of blood transfusion that are also rare include allergic reactions, severe lung injury, blood cell destruction, and cardiac consequences. The specific rates of blood transfusion for gender-related genitoplasty will be discussed in later sections.

3.5.5 Infection

Infection can occur with relation to surgery in any part of the body. Infections are most commonly caused by bacteria but can also be attributed to fungus. Surgical site infections are the most common perioperative infection type and occur in approximately 1 in 24 inpatient surgeries [22, 23]. Additional infection sites may be the urinary tract, lungs, blood, and heart.

3.5.6 Injury to Surrounding Structures

Genitoplasty surgery involves operating near important structures that, if injured, may cause complications. Anatomic variation in all people, scar tissue, and history of infection or injury may obscure the surgical areas that are necessary to access. When this occurs, an injury to a nearby organ, muscle, blood vessel, or nerve is possible. In gender-related genitoplasty, the structures that can potentially be injured are the bladder, rectum, urethra, ureters (tubes that bring urine from the kidneys to the bladder), muscles, blood vessels, and nerves in the region of surgery. If an organ is injured during surgery, it can generally be repaired at the time of surgery if the injury is recognized. Even with repair at the time of surgery, an injury can place the patient at higher risk for problems in the long or short term. The most concerning of these is a fistula or connection between the injured organ and a neighboring structure. Not all injuries are identified during surgery and may need to be repaired in a separate surgery.

3.5.7 Poor Wound Healing

Problems with wound healing may occur with any procedure and at any surgical site. In addition to the general risk factors associated with surgical complications previously discussed, other risks that are associated with poor wound healing include chronic steroid, immunosuppressant, chemotherapy treatment, malnutrition, and immobilization [24]. Wound problems are one of the more common complications associated with gender-related genitoplasty and can often be managed with topical creams or treatments. Occasionally, patients require additional stitches or a return to the operating room.

3.5.8 Repeat Surgeries

Several complications associated with gender-related genitoplasty may lead to a need to return to the operating room sooner than expected. These general complications include poor wound healing, infection, and hemorrhage, but there are many others that are surgery specific.

3.5.9 Anesthesia Risks

While modern anesthesia is considered extremely safe, it can also be associated with complications in even the healthiest of patients. General anesthesia is when a patient is placed completely asleep, does not feel pain or remember the procedure, and requires a breathing machine. While most risks overlap with surgery, including heart and lung problems, one does not and is of particular concern for aging patients. Cognitive-related concerns, including memory and thinking, can be impaired after general anesthesia. The risk is 10–15% and, if it occurs, is related to patient death within a year after surgery [25, 26]. Risk factors for this complication include advanced age, frailty, lower education level, and history of postoperative delirium (changes in mental status) [27, 28]. It is not clear that anesthesia or surgery itself causes this potential change in memory and thinking [29]. Additional studies need to be performed to better understand the cause of postoperative changes in cognition.

3.5.10 Perioperative Risks Associated with Gender-Related Genitoplasy

Research in the area of gender-related genitoplasty is lacking. While we gain more information every year, there is still no best method for performing these surgeries. Surgeons lack a "gold standard" after which procedures can be modeled. Because of the significantly varying techniques that exist, surgical risks also vary widely. Additionally, due to many patients traveling distances to have surgery, long-term patient follow-up that looks at complications related to surgery is unavailable. As a result of these significant gaps in knowledge secondary to the lack of available research, the degree to which risks can be attributed to surgery may not be accurate and is likely very dependent on the surgeon and technique applied to surgery. The data that does exist on complications related to genitoplasty also spans patients of all ages. Surgical complications can be expected to become more frequent as the patient's age increases due to changes in tissue quality, blood flow, and other complicating medical conditions that are more common in older age.

3.6 Top Surgeries

3.6.1 Breast Augmentation

For persons who seek to develop their breast tissue, there are two options, hormonal therapy including antiandrogens, estrogens, and, in some cases, progestagens and surgical breast augmentation. Hormone therapy typically includes a combination of antiandrogens, usually spironolactone, and estradiol. This regimen produces the development of secondary sex characteristics including breast growth, redistribution of fat, and softening of the skin [30]. Progestagens have not been shown to enhance breast development with certainty, yet some patients report affirming changes [30]. Surgical options include placement of bilateral saline or silicone breast implants. For older adults, this procedure is well-tolerated and is adapted to the individual's age, current breast size on hormones, and tissue elasticity [14]. Breast augmentation surgery is recommended to be completed prior to bottom surgery of any type [31].

3.6.2 Chest Surgery/Mastectomy

For persons seeking to reduce chest tissue, bilateral subcutaneous mastectomy is performed with liposuction and repositioning and reduction of the nipple/areolar area [31] in the manner decided by the patient and surgery team. Several surgical techniques are utilized and are well tolerated due to the limited invasion of the pectoral musculature compared to invasive radical mastectomy techniques. Surgical outcomes are based on appearance of a flat pectoral shelf with a well-placed nipple areolar complex and a small incisional scar in the pectoral-inframammary crease. Rare complications include tissue or incisional infection, nipple/areolar tissue loss, and venous thrombosis [31] with blood loss creating hematoma the most common cause of secondary surgical correction [32]. For older adults, the current amount of breast tissue, degree of ptosis and excess skin, and tissue frailty must be considered in the decision-making process [32]. This surgery is not comparable to radical mastectomy performed in cisgender women for removal of tissue for cancerous lesions.

3.7 Bottom Surgeries

3.7.1 Vaginoplasty

The World Professional Association for Transgender Health's (WPATH) Standards of Care (SOC) version 7 published in 2012 state criteria for genital surgery are (1) well-documented gender dysphoria, (2) ability to consent, (3) legal age of consent, (4) 12 months of HRT, (5) 12 months of living a gender role congruent with their gender identity, and 6) well-managed mental or medical concerns [33, 34]. Beyond the general health of a potential gender-affirming surgical candidate, each individual must achieve minimum medical criteria to proceed. This is consistent with preoperative standards yet often reflects the preference of the surgeon providing the procedure. Acceptable preoperative laboratory tests, complete blood count (CBC) and basic metabolic panel (BMP), electrocardiogram (ECG) results, temporary or permanent discontinuation of smoking, body mass index (BMI) evaluations, well-managed chronic health conditions, medication management, and addressing any issues related to polypharmacy are required prior to GAS procedures. BMI is assessed on a case-by-case basis due to individual levels of muscle mass in comparison to body fat, and, in certain cases, surgeons may require surgical candidates to achieve a BMI of 35 or less, to facilitate ease of access to intrapelvic anatomical landmarks, and to produce positive structural and cosmetic outcomes, though studies show BMI has little to no effect on surgical outcomes [35].

For our purposes, a brief examination of hormone replacement therapy must be explored. It must be stated that not all TGNC individuals who seek GAS have been prescribed and are taking hormone therapy, yet for those TGNC individuals who take estrogens, physiological changes may have an effect on readiness for GAS. Preoperative protocols for surgery require that hormones be temporarily discontinued or tapered to a lower dosage 2 weeks prior to surgery [14]. To reconcile the risk of postoperative deep vein thrombosis (DVT) or pulmonary embolism (PE), persons taking estrogens who also smoke tobacco are asked to stop smoking 6 weeks prior to surgery and delay restart of hormones until successful recovery at postoperative week two.

As surgical candidates age, their health status may strongly influence their ability to qualify for GAS. Though surgeons are sometimes reluctant to provide these services to older adults, there have been cases of persons up to 77 years of age that have been performed with great success. For these patients, stability of multiple chronic conditions is a priority, particularly hypertension and diabetes, and special attention to renal and hepatic tolerance is well-advised prior to surgery. Finally, for older patients, in some cases, tissue frailty may be the deciding factor as to what surgical options are available to individuals. Older patients seeking GAS may opt for a less invasive surgery than the 8–12-hour vaginoplasty procedure. Other viable options include bilateral orchiectomy, penectomy, zero-depth vaginoplasty, and labioplasty.

For persons seeking GAS to create a neovaginal space, several surgical methods for vaginoplasty may be employed; penile-scrotal skin flap (most frequently used), penile skin graft, non-genital skin graft (abdomen), non-genital skin flap (thigh), and pedicled intestinal transplant [36, 37]. Preparatory surgeries may include bilateral orchiectomy but is not required prior to vaginoplasty. Preoperative standards of care must be accomplished to prepare for the arduous procedure ahead. As mentioned previously, preoperative surgical preparation includes labs, ECG, and bowel prep [35]. Recent discussion adds preoperative physical therapy that focuses on strengthening of pelvic musculature, preparing the patient for postoperative physical restrictions, and pain management to ensure successful surgical outcomes.

Vaginoplasty is a complex surgery that is generally well-tolerated and successful [38]. Generally, vaginoplasty is the construction of a moist and elastic neovaginal space formed from autologous tissue, creating a hairless tube (achieved with recommended hair removal prior to surgery) filled with packing material (bolster) and positioned anterior to the rectum and posterior to the bladder while leaving the prostate intact [14]. Once the procedure is complete, the patient will recover immediately post-op in the ICU and will return with an intact bolster dressing, Foley catheter, penrose drains, IV, patient-controlled analgesia (PCA), and in some cases telemetry [14]. Postoperative recovery for the patient will include, most importantly, hourly inspection of blood loss at the bolster site and under the patient, monitoring urinary output, maintenance of a sequential compression device (SCD) to mitigate DVT and PE, and encouraging hourly incentive spirometry [34]. Regular venous duplex of the lower extremities will provide information indicating the presence or absence of DVT. Diet will progress from ice chips, clear, soft bland, to regular by postoperative day 3 or 4 depending on how this is being tolerated. Surgeons will utilize intraoperative antibiotics and in few cases, heparin, then will prescribe postoperative pain medications, antibiotics, antiemetics, stool softeners, antiulcer, and sleep aids [35].

Recovery from vaginoplasty includes beginning ambulation on the first postoperative day. Involvement of the physical therapy team is central to successful recovery. The patient will be instructed not to sit in their typical manner, on both ischial tuberosities, as this creates shear force to the perineum and surgical incisions, which is to be avoided. Patients will be instructed on how to sit to one side, how to walk stably with a walker, and how to log roll to get in and out of bed. Physical therapists will work with patients to aid with range of motion, core exercises, breathing, and pain management skills to aid their recovery. Of critical importance is to maintain cleanliness of the perineal area, especially the penrose drain opening where introduction of any fecal material greatly increases risk of infection. Patients will be instructed how to use the bedside commode, which includes learning to squeeze gluteal tissue together to decrease perineal shear, to not use valsalva maneuver (bearing down) and directionality of wiping. Nearing the end of the hospital stay, the patient will have the bolster removed; this may be painful and must be communicated to the patient. The following day, the Foley catheter will be removed, and voiding prior to release is required. Late in their hospital stay, patients will be instructed on how to use dilating devices to keep the opening to the neovagina (os) patent and tissue pliable. Hospital stays vary but average of 1 week with the possibility of further recovery at a long-term care facility [35].

Immediate postoperative complications for vaginoplasty regardless of method include bleeding, both incisional and retroperitoneal, granulation tissue, incisional dehiscence, rectovaginal fistula, urethral stenosis or deflected urine stream, and infection [39]. Later issues may be neovaginal prolapse, neovaginal stenosis, and prolonged pain. For granulation tissue, silver nitrate is kept at the bedside [35]. Depending on the surgical procedure performed and complication, some postoperative issues require a brief return to surgery.

Of the five methods of vaginoplasty utilized, penile inversion vaginoplasty has become the most commonly performed feminizing genitoplasty procedure. The surgery often involves removal of the penis and testicles, creation of a neovaginal canal with possible skin graft to assist in lining the neovagina, creation of clitoris and labia, as well as shortening of the urethra. This may be tailored based on patient goals for surgery. Thirty-three to eighty-seven percent of patients are able to have penetrative intercourse after this surgery, and 70–84% are able to orgasm. Most (76–100%) are satisfied with neovaginal length and only 2–6% reported pain with intercourse [40].

Some of the most serious complications related to penile inversion vaginoplasty include injury to surrounding organs including the bowel, bladder, and urethra. Rectal injury occurs in 2–4% of surgeries, urethral injury in 1% of surgeries, and bladder injury is significantly less common [39–44]. These injuries can lead to fistula formation, which is an aberrant connection between the injured area and a nearby structure. Fistulization can also occur without a known injury at the time of surgery. A connection between the rectum and the neovagina (rectoneovaginal fistula) occurs in 1–17% of surgeries. A fistula between the urethra and the neovagina (urethroneovaginal) is uncommon (2%). Vesiconeovaginal fistula or a connection between the bladder and the neovagina occurs even less frequently [39–44]. Fistulas can cause persistent and inadvertent leakage of stool or urine through the abnormal communication. If a rectoneovaginal fistula occurs, it usually requires a section of bowel to be brought out to the skin and for stool to drain into a bag at that site, so the rectum is bypassed. In the same way, a vesiconeovaginal or urethroneovaginal fistula often requires a long-term indwelling bladder catheter that may either traverse the urethra or be placed into the bladder through the skin just above the pubic bone.

Urinary issues that occur postoperatively are relatively common. The most frequently reported is urinary incontinence (19%) [40, 46]. Urinary retention (14%) is also commonly reported and tends to be an issue that occurs immediately after surgery but can occur at any point after the procedure is complete [41]. Narrowing of the urethra (5–10%) or the urethral opening (1–40%) can also occur [39–44]. Urinary tract infections become more common after vaginoplasty than prior to the procedure due to the shortening of the urethra and may happen in as many as 4–32% of patients [40, 41]. Splaying or spraying of the urine stream (10%) also occurs after surgery and tends to improve with time for many patients [41].

Wound healing may also be a problem for some patients postoperatively. Infections of the surgical area happen approximately 5% of the time [41]. Opening of the wound is the most frequent healing problem that patients encounter, occurring in 12–33% [39–44]. Death of the tissue in the surgical area may be severe or minor. Serious tissue death of the neovaginal graft is infrequent (2–4%) as is death of the neoclitoral tissue (1–3%) [40]. Tissue healing difficulties, the surgery itself, or nonadherence to dilation frequency and technique may lead to a narrowing of the neovagina in 1–12% of cases or neovaginal shortening in 2–10%. The opening of the neovagina can also be affected and become too narrow for dilation or intercourse (4–15%) [39–44].

Other postoperative complications that may occur are more bleeding than normal from the operative site (3–10%) and need for a blood transfusion (5%) [40, 41]. Reoperation due to bleeding happens in approximately 2% of patients [41]. Prolapse or a hernia of the neovaginal tissue where the neovaginal lining comes out of the neovaginal opening occurs infrequently (1–4%) and tends to happen many years after surgery [40, 41]. Postoperative pain is a normal occurrence immediately after surgery, but should not persist beyond 6 weeks. Three to nine percent may have persistent genital pain that is unresolved by 6 weeks postoperatively [43, 45].

Intestinal vaginoplasty is generally a surgery that is reserved for secondary procedures if the initial penile inversion vaginoplasty is unsuccessful. There are certain circumstances where this surgery is desirable as a primary procedure. This surgery involved taking a section of either large or small bowel and using it to line the neovaginal canal. The bowel that is not being used must then be reattached to allow normal bowel function to resume. Removal of the testicles, clitoris formation, labia construction, and urethral shortening is also involved. Although the complication rates appear lower with this surgery, it is likely that this is due to inability to follow-up with patients or other factors. This is a significantly more complicated procedure with many additional risks because surgery on the bowel is involved. Reported overall complication rates are approximately 6% for a large bowel procedure and 8% for a small bowel procedure. Blockage of the intestine occurs about 1% of the time, but has only been studied up to 2 years postoperatively, and so may be much higher. Foul smelling neovaginal discharge or odor occurs in 1–10% likely due to the presence of bowel bacteria and mucus inside the bowel-lined neovagina. Narrowing of the neovaginal opening happens 1–9% of the time, while narrowing of the neovagina itself occurs in 3–4% [46]. Prolapse of the bowel-lined neovagina is seen in 8% of patients [40, 47]. Inflammation or cancer of the bowel-lined neovagina is also possible; however, studies do not follow patients for long enough to know the rate at which this occurs. Lastly, 25% of patients experience pain during intercourse after intestinal vaginoplasty.

3.7.2 Phalloplasty

For transmasculine people, there are generally two options for genital reconstructive surgeries, phalloplasty and metoidioplasty, which will be covered below. Until recently, genital reconstructive surgeries for most transmasculine people in the United States were largely unobtainable due to high cost, lack of insurance coverage, and few capable surgeons. Over the last several years, expanding insurance coverage and better social awareness have increased interest in providing these procedures and improved overall accessibility to patients. Given historical limitations, however, relatively little research has been done about optimal technique, outcomes, and complications for these procedures. Existing information about outcomes is generally considered low-quality evidence, and no standardized measures exist to assess patient satisfaction [48]. Even less is known about these procedures in older adults. The average age of phalloplasty in most studies falls within the third decade of life, though procedures have been documented for patients at least well in their 60s [49].

Phalloplasty is the process of making a new phallus. The procedure typically involves several steps and multiple procedures. The overall structure of the phallus is made of tissue taken from a donor site elsewhere on the body, with a urethral extension created from mucosal tissue. Microsurgery is used to connect nerves and vasculature to the neophallus. Additional procedures are often performed to create a scrotum or glans and to achieve erectile capacity.

A variety of donor sites for the phallus have been used. Some of the most common sites include suprapubic, abdominal, inguinal, thoracodorsal, anterolateral thigh, calf, and radial forearm [50]. The radial forearm free-flap phalloplasty (RFFP) has emerged as the most common technique [50–53] and is increasingly the standard of care. The same flap is also commonly used for head and neck reconstruction, which may lead to overall comfort with its use [52]. The RFFP is thought to have a lower overall complication rate based on the available data and is less dependent on body habitus for appropriate donor tissue [52, 55, 56]. The subcutaneous fat in this area is typically thin, allowing for the tube within a tube design used to make the shaft of the phallus [52]. The flap includes the skin, subcutaneous tissue, fascia, vasculature, and nerve supply of the radial forearm. A small portion of the radius has been used in some techniques, though it is no longer common practice [52].

Although RFFP is increasingly prevalent, individual patient and surgeon factors may dictate a different choice of donor site [57]. In particular, older patients who have undergone surgery previously or in another country may have had an alternate procedure performed. Additional factors which may guide patient preference include scarring at the donor site, homogeneity of skin color between donor site and site of neophallus placement, and desired size and shape of the phallus. Although many of the complications are similar regardless of the exact procedure, outcomes, complication rates, and complications related to the donor site may vary.

Prior to the procedure, hair removal from the radial forearm with electrolysis or laser techniques is performed [58]. Topical anesthetic is often supplied in preparation for the extensive hair removal process [59, 60]. With use of the RFFP, prior to removal of the radial artery, testing for adequate ulnar vascular supply to the hand is often performed, using the Allen test and Doppler ultrasound [52]. Some techniques include a first step of preparing the neourethra by embedding it in the donor site for months prior to the planned procedure to encourage vascularization [52]. Some patients may also undergo hysterectomy with bilateral salpingo-oophorectomy at the time of phalloplasty; in other cases, this may be done previously [48].

Phalloplasty typically includes a vaginectomy and the creation of a scrotum. The outside scrotum is formed from the labia majora, through use of tissue expanders and testicular implants [61]. Phalloplasty is generally a multistage procedure by design, which is thought to produce better outcomes, although one-stage procedures have been performed [61–63]. The overall process can take 1 year or more [65]. The details of the procedure vary by specific technique and surgeon. Most commonly, a central stage involves formation and transfer of the phallus, along with anastomosing of vasculature and nerve supply. The donor site is covered with a skin graft, typically taken from the thigh [52].

Additional procedures, often occurring at separate stages, include connecting the native with the neourethra [52], hysterectomy, bilateral salpingo-oophorectomy, vaginectomy, scrotoplasty, sculpting of a glans, and insertion of an erectile prosthesis [54, 66]. To elongate the urethra, an extension of the native urethra is created from vaginal epithelial tissue, labia minora, and/or a buccal mucosal graft [55]. There are typically three sections to the neourethra, which from proximal to distal are often referred to as (1) the native urethra, (2) the fixed urethra (formed from local vaginal, labial, or extragenital tissue), and (3) the phallic urethra (portion running through the neophallus) [58]. Complications are most common at the sites of anastomosis between these different sections [52]. Some surgeons also incorporate medical tattooing or additional procedures for aesthetic value.

Several months to a year is usually required between stages, which allows for healing, observation for sufficient perfusion or complications, and development of protective tactile sensation in the phallus [58, 65]. Tactile sensation is considered a prerequisite for further procedures [65]. Additional interventions are often required to address complications. One long-term follow-up of 56 phalloplasty patients in France between 1986 and 2002 found a mean of 6 surgical procedures required, although surgical techniques have improved over time [67].

Available data on desired outcomes and complication rates are highly variable. Outcomes are reliant on provider report, and no standardized measures exist, making generalizability difficult [68]. However, below is a discussion of some of the more commonly assessed outcomes and reported complications.

Patients have individualized priorities when seeking genital reconstruction. The most common goals include appearance and sensation consistent with one's gender identity, desire to stand while urinating, desire to retain erogenous sensation, and ability to perform penetrative sex acts. These goals are achieved at variable rates and are affected by patient, surgeon, and technique-specific factors.

Many patients report satisfaction with aesthetic outcomes (>70% by some reports) [68], though a substantial number do not. Almost all patients are reported to develop tactile sensation of the neophallus [55], and the majority, although substantially less, also report erogenous sensation. In a review, pooling data from studies through 2015, of 545 patients who underwent RFFP, >98% reported tactile sensation, while 71% of patients reported erogenous sensation [55]. Time to initial sensation may take one to several months and may continue to improve for over a year. Different methods are used to promote erogenous sensation and retain ability to orgasm. Some techniques bury the retained clitoris at the base of the neophallus [48, 69]. Most techniques also include anastomosis of the clitoral dorsal nerve with the nerves of the donor site, which are included in neophallus. Both buried clitoris and anastomosis of the clitoral nerve appear to increase the likelihood of retained ability to orgasm [69]. Depending on these factors and others, reported rates of orgasmic ability following phalloplasty have varied widely, with rates as low as 20% and as high as 100% [68, 69].

With current surgical techniques, erection of the phallus is achieved via implantation of a prosthesis. This is usually done in a separate procedure, months to years after sufficient healing from phalloplasty. Different types of implants have been used, most commonly inflatable and semisolid malleable prostheses. Erection is achieved by a hydraulic pump, typically placed in the scrotum with an internal reservoir for filling the prosthesis, or by manual manipulation of the phallus containing a malleable device [55]. Following phalloplasty, most patients report the ability to urinate while standing, though the exact numbers vary. The native and phallic portions of the urethra are often anastomosed at a later procedure, with urine diverted via catheter between procedures. Definitive ability to urinate while standing may be dependent on urethral complications [55, 68].

The overall rate of complications for phalloplasty varies widely between individual surgeons and techniques but is frequently reported as greater than 50% [51,

55]. Major complications include infection, thrombosis, fistulas, urethral complications, and flap-related complications.

In the early postoperative period, within 1 month following the procedure, complications are most frequently related to infection, thrombosis, and/or ischemic flap loss [66]. Signs of infection are similar to infection elsewhere in the body, including warmth, erythema, pain, and purulence. Thrombosis can occur in either the arterial or venous systems. Arterial thrombosis is characterized by pallor, coldness, and loss of pulse. As with elsewhere in the body, arterial thrombosis is a threat to graft survival and must be treated emergently [66]. With venous thrombosis, the phallus may appear engorged, blue, or otherwise discolored, and the pulse may become progressively weakened with increasing venous congestion [66]. Venous thrombosis also must be evaluated for clot removal or treatment otherwise.

Flap complications range from hematoma to partial or total flap loss [58]. Drains are typically left in place prophylactically for a period of time to prevent collection of blood or serum. However, seromas and hematomas do occur and are characterized by swelling and increased turgor of the skin. These may resolve spontaneously or may be treated with drainage [58, 66]. Darkening or change in skin quality, along with change in odor may indicate flap necrosis, which presents as blackened tissue in later stages. Flap necrosis requires surgical evaluation.

Late postoperative complications, occurring 1 month or more following a procedure, are more commonly related to the urethra. The most common urethral complication is development of a fistula, occurring in up to 22–75% of phalloplasties [58, 69]. Fistulas most often occur at sites of anastomosis between the different sections of urethra, particularly between the phallic urethra and the fixed urethra, due to vascular insufficiency of the flap and change in lumen size. However, they can occur anywhere along the urethral path [70]. Fistulas are sometimes associated with increased pressure caused by a stricture [66]. Fistulas frequently close spontaneously within a few months; however, persistent fistulas may require urinary diversion or excision of the tract and repair with a graft [52, 56, 70]. Although urethral fistulas commonly communicate outward toward the skin, they may also communicate with remnant vaginal cavities, which can be seen with increased backward pressure from a stricture [70]. Persistent cavities are usually removed in entirety at the time of repair.

Urethral strictures, occluding or partially occluding the neourethra, are among the more serious complications. Reported rates of stricture range from 12% to more than 50% [55, 63, 70–72]. Strictures most frequently occur at the anastomosis between the fixed and phallic urethra and are thought to result from ischemia [70]. Strictures may be associated with urinary outlet obstruction, hydronephrosis, urinary leakage at a site of anastomosis, or urinary incontinence, due to urine trapping in the fixed and phallic parts of the urethra [69, 70]. Strictures are typically managed with endoscopic dilation and/or surgical repair; however, patients often experience recurrence [52, 56, 70]. Urethroplasty may occur in one or multiple stages, with months in between. When reconstruction fails, or patients prefer to avoid more interventions, a perineal urethrostomy may be performed, after which urine exits the body via the perineum [70].

Patients with urethral complications of phalloplasty will often present with urinary complaints, including increased strain to urinate, weak urinary stream, urinary incontinence, dysuria, or suprapubic pain. Drainage of urine or pus from a site other than the meatus may be seen in the presence of urethrocutaneous fistula [70]. Physical exam should include inspection of external structures for signs of infection and/or fistulas opening to the skin. The meatus can be assessed for patency. Ultrasound may also be utilized to assess for suspected collections or abscess [70]. If history and physical are consistent with urinary retention, a postvoid residual evaluation can be obtained. In the setting of a stricture, a suprapubic catheter may be required if unable to pass a urethral catheter [70]. Patients with suspected urethral complications should ideally follow up with their surgeon as soon as possible and may need further urological evaluation via urethrogram [70]. If the patient's surgeon is unavailable, consulting with a urologist familiar with post-phalloplasty anatomy would be optimal, given potential differences in evaluation and treatment (e.g., smaller caliber of neourethra vs. native urethra requiring different sized catheter/ureteroscope).

Specific complications and complication rates related to prostheses vary by type of procedure. Early complications, within 1 month of the procedure, are most often infectious, though infection can be seen later on [65, 73]. Later-onset complications also include erosion of the prosthesis into surrounding tissue, leak of the prosthetic device, malpositioning, and device dysfunction. The need for revision is common, and devices frequently need to be replaced after several years. By one report, the expected lifespan of a prosthesis is about 4 years [73].

Donor site complications can include infection, graft loss, and compartment syndrome [55, 66]. Most commonly, however, patients experience significant scarring. The scar associated with the radial forearm free-flap phalloplasty is large and highly visible. The scar tissue can be, though is typically not, associated with loss of mobility, decreased pinch and grip strength, sensory changes, and chronic swelling or lymphedema of the hand and arm [74].

Postoperatively, general restrictions to activity are consistent with surgeries of similar complexity. Some surgeons recommend elevation of the phallus when feasible. A suprapubic catheter is typically left in place for a period of weeks, until urination through the phallus can take place, the timing of which is determined by the surgeon [58, 66].

3.8 Metoidioplasty

Metoidioplasty is the process of creating a phallus by elongation and repositioning of an enlarged clitoris, following testosterone therapy [75]. In contrast to phalloplasty, metoidioplasty is typically planned as a one-stage procedure, though may require additional procedures to address complications or for desired revisions [75, 76].

Prior to metoidioplasty, the clitoris is held against the body by several ligaments and additional soft tissue, and the length of the urethra travels separately from the clitoris [77]. Metoidioplasty separates the clitoris from the ligamentous and soft tissue attachments to allow for straightening and repositioning of the neophallus to face outward from the body. A urethral extension is formed from a genital and/or a buccal mucosal graft and connected to the native urethra, extending the urethral meatus to the tip of the neophallus. This extension is meant to allow for urination from a standing position [78, 79]. A scrotum is typically formed from the labia majora, as with phalloplasty, into which testicular implants are placed. In contrast to phalloplasty, no tissue from distant donor sites is required, and the clitoris/neophallus maintains its original tactile and erogenous innervation and blood supply.

Pre- and postoperative techniques are sometimes used to optimize phallus length. Some surgeons recommend dihydrotestosterone (DHT) cream applied directly to the clitoris/neophallus for months prior to the procedure to optimize clitoral growth [78, 80]. Evidence for efficacy of doing so, however, remains unclear [81]. Pre- and postoperatively, some surgeons also use penile vacuum or traction devices to promote further elongation and prevent postoperative contraction of the neophallus [82]. Additional procedures, including hysterectomy, bilateral salpingo-oophorectomy, and vaginoplasty, are often performed prior to or at the time of metoidioplasty, per patient preference, and to negate the need for anatomy appropriate screening [83].

Desired outcomes for metoidioplasty are similar to those of phalloplasty: appearance and sensation consistent with one's gender identity, desire to stand while urinating, and desire to retain erogenous sensation and sexual satisfaction [84]. The resultant neophallus is typically between 4 and 10 cm in length, though longer phalluses (up to 12 cm) have been reported with use of a modified, more invasive metoidioplasty technique [83–86]. The vast majority of patients who undergo metoidioplasty report the ability to urinate while standing [76, 88]. Retention of tactile and erogenous sensation, along with erectile capacity, is consistently retained [76, 86, 87]. Overall sexual satisfaction rates are generally high [88]. However, for those wishing to perform penetrative sex, the length achieved with metoidioplasty is often reported as "inadequate" to do so [76, 89].

Metoidioplasty is overall associated with shorter hospitalization and operative times [78] and generally considered less expensive than phalloplasty [75]. Complication rates for metoidioplasty are also generally lower, in part owing to the shorter urethral length, and more reliable vascularization of the tissue [76, 79, 90]. Complications that do occur are often considered more minor [79].

Urethral complications are similar to those occurring in phalloplasty, primarily fistula and stricture or stenosis [87]. These complications typically present with urinary complaints, including difficulty urinating or spraying or dribbling with urination. These symptoms sometimes resolve spontaneously but should be evaluated by the patient's surgeon and/or urologist, as they may require further intervention [78]. Flap loss can occur at the site of the urethral extension, though again this is seemingly less likely than with phalloplasty [87]. Scarring is generally considered minimal and is limited to the immediate genital area [87]. Although patient satisfaction appears comparable from available data, patients wishing to do so may subsequently undergo phalloplasty, depending on the specifics of their anatomy.

Because of the lower complication rate, shorter operative time, and single-staged procedure, metoidioplasty may be a better option for patients with significant medical comorbidities, or those otherwise unable or unwilling to undergo the longer, more invasive procedure, and higher likelihood of complications associated with phalloplasty.

Following metoidioplasty, urinary diversion via catheter is often recommended for a number of weeks, prior to initiating urination through the urethral extension. The use of a vacuum device may also be recommended after appropriate recovery time to prevent postoperative shortening of the phallus [78].

3.9 Long-Term Complications

Historically, surgeons performing GAS have been limited in the United States (US) to the last 15–20 years, as such, long-term prospective studies of complications have not been observed. Existing study results vary based on the procedure performed and review of surgical outcomes with few including older transgender people. Immediate postoperative surgical complications have been previously examined earlier in this chapter, yet missing from the evidence base are studies following surgical outcomes over the life course into later years. As such, where available, incidence of surgical long-term complications of vaginoplasty, phalloplasty, and metoidioplasty will be briefly explored here.

Vaginoplasty has several potential complications that may occur over time: prolapse of the neovagina, reduction in size (depth and width) of the vaginal space, vaginal opening stenosis, and loss of satisfaction in sexual function. Systematic review of retrospective studies of vaginoplasty reports (93%) satisfaction and minimal (1%) regret [91] over time. Within this group of studies, one retrospective study of 475 patients in the Netherlands, where vaginoplasty has been performed for over three decades, has a significant length of surgical follow-up, averaging 7.8 years with the longest period being 15.9 years and an average age of patients 38.6 years with the oldest age 70.8 [92]. This research over the life course is rare and currently unavailable in US studies with genital surgery researchers agreeing that prospective studies with larger numbers and longer follow-up periods are essential [93].

Phalloplasty has few long-term complications that may occur over time, primarily related to the maintenance of the redirected and extended urethra. Urethral stricture has a 23–51% rate following radial forearm free-flap phalloplasty (RFFP) in the months immediately after surgery [94], yet data for older adults who have long recovered from phalloplasty is uncommon. For example, a 2017 study that compared two urethral lengthening techniques prior to phalloplasty, vaginectomy, or vaginal preservation, recorded outcomes in 224 patients with a mean age of 36 ± 11 years, 47 being the oldest age individual [95]. Metoidioplasty presents the fewest complications over time, though urethral stricture remains the most prevalent complication [96].

Conclusion Gender-affirming surgeries are viable options for older people who identify as transgender, gender nonconforming (TGNC) and non-binary. Surgeons will work with primary care and behavioral health providers to provide interdisciplinary patient-centered care to their TGNC patients. Older TGNC persons seeking gender confirmation who meet WPATH preoperative criteria, are medically fit, and have chronic conditions well- managed will often be approved for gender-affirming surgical procedures.

References

1. Flores AR, Herman JL, Gates GJ, Brown TNT How many adults identify as transgender in the United States? Los Angeles, CA: The Williams Institute. 2016; Flores AR, Herman JL, Brown TNT. Race and ethnicity of adults who identify as transgender in the United States. Los Angeles, CA: The Williams Institute. 2016.
2. Civic Impulse. H.R. 3590 — 111th congress: patient protection and affordable care act. 2017. Retrieved from https://www.govtrack.us/congress/bills/111/hr3590.
3. Coleman E, Bockting W, Botzer M, et al. Standards of care for the health of transsexual, transgender, and gender-nonconforming people, version 7. Int J Transgenderism. 2012;13:165–232.
4. Baker KE. The future of transgender coverage. N Engl J Med. 2017;376(19):1801–4.
5. Human Rights Campaign Foundation (HRC). Corporate equality index 2017: rating workplaces on lesbian, gay, bisexual and transgender equality. Washington, DC: Human Rights Campaign Foundation; 2017. http://www.hrc.org/campaigns/corporate-equality-index?_ga=1.155475583.579950537.1457713105
5. Veterans Health Administration (VHA). Veterans Health Administration Directive 2011-024: Providing health care for transgender and intersex veterans. Veterans Health Administration. 2011. Replaced by Veterans Health Administration Directive 2013–003: Providing health care for transgender and intersex veterans. 2013. Available at: http://www.va.gov/vhapublications/ViewPublication.asp?pub_ID=2863. Accessed 31 Dec 2017.
6. Kauth MR, Shipherd JC, Lindsay J, Blosnich JR, Brown GR, Jones KT. Access to care for transgender veterans in the veterans health administration: 2006–2013. Am J Public Health. 2014;104(Suppl 4):S532–4. https://doi.org/10.2105/AJPH.2014.302086
7. Rabin RC. Medicare to now cover sex-change surgery. The New York Times, PP. A14. 2014, May 31. Retrieved from https://www.nytimes.com/2014/05/31/us/ban-on-medicare-coverage-of-sex-change-surgery-is-lifted.html.
8. Berli JU, Knudson G, Fraser L, et al. What surgeons need to know about gender confirmation surgery when providing care for transgender individuals: a review. JAMA Surg. 2017;152(4):394–400. https://doi.org/10.1001/jamasurg.2016.5549.
9. James SE, Herman JL, Rankin S, Keisling M, Mottet L, Ana M. The report of the 2015 U.S. transgender survey. Washington, DC: National Center for Transgender Equality; 2016.
10. Proctor K, Haffer SC, Ewald E, Hodge C, James CV. Identifying the transgender population in the Medicare program. Transgender Health. 2016;1(1):250–65. https://doi.org/10.1089/trgh.2016.0031.
11. Dragon CN, Guerino P, Ewald E, Laffan AM. Transgender Medicare beneficiaries and chronic conditions: exploring fee-for-service claims data. LGBT Health. 2017;4(6):404–11.
12. Blosnich JR, Brown GR, Shipherd P, et al. Prevalence of gender identity disorder and suicide risk among transgender veterans utilizing veterans health administration care. Am J Public Health. 2013;103:e27–32.
13. Schechter LS. Gender confirmation surgery: an update for the primary care provider. Transgender health. 2016;1(1):32–40.

14. Lee TH, Marcantonio ER, Mangione CM, et al. Derivation and prospective validation of a simple index for prediction of cardiac risk of major noncardiac surgery. Circulation. 1999;100:1043–9.
15. Smetana GW, Lawrence VA, Cornell JE, American College of Physicians. Preoperative pulmonary risk stratification for noncardiothoracic surgery: systematic review for the American College of Physicians. Ann Intern Med. 2006;144:581–95.
16. Geerts WH, Bergqvist D, Pineo GF, et al. Prevention of venous thromboembolism: American College of Chest Physicians Evidence-Based Clinical Practice Guidelines (8th edition). Chest. 2008;133:381S–453S.
17. Geerts WH, Pineo GF, Heit JA, et al. Prevention of venous thromboembolism: the seventh ACCP conference on antithrombotic and thrombolytic therapy. Chest. 2004;126:338S–400S.
18. Kuehnert MJ, Roth VR, Haley NR, et al. Transfusion-transmitted bacterial infection in the United States, 1998 through 2000. Transfusion. 2001;41:1493–9.
19. Zou S, Dorsey KA, Notari EP, et al. Prevalence, incidence, and residual risk of human immunodeficiency virus and hepatitis C virus infections among United States blood donors since the introduction of nucleic acid testing. Transfusion. 2010;50:1495–504.
20. Pomper GJ, Wu Y, Snyder EL. Risks of transfusion-transmitted infections: 2003. Curr Opin Hematol. 2003;10:412–8.
21. Consensus paper on the surveillance of surgical wound infections. The Society for Hospital Epidemiology of America; The Association for Practitioners in Infection Control; The Centers For Disease Control; The Surgical Infection Society. Infect Control Hosp Epidemiol 1992;13:599–605.
22. Horan TC, Gaynes RP, Martone WJ, Jarvis WR, Emori TG. CDC definitions of nosocomial surgical site infections, 1992: a modification of CDC definitions of surgical wound infections. Infect Control Hosp Epidemiol. 1992;13:606–8.
23. Jones HW, Rock JA. Te Linde's operative gynecology. 2015; Philadelphia: Wolters Kluwer.
24. O'Brien H, Mohan H, Hare CO, Reynolds JV, Kenny RA. Mind over matter? The hidden epidemic of cognitive dysfunction in the older surgical patient. Ann Surg. 2017;265:677–91.
25. Moller JT, Cluitmans P, Rasmussen LS, et al. Long-term postoperative cognitive dysfunction in the elderly ISPOCD1 study. ISPOCD investigators. International Study of Post-Operative Cognitive Dysfunction. Lancet. 1998;351:857–61.
26. Monk TG, Weldon BC, Garvan CW, et al. Predictors of cognitive dysfunction after major noncardiac surgery. Anesthesiology. 2008;108:18–30.
27. Sprung J, Roberts RO, Weingarten TN, et al. Postoperative delirium in elderly patients is associated with subsequent cognitive impairment. Br J Anaesth. 2017;119:316–23.
28. Hughes CG, Patel MB, Jackson JC, et al. Surgery and anesthesia exposure is not a risk factor for cognitive impairment after major noncardiac surgery and critical illness. Ann Surg. 2017;265:1126–33.
29. Wesp LM, Deutsch MB. Hormonal and surgical treatment options for transgender women and transfeminine spectrum persons. Psychiatric Clinics. 2017;40(1):99–111.
30. Schechter LS, D'Arpa S, Cohen MN, Kocjancic E, Claes KE, Monstrey S. Gender confirmation surgery: guiding principles. J Sex Med. 2017;14(6):852–6.
31. Kääriäinen M, Salonen K, Helminen M, Karhunen-Enckell U. Chest-wall contouring surgery in female-to-male transgender patients: a one-center retrospective analysis of applied surgical techniques and results. Scand J Surg. 2017;106(1):74–9.
32. World Professional Association for Transgender Health (WPATH). Standards of care for the health of transsexual, transgender, and gender nonconforming people, Version 7. 2011. American Journal of Public Health, Minneapolis, MN, October 2013, Vol 103, No. 10.
33. Wylie K, Knudson G, Khan SI, Bonierbale M, Watanyusakul S, Baral S. Serving transgender people: clinical care considerations and service delivery models in transgender health. Lancet. 2016;388(10042):401–11.
34. King M, Bachra J, Johnson R, Sullivan P, McKeague K. Cultural competence and the LGBTQ community/surgical procedures/quiz [PowerPoint slides]. 2018.

35. Monstrey S, Hoebeke P, Dhont M, et al. Surgical therapy in transsexual patients: a multi-disciplinary approach. Acta Chir Belg. 2001;101:200–9.
36. Horbach SE, Bouman MB, Smit JM, Özer M, Buncamper ME, Mullender MG. Outcome of vaginoplasty in male-to-female transgenders: a systematic review of surgical techniques. J Sex Med. 2015;12(6):1499–512.
37. Gaither TW, Awad MA, Osterberg EC, Murphy GP, Romero A, Bowers ML, et al. Postoperative complications following primary penile inversion vaginoplasty among 330 male-to-female transgender patients. J Urol. 2018;199(3):760–5.
38. Dreher PC, Edwards D, Hager S, Dennis M, Belkoff A, Mora J, et al. Complications of the neovagina in male-to-female transgender surgery: a systematic review and meta-analysis with discussion of management. Clin Anat. 2017;31(2):191–9.
39. Horbach SE, Bouman MB, Smit JM, Ozer M, Buncamper ME, Mullender MG. Outcome of vaginoplasty in male-to-female transgenders: a systematic review of surgical techniques. J Sex Med. 2015;12:1499–512.
40. Buncamper ME, van der Sluis WB, van der Pas RS, et al. Surgical outcome after penile inversion vaginoplasty: a retrospective study of 475 transgender women. Plast Reconstr Surg. 2016;138:999–1007.
41. Gaither TW, Awad MA, Osterberg EC, et al. Postoperative complications following primary penile inversion vaginoplasty among 330 male-to-female transgender patients. J Urol. 2017;197:e1258.
42. Lawrence AA. Patient-reported complications and functional outcomes of male-to-female sex reassignment surgery. Arch Sex Behav. 2006;35:717–27.
43. Manrique OJ, Adabi K, Martinez-Jorge J, Ciudad P, Nicoli F, Kiranantawat K. Complications and patient-reported outcomes in male-to-female vaginoplasty-where we are today: a systematic review and meta-analysis. Ann Plast Surg. 2018;80:684.
44. Rossi Neto R, Hintz F, Krege S, Rubben H, Vom Dorp F. Gender reassignment surgery–a 13 year review of surgical outcomes. Int Braz J Urol. 2012;38:97–107.
45. Hoebeke P, Selvaggi G, Ceulemans P, et al. Impact of sex reassignment surgery on lower urinary tract function. Eur Urol. 2005;47:398–402.
46. Bouman MB, van Zeijl MC, Buncamper ME, Meijerink WJ, van Bodegraven AA, Mullender MG. Intestinal vaginoplasty revisited: a review of surgical techniques, complications, and sexual function. J Sex Med. 2014;11:1835–47. JULES Phalloplasty
47. Frey JD, Poudrier G, Chiodo MV, Hazen A. An update on genital reconstruction options for the female-to-male transgender patient: a review of the literature. Plast Reconstr Surg. 2017;139(3):728–37.
48. Hage JJ, Bout CA, Bloem JJ, Megens JA. Phalloplasty in female-to-male transsexuals: what do our patients ask for? Ann Plast Surg. 1993;30(4):323–6.
49. Courtois F, Terrier JÉ, Brassard P, Ruffion A, Morel-Journel N. Development of surgical phalloplasty techniques: is there a gold standard? Theol Sex. 2012;21(2):55–9.
50. Santucci RA. Urethral complications after transgender phalloplasty and strategies to treat them and minimize their occurrence. Clinical Anat. 2017;31(2):187–90.
51. Kim S, Dennis M, Holland J, Terrell M, Loukas M, Schober J. The anatomy of forearm free flap phalloplasty for transgender surgery. Clin Anat. 2017; 31(2):145–51.
52. Monstrey S, Hoebeke P, Selvaggi G, Ceulemans P, Van Landuyt K, Blondeel P, et al. Penile reconstruction: is the radial forearm flap really the standard technique? Plast Reconstr Surg. 2009;124:510–8.
53. Garaffa G, Ralph DJ. Free flap phalloplasty for female to male gender dysphoria. J Sex Med. 2016;13(12):1942–7.
54. Morrison S, Shakir A, Vyas KS, Kirby J, Crane CN, Lee GK. Phalloplasty: a review of techniques and outcomes. Plast Reconstr Surg. 2016;138:594–615.
55. Ascha M, Massie JP, Morrison SD, Crane CN, Chen ML. Outcomes of single stage phalloplasty by pedicled anterolateral thigh flap versus radial forearm free flap in gender confirming surgery. J Urol. 2018;199(1):206–14.
56. Terrier JE, Courtois F, Ruffion A, Morel JN. Surgical outcomes and patients' satisfaction with suprapubic phalloplasty. J Sex Med. 2014;11(1):288–98.

57. Morrison SD, Perez MG, Carter CK, Crane CN. Pre- and post-operative care with associated intra-operative techniques for phalloplasty in female-to-male patients. Urol Nurs. 2015;35(3):134–8.
58. Guardiano RA, Norwood CW. Direct comparison of EMLA versus lidocaine for pain control in Nd:YAG 1,064 nm laser hair removal. Dermatol Surg. 2005;31(4):396–8.
59. Akinturk S, Eroglu A. A clinical comparison of topical piroxicam and EMLA cream for pain relief and inflammation in laser hair removal. Lasers Med Sci. 2008;24(4):535.
60. Sengezer M, Sadove RC. Scrotal construction by expansion of labia majora in biological female transsexuals. Ann Plast Surg. 1993;31(4):372–6.
61. Kojovic V, Bizic M, Majstorovic M, Kojic S, Stanojevic D, Korac G, et al. Combined total phalloplasty and metoidioplasty as a single stage procedure in female to male gender reassignment surgery. Eur Urol Suppl. 2009;8(8):648.
62. Stojanovic B, Bizic M, Bencic M, Kojovic V, Majstorovic M, Jeftovic M, et al. One-stage gender-confirmation surgery as a viable surgical procedure for female-to-male transsexuals. J Sex Med. 2017;14(5):741–6.
63. van der Sluis W, Smit JM, Pigot GLS, Buncamper ME, Bouman MB. One-stage pedicled anterolateral thigh flap phalloplasty combined with free radial forearm flap urethral reconstruction in transgender men: surgical technique and outcome in nineteen patients. J Sex Med. 2016;13:S223–S4.
64. Zuckerman JM, Smentkowski K, Gilbert D, Storme O, Jordan G, Virasoro R, et al. Penile prosthesis implantation in patients with a history of total phallic construction. J Sex Med. 2015;12(12):2485–91.
65. Garaffa G, Christopher NA, Ralph DJ. Total phallic reconstruction in female-to-male transsexuals. Eur Urol. 2010;57(4):715–22.
66. Leriche A, Timsit M-O, Morel-Journel N, Bouillot A, Dembele D, Ruffion A. Long-term outcome of forearm free-flap phalloplasty in the treatment of transsexualism. Reconstr Urol. 2008;101:1297–300.
67. Frey JD, Poudrier G, Chiodo MV, Hazen A. A systematic review of metoidioplasty and radial forearm flap phalloplasty in female-to-male transgender genital reconstruction: is the "ideal" neophallus an achievable goal? Plastic Reconstr Surg Glob Open. 2016;4(12):e1131.
68. Garcia M, Christopher N, D'eLuca F, Spilotros M, Garaffa G, Ralph D. PD3-03 light-touch, erogenous sensation, and sexual function among transgender men undergoing suprapubic pedicle and radial artery forearm free-flap phalloplasty. J Urol. 2014;191(4S):e20–e1.
69. Nikolavsky D, Yamaguchi Y, Levine JP, Zhao LC. Urologic sequelae following phalloplasty in transgendered patients. Urol Clin North Am. 2017;44(1):113–25.
70. Schechter LS. Gender confirmation surgery: an update for the primary care provider. Transgender Health. 2016;1(1):32–40.
71. van de Grift TC, Pigot GLS, Boudhan S, Elfering L, Kreukels BPC, Gijs L, et al. A longitudinal study of motivations before and psychosexual outcomes after genital gender-confirming surgery in transmen. J Sex Med. 2017;14(12):1621–8.
72. Neuville P, Morel-Journel N, Maucoutr-Boulch D, Ruffion A, Paparel P, Terrier JE. Surgical outcomes of erectile implants after phalloplasty: retrospective analysis of 95 procedures. J Sex Med. 2016;13:1758–64.
73. Van Caenegem E, Verhaeghe E, Taes Y, Wierckx K, Toye K, Goemaere S, et al. Long-term evaluation of donor-site morbidity after radial forearm flab phalloplasty for transexual men. J Sex Med. 2013;10:1644–51.
74. Frey JD, Poudrier G, Chiodo MV, Hazen A. An update on genital reconstruction options for the female-to-male transgender patient: a review of the literature. Plast Reconstr Surg. 2017;139(3):728–37.
75. Frey JD, Poudrier G, Chiodo MV, Hazen A. A systematic review of metoidioplasty and radial forearm flap phalloplasty in female-to-male transgender genital reconstruction: is the "ideal" Neophallus an achievable goal? Plastic Reconstr Surg Global Open. 2016;4(12):e1131.
76. Vukadinovic V, Stojanovic B, Majstorovic M, Milosevic A. The role of clitoral anatomy in female to male sex reassignment surgery. The Scientific World Journal. 2014;2014:437378.

77. Djordjevic ML, Stanojevic D, Bizic M, Kojovic V, Majstorovic M, Vujovic S, et al. Metoidioplasty as a single stage sex reassignment surgery in female transsexuals: belgrade experience. J Sex Med. 2009;6(5):1306–13.
78. Nikolavsky D, Yamaguchi Y, Levine JP, Zhao LC. Urologic sequelae following phalloplasty in transgendered patients. Urol Clin North Am. 2017;44(1):113–25.
79. Kaya C, Bektic J, Radmayr C, Schwentner C, Bartsch G, Oswald J. The efficacy of dihydrotestosterone transdermal gel before primary hypospadias surgery: a prospective, controlled, randomized study. J Urol. 2008;179(2):684–8.87.
80. Roth CC, Frimberger D, Kropp BP. Re: the efficacy of dihydrotestosterone transdermal gel before primary hypospadias surgery: a prospective, controlled, randomized study. J Urol. 2008;180(2):786. author reply -7
81. Cohanzad S. Penile improvement protocol in postoperative management of patients undergoing metoidioplasty. Aesthet Plast Surg. 2016;40(6):947–53.
82. Perovic SV, Djordjevic ML. Metoidioplasty: a variant of phalloplasty in female transsexuals. BJU Int. 2003;92(9):981–5.
83. Rachlin K. Factors which influence individual's decisions when considering female-to-male genital reconstructive surgery. Int J Transgenderism. 1999;3(3):97–03.
84. Cohanzad S. Extensive metoidioplasty as a technique capable of creating a compatible analogue to a natural penis in female transsexuals. Aesthet Plast Surg. 2016;40(1):130–8.
85. Hage J, van Tunrhout A. Long-term outcome of metaidioplasty in 70 female-to-male transexuals. Ann Plast Surg. 2006;57:312–6.
86. Morrison S, Shakir A, Vyas KS, Kirby J, Crane CN, Lee GK. Phalloplasty: a review of techniques and outcomes. Plastic Reconstr Surg. 2016;138:594–615.
87. Stojanovic B, Bizic M, Bencic M, Kojovic V, Majstorovic M, Jeftovic M, et al. One-stage gender-confirmation surgery as a viable surgical procedure for female-to-male transsexuals. J Sex Med. 2017;14(5):741–6.
88. Djordjevic ML, Bizic M, Stanojevic D, Bumbasirevic M, Kojovic V, Majstorovic M, et al. Urethral lengthening in metoidioplasty (female-to-male sex reassignment surgery) by combined buccal mucosa graft and labia minora flap. Urology. 2009;74(2):349–53.
89. Garcia M, Christopher N, D'eLuca F, Spilotros M, Garaffa G, Ralph D. PD3-03 light-tough, erogenous sensation, an sexual function among transgender men undergoing suprapubic pedicle and radial artery forearm free-flap phalloplasty. J Urol. 2014;191(4S):e20–e1.
90. Manrique OJ, Adabi K, Martinez-Jorge J, Nicoli F, Kiranantawat K. Complications and patient-reported outcomes in male-to-female vaginoplasty-where we are today: a systematic review and meta-analysis. Ann Plast Surg. 2018;80:684.
91. Buncamper ME, van der Sluis WB, van der Pas RS, Özer M, Smit JM, Witte BI, et al. Surgical outcome after penile inversion vaginoplasty: a retrospective study of 475 transgender women. Plast Reconstr Surg. 2016;138(5):999–1007.
92. Horbach SE, Bouman MB, Smit JM, Özer M, Buncamper ME, Mullender MG. Outcome of vaginoplasty in male-to-female transgenders: a systematic review of surgical techniques. J Sex Med. 2015;12(6):1499–512.
93. Santucci RA. Urethral complications after transgender phalloplasty: strategies to treat them and minimize their occurrence. Clin Anat. 2018;31(2):187–90.
94. Massie JP, Morrison SD, Wilson SC, Crane CN, Chen ML. Phalloplasty with urethral lengthening: addition of a vascularized Bulbospongiosus flap from vaginectomy reduces postoperative urethral complications. Plastic Reconstr Surg. 2017;140(4):551e–8e.
95. Nikolavsky D, Yamaguchi Y, Levine JP, Zhao LC. Urologic sequelae following phalloplasty in transgendered patients. Urol Clin. 2017;44(1):113–25.

The Intersection of Transgender Identities, HIV, and Aging

4

Kristen E. Porter and Mark Brennan-Ing

4.1 HIV in Older Adults

Infection with the human immunodeficiency virus (HIV) is one of the most significant health disparities faced by the transgender and gender nonconforming (TGNC) community. Until the advent of highly active antiretroviral therapy (HAART) in the mid-1990s, HIV infection inevitably progressed to acquired immune deficiency syndrome (AIDS) and subsequent early death due to opportunistic infections with AIDS-associated conditions [1, 2]. Because of HAART, HIV has been transformed into a chronic, although serious, manageable condition [3]. People with HIV who are diagnosed soon after infection, initiate and are adherent to HAART, and achieve viral suppression can achieve life expectancies comparable to those who do not have the virus [4]. As a result, the population with HIV, including those with TGNC identities, is aging. As of 2015, approximately 50% of the HIV population in the United States was aged 50 or older [2], and this proportion is expected to reach 70% by the year 2020 [5].

Although risk factors for HIV are the same regardless of age, older adults may not be as aware of their HIV risk. The current generation of older adults came of age during the pre-HIV era and may now be sexually active with new partners following divorce or death of a spouse. Postmenopausal older women are less likely to use condoms since they are not at risk of pregnancy. However, age-related changes to the vaginal tissue (e.g., thinning and dryness) increase women's risk for HIV [6]. Older adults may not be educated in safer sex practices or understand their risk and

K. E. Porter, PhD (✉)
Zen Executive LLC, Boston, MA, USA

M. Brennan-Ing, PhD
Brookdale Center for Healthy Aging, Hunter College, The City University of New York, New York, NY, USA

Rory Meyers College of Nursing, New York University, New York, NY, USA
e-mail: mark.ing@hunter.cuny.edu

M. Houlberg et al. (eds.), *Transgender and Gender Nonconforming Health and Aging*,
https://doi.org/10.1007/978-3-319-95031-0_4

are not often targeted in HIV prevention or testing efforts [7, 8]. The ageist belief that older adults are not sexually active is reinforced by health-care providers who are unlikely to discuss sexual health and safe sex practices with older patients [6, 8]. As a result of failure to screen for HIV and other sexually transmitted infections, older adults are more likely to receive a HIV diagnosis later in the course of the disease compared to younger adults, which may result in more immune system damage, cardiovascular damage, and central nervous system complications, predicting higher mortality and morbidity [9].

4.2 HIV and Transgender Health Disparities

HIV is just one example of the numerous health disparities faced by TGNC individuals best evidenced by comparing transgender and cisgender populations. Dragon and colleagues [10] found a higher proportion of transgender beneficiaries were receiving Medicare due to disability rather than age when compared to their cisgender peers (71% and 17%, respectively), indicating greater disability among TGNC individuals. TGNC beneficiaries had greater prevalence of a number of chronic conditions compared to their cisgender peers, including asthma, chronic obstructive pulmonary disease, and hepatitis. In a similar study, Brown and Jones [11] examined health disparities based on gender identity among veterans and found transgender veterans were more likely to have 16 of 17 health conditions, had higher rates of incarceration and a history of homelessness, and were more likely to report sexual victimization on duty compared to cisgender veterans.

Behavioral Health Behavioral health issues have been identified as a driver of the HIV epidemic by increasing risky activities associated with HIV transmission. For example, a study of patients with sexually transmitted infections found that those who were depressed were more likely to have engaged in transactional sex, had a greater number of sex partners, and were more likely to have had sex while using substances [12]. Depression is also correlated with engaging in unprotected sex, increasing risk of HIV transmission as condom use is one of the most effective ways of preventing HIV [13]. Risky sexual behavior has also been found to be more common among victims of childhood sexual or physical abuse or those who have experienced violence [14, 15].

The literature points to behavioral health disparities among TGNC individuals as one contributor to HIV infection in this population. Brown and Jones [11] found that transgender veterans had a higher prevalence of all ten mental health conditions examined (e.g., depression, panic disorder, post-traumatic stress disorder) compared with cisgender veterans. Dragon and colleagues [10] found transgender Medicare beneficiaries had higher rates of mental and behavioral health conditions compared to their cisgender peers, including anxiety disorders (39% and 17%, respectively), bipolar disorder (12% and 2%, respectively), depression (54% and 25%, respectively), personality disorders (8% and 1%, respectively), post-traumatic stress disorder (6% and 1% respectively), substance use disorders (8% and 2%, respectively), and schizophrenia and other psychotic disorders (13% and 4%, respectively). Suicidal ideation is also high among transgender adults [16]. One study found that 40% of transgender adults aged 18 or older had attempted suicide in their lifetime—nearly nine times the rate of attempted suicide in the general population [16].

Transgender older adults are more likely to have children and larger social networks and are less likely to live alone when compared to their cisgender and lesbian, gay, and bisexual (LGB) counterparts. Yet, they report lower levels of social support and higher levels of depression when compared to both their cisgender and LGB peers [17]. Fear of rejection, and anxiety around not "passing" as their identified gender, limits social interaction, which increases feelings of loneliness and isolation. Levels of social support and depression may be even more disparate in transgender older adults with HIV as the population is largely transgender women who report high rates of family rejection [18].

Transgender health disparities are driven by a number of structural and personal factors, including barriers to accessing health-care services, high rates of tobacco use, obesity and sedentary lifestyles, inadequate social supports, internalized stigma, victimization, and fear of disclosing their TGNC identities [17]. Discrimination by health-care providers may be both anticipated and experienced, which results in TGNC people delaying or avoiding medical care. This in turn exacerbates TGNC health disparities and interferes with preventative measures like HIV testing [16, 19, 20].

HIV and Transgender Adults While there is an emerging literature on older adults with HIV, little has focused specifically on people of TGNC experience, contributing to the invisibility of this population. The Centers for Disease Control and Prevention (CDC) surveillance methods have historically used sex assigned at birth as part of the formula to classify HIV transmission category [21]. Including transgender women in the category of men who have sex with men (MSM) also contributes to the invisibility of this population in the HIV epidemic. The CDC assessed the inclusion of "transgender" as a response option in more recent HIV surveillance data and found higher HIV infection rates among transgender individuals (range = 1.7%–4.7%) when compared to both cisgender men (range = 0.9%–1.4%) and cisgender women (range = 0.2%–0.4%) [21]. In Dragon and colleagues' study of Medicare beneficiaries [10], transgender individuals were also more likely to be diagnosed with HIV compared to cisgender beneficiaries (11% and 0.4%, respectively). In Brown and Jones' assessment of transgender veterans [11], HIV prevalence was the largest observed health disparity based on gender identity (2.9% of transgender veterans compared with 0.51% of cisgender veterans).

4.3 Intersectionality and HIV Risk

The intersectionality framework provides a vantage point to the complex convergence of interrelated stigma and resultant social inequality that have the potential to affect a transgender individual's lived experience [22]. For transgender older adults with HIV, these intersecting identities include age, gender identity, HIV stigma, sexual orientation, class, and race [23, 24]. Thus, we cannot understand the experience of a transgender person with HIV solely through the lens of gender identity, nor their marginalization solely through transphobia.

In its earliest conceptions, ageism (i.e., stigma based upon age) was understood to be "...particularly virulent against those who are already vulnerable to other kinds of discrimination" [25]. Race, specifically being Black/African-American, is consistently the greatest risk factor and predictor of HIV infection among transgender and cisgender persons of all ages. More than half of all transgender people with HIV are Black/African-American [26, 27]. HIV stigma is well-documented as a pernicious and pervasive phenomenon rooted within social inequality [3, 28, 29]. The term "multiple jeopardy" in the HIV literature has been used to describe both an additive model of disadvantage and an interlocking convergence of oppression based upon race, class, age, and gender [30]. The multiplicative model of intersectionality we describe below posits that a transgender older adult with HIV would experience racism, classism, ageism, HIV stigma, and sexism differently than a cisgender older adult with HIV and must cope with transphobia as well.

We propose a new phrase to express the unique experiences of transgender older adults with HIV that expands the multiple jeopardy framework and embraces an intersectional perspective—*Five Corners*. Five Corners captures the crossroads of race, class, gender identity, sexual orientation, age, and HIV stigma that shape the experience of transgender older adults with HIV. The Five Corners intersectionality model can help us understand the convergence of multiple aspects of identity that contribute to stigma and discrimination, which provides a more nuanced perspective on health equity affecting TGNC older adults with HIV (Fig. 4.1).

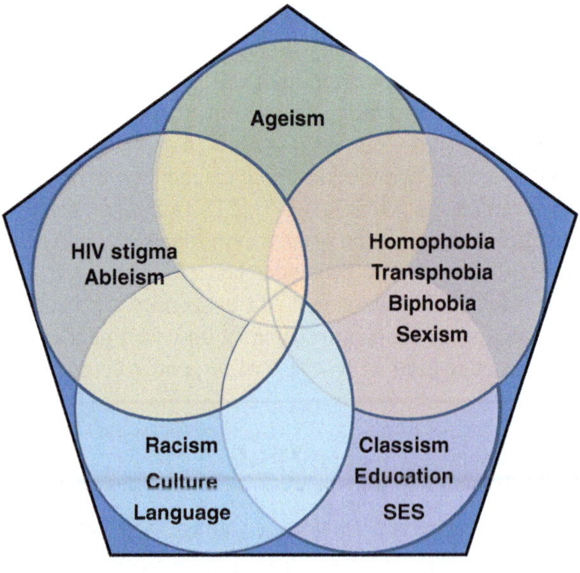

Fig. 4.1 The Five Corners intersectionality model

The stigma and discrimination experienced at the Five Corners intersection of these marginalized identities result in various risks to mental and physical health. HIV stigma is correlated with increased isolation, higher rates of depression, lower self-esteem, lower rates of HIV disclosure, and engagement in more risky sexual behavior, which all negatively impacts psychological well-being [1]. Stigma and discrimination based upon transphobia and homophobia result in much higher rates of violence and abuse experienced by transgender people when compared to the general population [16, 17, 31]. Nearly half (47%) of transgender people have been sexually assaulted [16]. At home, more than half (54%) of transgender people experience intimate partner violence [16]. When compared to their cisgender LGB counterparts, transgender older adults report higher rates of discrimination, lifetime victimization, and internalized stigma [17].

The experiences and consequences of stigma and the resultant psychological vulnerability intersect with other social determinants. For transgender persons, these include high lifetime rates of homelessness (30%), high lifetime rates of incarceration (33%), and higher rates of sexual assault while incarcerated [16, 27]. Transgender adults have lower rates of health insurance compared to the general population and are more likely to experience health-care discrimination. Higher rates of under- or unemployment are found among transgender adults with 30% reporting they lost a job due to their gender identity [16]. Furthermore, societal ageism may interfere with older TGNC adults accessing HIV testing and supportive services and may have a direct detrimental effect on their health through the internalization of ageist beliefs [32].This intersectionality results in greater HIV disease burden and added challenges to testing and treatment, especially for older adults [1].

Transgender Women and HIV Baral and colleagues' [33] meta-analysis reports that transgender women have the highest rates of HIV of any group and 34 times higher odds of infection when compared to comparable adult groups of reproductive age in the USA. Mizuno and colleagues [34] produced nationally representative estimates of people with HIV receiving medical care in the United States from 2009 to 2011, reporting that transgender women comprised 1.3% of adults with HIV, 13% of them were aged 55 and older, and 87% were people of color. African-American transgender women bear the greatest HIV burden [26, 27]. National-level data on new HIV infections from 2009 to 2014 found that of newly diagnosed transgender women, 51% were African-American, 29% Latinx, 11% White, 6% multiple races, 2% Asian, 0.7% American Indian/Alaskan Native, and 0.6% Native Hawaiian/other Pacific Islander [26].

Transgender women with HIV are socially and economically disadvantaged and report low rates of employment, health insurance coverage, HIV-related health care, HAART use, and HAART adherence [35, 36]. They also report higher prevalence of incarceration, victimization, homelessness, and employment discrimination [36]. These disadvantages predispose participation in the underground economy, with 19% of transgender women engaging in some type of sex work, exchange sex, or survival sex [16]. A review of 29 studies found an average lifetime rate of sex work to be 42% among transgender women [27].

Among transgender women with a history of sex work, a risk factor for HIV infection, a staggering majority have endured intimate partner violence (77%) or have been sexually assaulted (72%) [16]. One meta-analysis found a significant difference in HIV prevalence rates between transgender women engaging in sex work (27%) and transgender women not engaging in sex work (15%), although whether the HIV infection was related to sex work itself could not be determined [37]. Most transgender women were infected with HIV through sexual contact (87%), and many report inconsistent condom use while engaging in receptive anal sex [26, 36].

HIV in transgender women is not effectively medically managed. Suppression of the HIV viral load (i.e., "undetectable viral load") is the goal of HAART. Transgender women with HIV have viral load counts almost three times higher than cisgender adults with HIV [38]. Transgender women with HIV are less likely to use HAART and have lower rates of HAART adherence, thus increasing the probability of disease progression. In a study of Ryan White Program participants, while transgender individuals had similar rates of retention in care compared to their cisgender counterparts (approximately 80% in both groups), they were less likely to achieve viral suppression (74% and 81%, respectively) [39]. A cross-sectional population-based study using Medical Monitoring Project data reported that only 51% of transgender women had an undetectable viral load during the past year compared to 61% of cisgender men [34]. Effective viral suppression via HAART keeps the individual with HIV healthy and virtually eliminates the risk of transmitting HIV to others, making effective HIV treatment in transgender women a critical public health initiative [40]. Contributing factors to the ineffective management of HIV among transgender women include negative past experiences with health-care providers, high rates of housing insecurity, and concerns that HAART may interrupt or inhibit feminizing hormone therapy [36, 41].

Transgender Men and HIV Clark and colleagues [26] conducted a national-level analysis of transgender people newly diagnosed with HIV. Of the transgender men newly diagnosed with HIV in their study, 58% were African-American, 15% Latinx, 16% White, 9% multiple races, 1% Asian, and less than 1% American Indian/Alaska Native. Over half of transgender men were diagnosed by the age of 34, 8% were aged 55 and older, and 57% had an unknown transmission category with 34% infected through sexual contact and 9% through injection drug use. Transgender men with HIV also faced other disadvantages; almost half (47%) lived in poverty, and almost a quarter (23%) were clinically depressed. However in stark comparison to transgender women, transgender men accounted for only 0.2% of adults with HIV and 11% of all transgender adults with HIV in the United States [26]. HIV in transgender men appears better managed compared to transgender women; one study reported 60% of transgender men had an undetectable viral load during the past year [42]. Yet, transgender men, transgender women, and non-binary adults with HIV fall far short of the National HIV/AIDS Strategy: updated to 2020 goal of 80% viral suppression [40].

4.4 Health Concerns for Transgender People Aging with HIV

While there is a growing literature regarding the implications of aging with HIV on health, we know very little about the health consequences of growing older as a transgender individual regardless of HIV status. In particular, we have scant understanding of how gender-affirming medications and surgeries affect one's health in the long term, if there are differences in these effects depending on the age of transition or how the use of sex hormones might interact with medications commonly taken for age-related chronic conditions. This picture is further complicated for those growing older with HIV which, like aging, promotes states of chronic inflammation and immunosenescence, even when the virus is well-controlled and viral loads are undetectable [43]. In the absence of scientific literature that addresses this topic, this section will explore how some of the health concerns and disparities endemic to TGNC populations might be manifested in the health concerns common to HIV and aging, namely, multimorbidity, polypharmacy, and models of care.

Multimorbidity One of the first recognized consequences of aging with HIV is multimorbidity, or having multiple chronic conditions. In practical terms, multimorbidity represents the accumulation of serious health conditions that have the potential to negatively affect one's functional ability or cognitive status [44]. While multimorbidity is often observed in HIV-negative aging individuals, people with HIV are experiencing multimorbidity decades earlier than their non-infected peers [45]. Further, data show that older people with HIV are more likely to die of a non-AIDS-defining illness (i.e., noncommunicable diseases) rather than complications of HIV, and risk of these other conditions is related to nadir CD4 count (i.e., the lowest t-cell count observed), time from HIV infection to the initiation of HAART, and viral load suppression [46].These observations have led many to postulate that people growing older with HIV are experiencing accelerated aging [47].

However, the scientific evidence to support the accelerated aging hypothesis is equivocal. As Karpiak and Havlik observe, one of the confounds in addressing this issue is the lack of valid comparison groups to HIV-positive populations studied, given higher rates of substance use, tobacco use, hepatitis C, sexually transmitted infections, and structural inequalities (housing, employment, discrimination) are more common among people with HIV [47]. Biological processes correlated with aging are occurring earlier in HIV-infected individuals, but clinical presentation of disease conditions does not necessarily happen earlier for this population. Some have proposed that the high levels of multimorbidity observed in those aging with HIV are the result of accentuated aging [48]. That is, disease incidence is not happing at earlier ages in HIV-infected populations but that people with HIV are experiencing an early onset of multiple chronic conditions [47, 49].

Certain physical comorbidities are common in people aging with HIV, including cardiovascular disease, certain cancers (lung, oral, anal, Hodgkin's disease, and Kaposi's sarcoma), renal failure, geriatric syndromes (falls, fractures), and hepatitis C [47]. Multivariate analyses found that the number of comorbid conditions among older people with HIV is related to female gender, inadequate incomes, a history of substance use, prior AIDS diagnosis, longer time since HIV diagnosis, poor self-rated health, and depression [45]. Given the overall health disparities faced by TGNC individuals compared to both heterosexual and sexual minority cisgender populations, the additional risk for comorbidity and multimorbidity in the context of HIV disease is a cause for concern. At present we do not have data to assess whether TGNC individuals with HIV have even greater risk for comorbid conditions and multimorbidity than cisgender people with HIV and, if this risk is present, whether it poses an additive or multiplicative effect.

One of the most prevalent comorbidities in people aging with HIV is depression. Studies on older adults with HIV have found levels of depressive symptoms three to five times higher than in the general population, with over 40% scoring in the severe range of depressive symptoms [50]. The etiology of depression in older adults with HIV is not well-understood given the lack of longitudinal data that could address causality. Cross-section studies find that severe levels of depressive symptoms among older adults with HIV are related to younger age, self-reported cognitive impairment, self-reported fatigue, greater HIV stigma, and loneliness [51]. Considering the greater likelihood of experiencing depression and a history of substance use, TGNC individuals experience significant stigma due to their gender identities and have poor social support resources [10, 11, 17]. Thus, depression may be even more critical for TGNC individuals with regard to managing HIV compared to those who are cisgender and HIV-positive. Depression is one of the best predictors of HIV medication nonadherence [52]. Thus, successful management of depression and other behavioral health issues (e.g., substance use) is key to managing HIV for TGNC populations. However, in a survey of psychologists and graduate students, only half reported training on TGNC populations, and only one-quarter felt they were competent in providing services to this population [53]. The scarcity of behavioral health providers who are trained and competent to serve the TGNC population could present a barrier to achieving viral suppression for HIV-positive individuals.

Polypharmacy Due to the increase in comorbid conditions and multimorbidity in later life, polypharmacy may be an inevitable consequence of growing older and becomes more complex in the context of HIV treatment. Polypharmacy is defined as needing five or more medications. Thus, the combination of HAART with medications for other chronic conditions places considerable additional medication burden on people aging with HIV [54]. In addition, HAART may have negative interactions with other medications and lead to adverse effects that are exacerbated by changes in kidney and liver function associated with aging. Polypharmacy can also precipitate problems with adherence to HAART and other medications needed to control HIV and treat other comorbidities [54].

Polypharmacy in older TGNC adults with HIV is further complicated due to potential interactions of gender-affirming hormone treatment, HAART, and medications for other comorbidities. Hormone levels may be depressed in the presence of

HAART, and there is the potential for side effects, drug failures, and other health problems [41, 55]. Unfortunately, data on the interactions between hormones and HAART have been based on cisgender women taking oral contraception, and we lack good evidence in this domain from TGNC individuals with HIV. Finally, using over-the-counter and recreational drugs, which is common among TGNC people with HIV, can also exacerbate polypharmacy issues [54]. Problems related to polypharmacy can be ameliorated through careful patient monitoring and through the reformulation of medications, including long-lasting medications that can minimize problems with adherence [54, 55].

Models of Care Providing appropriate health care for TGNC people aging with HIV in the context of multimorbidity, geriatric syndromes and polypharmacy presents challenges to the clinical management of this population. While these challenges are frequently observed in older patients and are familiar to the geriatricians who care for them, they may not be recognized by the HIV-treating provider [56]. An appropriate response may be the incorporation of geriatric care principles and models into the care of the older person with HIV [56–58]. Singh and colleagues [56] elucidate several principles of geriatric care which include (1) aging is not defined or measured by the presence of disease, (2) the impact of multimorbidity is qualitatively different than the additive effects of individual disease conditions, (3) geriatric syndromes are different than non-age-related medical conditions, and (4) geriatric syndromes are observed in people aging with HIV before they are chronologically old.

Sangarlangkarn and colleagues [58] describe how multimorbidity and the synergistic interactions of multiple disease conditions increase the risk for iatrogenic illnesses and care fragmentation as multiple providers in multiple settings become involved in patient care. Simply put, providers who treat one condition without considering the other comorbidities may initiate single-disease treatment regimens that worsen the other conditions or may be at odds with the treatment of these conditions. For example, as discussed above, for TGNC individuals with HIV, HAART may interfere with gender-affirming hormone therapy. Geriatric care models focus on the patient's overall functional ability and quality of life, namely, patient-centered outcomes, and employ care coordination to avoid iatrogenic disorders and integrate medical and social services. Care integration lies on a continuum from linkage (combining existing services with minimal communication among providers), to coordination (creating structures and policies that facilitate transitions across systems), to full integration (using pooled resources to develop new programs) [57].

While the specifics of geriatric care models are variable, they tend to share certain common features [59]. To begin, these models assess all domains of patient functioning (disease, disability, functional ability, cognitive function, medications, self-care activities, lifestyle behaviors, psychological functioning, social supports, patient values, and care preferences). Second, these models address the development, implementation, and monitoring of a patient-centered care plan in line with patient values and preferences. Third is that communication and coordination among all of a patient's health-care and social service providers are emphasized. Finally, geriatric care models promote and facilitate the involvement of the patient and their significant others in health-care planning and decision-making, which may include patient self-management and the active support of health and social service providers.

The implementation of geriatric care models for TGNC individuals growing older with HIV could have significant promise in optimizing clinical and psychosocial outcomes. The component of global assessment of patient domains for this population would include gender identity, as well as medical and social transitioning. Given the physical and mental health disparities faced by TGNC people, the assessment of multiple comorbid conditions and treatment goals to maximize function could bolster quality of life. Further, in the context of the distrust that many TGNC people feel toward the medical community [16, 19, 20], an emphasis on patient-centered care that is in line with patient values and preferences could act to restore trust between these patients and their health-care providers. Coordination and communication between service providers would be extremely beneficial, for example, in cases where hormone therapy and other medical treatments are not compatible or contraindicated.

Siegler and Brennan-Ing [57] posit that geriatric principles and models could be infused into the care of the patient aging with HIV in two ways. The first is adapting systems of HIV care for the aging patient, which would involve provider education on aging issues, blending access to geriatric- and community-based social services and supports, creating linkages with community agencies, and incorporating geriatric expertise into HIV services (i.e., embedding a geriatrician in an HIV clinic). The alternative is to adapt existing geriatric care systems to patients aging with HIV. For example, existing payment structures are geared toward end-of-life care and may not provide sufficient resources to address the ongoing chronic conditions common to the older person with HIV. Reimbursement models also need to account for the added expense of caring for a patient with HIV and other multiple comorbid conditions.

Of course, the application of geriatric care models to the aging HIV-positive TGNC population must have as its foundation culturally competent and nonjudgmental care, both with regard to gender identity and HIV serostatus. Many TGNC patients find themselves in the situation of having to educate providers on transgender issues [60]. This problem results from the lack of attention to sexual minority and gender diverse individuals in medical education; one study reported that medical undergraduates received only 7 hours of training on average on these populations. To further complicate the problem, some providers consider a TGNC identity itself as an indicator of mental illness, which immediately erects barriers to patient-provider rapport [60].

Although not specific to those aging with HIV, a number of innovative care models specific to the TGNC population are in development [39]. In response to a community consultation, the US Health Resources and Service Administration provided funding to enhance care engagement and retention in four community and five clinical demonstration sites. These programs involved enhancements of existing service structures as well as the creation of new programs based on conceptual models of TGNC care. Although the nine sites were independent, most incorporated three key concepts: provision of culturally competent care, inclusion of supportive messages to support personal and community development as well as health literacy, and improving social support by facilitating caring relationships between providers and patients and between patients and their communities [39].

Other models of care for TGNC people with HIV have been developed at that community level. Amida Care, a community-sponsored HIV Medicaid special needs managed care plan in New York City, is developing a specialized program for its TGNC members [61]. Amida Care has provided services for TGNC people with HIV since its founding in 2003. At present, 7% or approximately 400 Amida Care members are people of TGNC experience. In 2015, the New York State Medicaid program initiated coverage of gender-affirming hormone therapy and surgical treatment, and Amida Care is able to offer these services as part of this program. It is notable that the Amida Care program incorporates many of the elements of geriatric care models including specialized care coordination through integrated multidisciplinary care teams, treatment adherence services, HIV prevention and risk reduction education, and behavioral health services. Data mining is used to monitor member utilization and clinical outcomes, while health navigators promote engagement in care and treatment adherence. Amida Care also addresses the larger context of TGNC members' lives by assisting with job training and vocational placement, as well as elements of social transitioning such as name changes or gender markers on identity documents. This program is guided by a Transgender Clinical Advisory Committee. The success of this program is also fostered by reducing stigma through regular staff trainings to insure cultural competency, building a culturally competent provider network, and making the physical environment welcoming, for example, by having all-gender restrooms for members.

Long-Term Care Services and Supports (LTCSS) The topics of informal and formal LTCSS are discussed in detail elsewhere in this volume. However, the issue of the Five Corners intersectionality of identities further complicates LTCSS access for older TGNC people with HIV. That is, beyond issues of lack of family and friends, disclosure, detransitioning, discrimination, and abuse due to gender identity [62], older TGNC people with HIV face the added problem of HIV-related stigma and discrimination. Discrimination in nursing home admissions for having an HIV-positive serostatus is still being reported, despite the fact that such discrimination is illegal according to the Fair Housing Act, the Americans with Disabilities Act, and for Medicaid or Medicare patients under the federal Rehabilitation Act [63].

Unfortunately, research on the experience of HIV-positive patients and institutional care placement is limited [64]. One of the only papers on this topic reports on a testing study of health-care services in Los Angeles County, CA. With regard to skilled nursing facilities, Sears [65] found only 36% provided an unquailed "yes" when asked if they would take HIV-positive patients. Of those that would not accept patients with HIV, many did not provide any justification for their response. When refusal was justified, some said that they had no prior experience with HIV patients, and others cited a lack of isolation rooms or units, that protocols for HIV patients were not in place, or that they would refer a patient with HIV to another facility. Some cited the desire to protect their sexually active residents from someone with HIV. Part of the resistance to accepting individuals with HIV into long-term care settings inevitably stems from stigmatizing beliefs about HIV held by health-care workers. In a study of these workers in the Deep South, 93% of social and community workers, 89% of clinical staff, and 90% of other staff endorsed at least one stigmatizing attitude [66]. In multivariate analysis, stigmatizing attitudes were significantly related to Protestant religious affiliation, White race, working in an HIV/STI clinic, unavailability of postexposure prophylaxis for HIV, and lax enforcement of antidiscrimination policies. Given the uphill battle older TGNC people face in accessing culturally competent and nondiscriminatory LTCSS in their communities, adding HIV to the mix will surely present additional challenges that will need to be ameliorated through policy and programmatic remedies.

4.5 Conclusions and Implications

While this chapter has focused on the myriad challenges faced by older TGNC individuals with HIV, it is important to acknowledge that older adults with HIV show great resilience in the face of adversity, and the majority of TGNC older adults report they are aging successfully despite health challenges [28, 67]. Resilience in both TGNC older adults, and in older adults with HIV, has been associated with self-care health behaviors, productivity and community engagement (e.g., volunteering), social engagement with the transgender community and the HIV community, and involvement with and participation in spiritual activities and communities [17, 62, 67]. TGNC older adults with HIV reveal a resilience plasticity by which protective behaviors and beliefs can interrupt transphobia and HIV stigma by nurturing gender pride and building self-esteem, empowering the reclamation of sexual power, and fostering gerotranscendence. Within our current society and culture, where the struggle to accept those who do not identify as cisgender lingers, TGNC older adults have demonstrated remarkable hardiness, which provides an important personal resource that can be leveraged in clinical settings and psychosocial interventions.

It is clear that the evidence base around aging with HIV for people of transgender experience is sorely lacking. Not only does this contribute to the invisibility of this population, but it severely limits our ability to develop an informed policy and programmatic response to HIV infection in the aging TGNC community. Gaps in our knowledge concerning how gender-affirming medical treatment affects health as we age, and how this interacts with other disease conditions like HIV, can only serve to increase the health inequalities faced by TGNC individuals. More research is also needed on psychosocial challenges and remedies faced by those who are aging with HIV and TGNC, given the interplay between psychosocial concerns and health.

A consistent message in this chapter has been the vital role that culturally competent services play in ensuring decent quality of life and optimal clinical outcomes for the older TGNC individual with HIV. But this demands a Five Corners cultural competency, involving gender identity, HIV status, race/ethnicity, social class, and age. The foundations of this multidimensional competency must be laid in medical and professional education, which would benefit providers as well as the diverse patients and clients that they serve. As our communities become increasingly diverse, our providers must have the ability to serve an increasingly heterogeneous population. This will benefit not only older TGNC individuals with HIV but our larger society as well.

4.6 Summary

- TGNC health disparities are driven by a number of structural and personal factors, including barriers to accessing health-care services, high rates of tobacco use, obesity and sedentary lifestyles, inadequate social supports, internalized stigma, victimization, and fear of disclosing their TGNC identities.
- HIV is one of numerous health disparities found in the TGNC population; the highest rates of HIV infection are found in the TGNC population.
- African-American transgender women are particularly at risk.
- Five Corners intersectionality approach considers the crossroads of race, class, gender identity, age, and HIV stigma that influence the experience of TGNC older adults with HIV.
- HIV is not well-managed medically in TGNC adults with HIV.
- Mental and behavioral health, multimorbidity, and polypharmacy all pose unique challenges for TGNC older adults with HIV.
- Several models of care are being developed around aging with HIV and TGNC identities, which have at their core culturally competent and patient-centered care.
- TGNC older adults with HIV reveal a resilience plasticity by which protective behaviors and beliefs can interrupt transphobia and HIV stigma by nurturing gender pride and building self-esteem, empowering the reclamation of sexual power, and fostering gerotranscendence.

References

1. Karpiak SE, Brennan M. The emerging population of older adults with HIV and introduction to the ROAH study. In: Older adults with HIV: an in-depth examination of an emerging population. New York: Nova Science Publishers; 2009. p. 1–2.
2. High KP, Brennan-Ing M, Clifford DB, Cohen MH, Currier J, Deeks SG, Deren S, Effros RB, Gebo K, Goronzy JJ, Justice AC. HIV and aging: state of knowledge and areas of critical need for research. A report to the NIH Office of AIDS Research by the HIV and Aging Working Group. J Acquir Immune Defic Syndr (1999). 2012;60(Suppl 1):S1–18.

3. amfAR: Thirty years of HIV/AIDS: Snapshots of an epidemic [Internet]. http://www.amfar.org/thirty-years-of-hiv/aids-snapshots-of-an-epidemic/ 2013. Accessed 27 Jan 2018.
4. Nakagawa F, May M, Phillips A. Life expectancy living with HIV: recent estimates and future implications. Curr Opin Infect Dis. 2013;26(1):17–25.
5. Diverse Elders Coalition. Eight policy recommendations for improving the health and wellness of older adults with HIV [Internet]. 2014. https://www.sageusa.org/files/DEC-HIV-and-Aging-Policy-Report_web.pdf. Accessed 27 Jan 2018.
6. Centers for Disease Control and Prevention. HIV among people aged 50 and 0lder [Internet]. 2017. https://www.cdc.gov/hiv/group/age/olderamericans/index.html. Accessed 27 Jan 2018.
7. ACRIA. Age is not a condom [Internet]. www.ageisnotacondom.org. Accessed 27 Jan 2018.
8. Brennan-Ing M, Seidel L, Ansell P, Raik BL, Greenberg D, Nicastri C, Breznay J, Karpiak SE, Adelman RD. Addressing sexual health in geriatrics education. Gerontol Geriatr Educ. 2017;17:1–5.
9. Stoff DM, Khalsa JH, Monjan A, Portegies P. Introduction. AIDS [Internet]. Ovid Technol (Wolters Kluwer Health). 2004;18(Supplement 1):1–2. Available from: https://doi.org/10.1097/00002030-200401001-00001
10. Dragon CN, Guerino P, Ewald E, Laffan AM. Transgender Medicare beneficiaries and chronic conditions: exploring fee-for-service claims data. LGBT health. 2017;4(6):404–11.
11. Brown GR, Jones KT. Mental health and medical health disparities in 5135 transgender veterans receiving healthcare in the veterans health administration: a case–control study. LGBT health. 2016;3(2):122–31.
12. Hutton HE, Lyketsos CG, Zenilman JM, Thompson RE, Erbelding EJ. Depression and HIV risk behaviors among patients in a sexually transmitted disease clinic. Am J Psychiatr. 2004;161(5):912–4.
13. Shrier LA, Harris SK, Sternberg M, Beardslee WR. Associations of depression, self-esteem, and substance use with sexual risk among adolescents. Prev Med. 2001;33(3):179–89.
14. Plotzker RE, Metzger DS, Holmes WC. Childhood sexual and physical abuse histories, PTSD, depression, and HIV risk outcomes in women injection drug users: a potential mediating pathway. Am J Addict. 2007;16(6):431–8.
15. Johnson SD, Cunningham-Williams RM, Cottler LB. A tripartite of HIV-risk for African American women: the intersection of drug use, violence, and depression. Drug Alcohol Depend. 2003;70(2):169–75.
16. James SE, Herman JL, Rankin S, Keisling M, Mottet L, Anafi MA. The report of the 2015 US transgender survey. Washington, DC: National Center for Transgender Equality; 2016.
17. Fredriksen-Goldsen KI, Cook-Daniels L, Kim HJ, Erosheva EA, Emlet CA, Hoy-Ellis CP, Goldsen J, Muraco A. Physical and mental health of transgender older adults: an at-risk and underserved population. The Gerontologist. 2013;54(3):488–500.
18. Erenrich R, Seidel L, Karpiak S, Brennan-Ing M, Lunievicz J. Research on older adults with HIV: Bay Area focus group report: Alameda County and San Francisco. New York: ACRIA; 2017.
19. Bauer GR, Hammond R, Travers R, Kaay M, Hohenadel KM, Boyce M. "I don't think this is theoretical; this is our lives": how erasure impacts health care for transgender people. J Assoc Nurses AIDS Care. 2009;20(5):348–61.
20. Walker RV, Powers SM, Witten TM. Impact of anticipated bias from healthcare professionals on perceived successful aging among transgender and gender nonconforming older adults. LGBT Health. 2017;4(6):427–33.
21. Centers for Disease Control and Prevention. CDC-funded HIV testing: United States, Puerto Rico, & the U.S. Virgin Islands. 2014. MMWR Morb Mortal Wkly Rep. 2016;65(40):1099–103.
22. Crenshaw, K. Demarginalizing the intersection of race and sex: a black feminist critique of antidiscrimination doctrine, feminist theory and antiracist politics, U Chic Legal F. 1989:139(1), Article 8. Available at: http://chicagounbound.uchicago.edu/uclf/vol1989/iss1/8.
23. Taskforce AL, Harper A, Finnerty P, Martinez M, Brace A, Crethar HC, Loos B, Harper B, Graham S, Singh A, Kocet M. Association for Lesbian, gay, bisexual, and transgender issues in counseling competencies for counseling with lesbian, gay, bisexual, queer, questioning,

intersex, and ally individuals: approved by the ALGBTIC board on June 22, 2012. J LGBT Issues Couns. 2013;7(1):2–43.
24. Witten TM. The intersectional challenges of aging and of being a gender non-conforming adult. Generations. 2016;40(2):63–70.
25. Kleyman P. Senior power: growing old rebelliously: Glide Publications; San Francisco. 1974.
26. Clark H, Babu AS, Wiewel EW, Opoku J, Crepaz N. Diagnosed HIV infection in transgender adults and adolescents: results from the national HIV surveillance system, 2009–2014. AIDS Behav. 2017;21(9):2774–83.
27. Herbst JH, Jacobs ED, Finlayson TJ, McKleroy VS, Neumann MS, Crepaz N. HIV/AIDS prevention research synthesis team. Estimating HIV prevalence and risk behaviors of transgender persons in the United States: a systematic review. AIDS Behav. 2008;12(1):1–7.
28. Porter KE, Brennan-Ing M, Burr JA, Dugan E, Karpiak SE. Stigma and psychological well-being among older adults with HIV: the impact of spirituality and integrative health approaches. The Gerontologist. 2015;57(2):219–28.
29. Emlet CA. Stigma in an aging context. In: HIV and aging, vol. 42: Karger Publishers; San Francisco. 2017. p. 144–58.
30. Brown TH, Richardson LJ, Hargrove TW, Thomas CS. Using multiple-hierarchy stratification and life course approaches to understand health inequalities: the intersecting consequences of race, gender, SES, and age. J Health Soc Behav. 2016;57(2):200–22.
31. Witten TM, Eyler AE, editors. Gay, lesbian, bisexual, and transgender aging: challenges in research, practice, and policy: JHU Press; San Francisco. 2012.
32. DeMarco RF, Brennan-Ing M, Sprague C, Brown SM. Ageism, aging and HIV: community responses to prevention, treatment, care and support. In: HIV and aging, vol. 42: Karger Publishers; San Francisco. 2017. p. 234–9.
33. Baral SD, Poteat T, Strömdahl S, Wirtz AL, Guadamuz TE, Beyrer C. Worldwide burden of HIV in transgender women: a systematic review and meta-analysis. Lancet Infect Dis. 2013;13(3):214–22.
34. Mizuno Y, Frazier EL, Huang P, Skarbinski J. Characteristics of transgender women living with HIV receiving medical care in the United States. LGBT health. 2015;2(3):228–34.
35. Clements-Nolle K, Marx R, Guzman R, Katz M. HIV prevalence, risk behaviors, health care use, and mental health status of transgender persons: implications for public health intervention. Am J Public Health. 2001;91(6):915.
36. Denson DJ, Padgett PM, Pitts N, Paz-Bailey G, Bingham T, Carlos JA, McCann P, Prachand N, Risser J, Finlayson T. Health care use and HIV-related behaviors of black and Latina transgender women in 3 US metropolitan areas: results from the transgender HIV behavioral survey. J Acquir Immune Defic Syndr. 2017;75:S268–75.
37. Operario D, Soma T, Underhill K. Sex work and HIV status among transgender women: systematic review and meta-analysis. J Acquir Immune Defic Syndr. 2008;48(1):97–103.
38. Das M, Chu PL, Santos GM, Scheer S, Vittinghoff E, McFarland W, Colfax GN. Decreases in community viral load are accompanied by reductions in new HIV infections in San Francisco. PLoS One. 2010;5(6):e11068.
39. Rebchook G, Keatley J, Contreras R, Perloff J, Molano LF, Reback CJ, Ducheny K, Nemoto T, Lin R, Birnbaum J, Woods T. The transgender women of color initiative: implementing and evaluating innovative interventions to enhance engagement and retention in HIV care. Am J Public Health. 2017;107(2):224–9.
40. Centers for Disease Control and Prevention. National HIV/AIDS strategy: updated to 2020 2015. Retrieved from https://www.aids.gov/federal-resources/national-hiv-aids-strategy/nhas-update.pdf.
41. Sevelius JM, Carrico A, Johnson MO. Antiretroviral therapy adherence among transgender women living with HIV. J Assoc Nurses AIDS Care. 2010;21(3):256–64.
42. Lemons A, Beer L, Finlayson T, McCree DH, Lentine D, Shouse RL. Medical monitoring project. Characteristics of HIV-positive transgender men receiving medical care: United States, 2009–2014. Am J Public Health. 2018;108(1):128–30.

43. Nasi M, Pinti M, De Biasi S, Gibellini L, Ferraro D, Mussini C, Cossarizza A. Aging living with HIV infection: a journey to the center of inflammAIDS, immunosenescence and neuro-HIV. Immunol Lett. 2014;162(1):329–33.
44. Brown TT, Guaraldi G. Multimorbidity and burden of disease. In: HIV and aging, vol. 42: Karger Publishers; San Francisco. 2017. p. 59–73.
45. Havlik RJ, Brennan M, Karpiak SE. Comorbidities and depression in older adults with HIV. Sex Health. 2011;8(4):551–9.
46. Marin B, Thiébaut R, Bucher HC, Rondeau V, Costagliola D, Dorrucci M, Hamouda O, Prins M, Walker AS, Porter K, Sabin C. Non-AIDS-defining deaths and immunodeficiency in the era of combination antiretroviral therapy. AIDS (London, England). 2009;23(13):1743.
47. Karpiak SE, Havlik R. Are HIV-infected older adults aging differently? In: HIV and aging, vol. 42: Karger Publishers; San Francisco. 2017. p. 11–27.
48. Pathai S, Bajillan H, Landay AL, High KP. Is HIV a model of accelerated or accentuated aging? J Gerontol A: Biomed SciMed Sci. 2013;69(7):833–42.
49. Althoff KN, McGinnis KA, Wyatt CM, Freiberg MS, Gilbert C, Oursler KK, Rimland D, Rodriguez-Barradas MC, Dubrow R, Park LS, Skanderson M. Comparison of risk and age at diagnosis of myocardial infarction, end-stage renal disease, and non-AIDS-defining cancer in HIV-infected versus uninfected adults. Clin Infect Dis. 2014;60(4):627–38.
50. Applebaum A, Brennan M. Mental health and depression. In: Older adults with HIV: An in-depth examination of an emerging population. New York: Nova Science Publishers; 2009. p. 27–34.
51. Grov C, Golub SA, Parsons JT, Brennan M, Karpiak SE. Loneliness and HIV-related stigma explain depression among older HIV-positive adults. AIDS Care. 2010;22(5):630–9.
52. Safren SA, Hendriksen ES, Mayer KH, Mimiaga MJ, Pickard R, Otto MW. Cognitive-behavioral therapy for HIV medication adherence and depression. Cogn Behav Pract. 2004;11(4):415–24.
53. American Psychological Association. Task Force on Gender Identity and Gender Variance. Report of the task force on gender identity and gender variance. Washington, DC: Author; 2009. Retrieved from https://www.apa.org/pi/lgbt/resources/policy/gender-identity-report.pdf
54. Alberts LH. Polypharmacy, using new treatments to customize care for aging patients and adherence present and future. In: HIV and aging, vol. 42: Karger Publishers; San Francisco. 2017. p. 74–84.
55. Williamson C. Providing care to transgender persons: a clinical approach to primary care, hormones, and HIV management. J Assoc Nurses AIDS Care. 2010;21(3):221–9.
56. Singh HK, Del Carmen T, Freeman R, Glesby MJ, Siegler EL. From one syndrome to many: incorporating geriatric consultation into HIV care. Clin Infect Dis. 2017;65(3):501–6.
57. Siegler EL, Brennan-Ing M. Adapting systems of care for people aging with HIV. J Assoc Nurses AIDS Care. 2017;65(3):501–6.
58. Sangarlangkarn A, Avihingsanon A, Appelbaum JS. Application of geriatric principles and care models in HIV and aging. In: HIV and aging, vol. 42: Karger Publishers; San Francisco. 2017. p. 119–33.
59. Boult C, Wieland GD. Comprehensive primary care for older patients with multiple chronic conditions: "nobody rushes you through". JAMA. 2010;304(17):1936–43.
60. Dickey LM. Toward developing clinical competence: improving health care of gender diverse people. Am J Public Health. 2017;107(2):222–3.
61. Ernst J, Fusaris E. Providing access to medical, surgical, and behavioral health services for people of transgender experience in Medicaid managed care: A case study. Paper presented at the Gay and Lesbian Medical Association annual conference on LGBT health. 2017 Sept. 16.
62. Porter KE, Brennan-Ing M, Chang SC, Dickey LM, Singh AA, Bower KL, Witten TM. Providing competent and affirming services for transgender and gender nonconforming older adults. Clin Gerontol. 2016;39(5):366–88.
63. Lambda Legal. Long-term care and people living with HIV. 2010. Retrieved from: https://www.lambdalegal.org/sites/default/files/publications/downloads/fs_long-term-care-and-people-living-with-hiv_1.pdf.

64. Hughes A, Davies B, Gudmundsdottir M. "Can you give me respect?" experiences of the urban poor on a dedicated AIDS nursing home unit. J Assoc Nurses AIDS Care. 2008;19(5):342–56.
65. Sears B. HIV discrimination in health care services in Los Angeles County: the results of three testing studies. Wash Lee J Civil Rts Soc Just. 2008;15:85.
66. Stringer KL, Turan B, McCormick L, Durojaiye M, Nyblade L, Kempf MC, Lichtenstein B, Turan JM. HIV-related stigma among healthcare providers in the deep south. AIDS Behav. 2016;20(1):115–25.
67. Porter KE, Ronneberg CR, Witten TM. Religious affiliation and successful aging among transgender older adults: findings from the trans MetLife survey. J Relig Spiritual Aging. 2013;25(2):112–38.

Recommended Reading

American Psychological Association. Guidelines for psychological practice with transgender and gender nonconforming people. Am Psychol. 2015;70(9):832–64.

Brennan-Ing M, DeMarco RF, editors. HIV and aging: Karger Medical and Scientific Publishers; 2017.

Porter KE, Brennan-Ing M, Chang SC, Dickey LM, Singh AA, Bower KL, Witten TM. Providing competent and affirming services for transgender and gender nonconforming older adults. Clin Gerontol. 2016;39(5):366–88.

Transgender Intimate Partner Violence and Aging

5

Adam M. Messinger and Jennifer Roark

> In the support group, I found comfort and solidarity, but I also had to sacrifice pieces of who I was to access the space. Statements were regularly exchanged about how we were all women and that made the space so safe, while I bit my lip and stared at my hands. It took me a full year after coming out as trans to tell the group. I didn't think I could be there anymore if they knew I was a guy. ([1], 178)

The story above details the experience of Timothy Colm, a survivor of intimate partner violence (IPV), that is, psychological, physical, or sexual abuse within romantic and sexual relationships. Like many IPV survivors, Colm found a safe space designed for cisgender women to escape from and cope with abuse. Unfortunately, as is particularly common for transgender survivors, Colm felt he had to hide his identity as a transgender man, lest he be discriminated against and barred from services [1]. Despite the research literature on IPV in relationships involving a transgender survivor or abuser (T-IPV) emerging only a decade ago (e.g., [2–4]), studies have now repeatedly confirmed that transphobia plays an integral role in shaping the etiology, dynamics, and outcomes for abuse within these relationships [5]. What is less clear in this literature is whether T-IPV is homogeneous across the lifespan or if, instead, it presents additional challenges among aging populations.

To begin filling this knowledge gap, this chapter draws on the respective T-IPV literature and aging cisgender IPV literature to review what is known and may be inferred about T-IPV among older individuals (e.g., 55 and older). In addition to detailing methodological challenges inherent in studying this topic, this chapter discusses the prevalence, tactics, and outcomes of T-IPV and IPV among aging

A. M. Messinger (✉)
Justice Studies Department, Northeastern Illinois University, Chicago, IL, USA
e-mail: a-messinger@neiu.edu

J. Roark
Department of Sociology, Social Work, and Anthropology, Utah State University, Logan, UT, USA

M. Houlberg et al. (eds.), *Transgender and Gender Nonconforming Health and Aging*,
https://doi.org/10.1007/978-3-319-95031-0_5

populations, as well as help-seeking and help-giving issues regarding these populations. Implications for future research and service provision are discussed.

5.1 Methodological Challenges

Although there are many reasons why research about T-IPV among aging populations remains relatively scarce, a key factor is that methodological challenges can hinder exploration of this issue. As Messinger [5] notes, there are numerous challenges in studying IPV among any population type, many of which are not specific to T-IPV studies. These general challenges include resolving the inherent trade-off of enhanced convenience and decreased accuracy in sampling from survivor-saturated sites like shelters rather than more general population sites (a concern only exacerbated for difficult-to-reach populations like older transgender individuals). Additional challenges include designing IPV survey measures that balance the needs for sensitivity (identifying all IPV survivors in a sample) with specificity (excluding "false positives"), as well as being inclusive of a broad variety of IPV tactics and forms. A final set of challenges in studying IPV among any population type includes using appropriate IPV recall time frames, in addition to clearly distinguishing victimization from perpetration [5]. On top of this, researching T-IPV among older individuals presents a host of unique challenges: (1) defining the population, (2) designing IPV measures that adequately distinguish IPV from other violence types, and (3) designing culturally specific IPV measures. Each of these challenges is detailed in this section.

5.1.1 Defining the Population

Researchers often define transgender populations as consisting of people whose gender identity differs from their biological sex assigned at birth. Where researchers are more divided is in whether it is best to use identity or behavioral measures to operationalize this definition in a study. Self-identity measures entail directly inquiring as to whether participants identify as transgender, nonbinary, genderqueer, and so forth, along with a "fill-in-the-blank" option to account for unlisted identities. This may be valuable on one hand because self-identity can impact experiences with transphobia-related IPV factors and, on the other hand, because ignoring identity may be viewed by some participants as disrespectful [5]. At the same time, many transgender people whose gender identity differs from their biological sex assigned at birth may identify only as a "woman" or as a "man," *not* as "transgender." Because these individuals would be overlooked by such a self-identity measure, many researchers opt to instead or also use a behavioral definition of transgender populations. Specifically, researchers may inquire in separate questions about participants' biological sex assigned at birth and current gender identity [6]. While some researchers have required participants to select from binary sex at birth (female, male) and binary gender identities (woman, man; e.g., [7]), a more inclusive approach would be to permit answers beyond these binaries. Studies utilizing both self-identity and behavioral measures may offer a more accurate picture of transgender participants, and findings from such studies will also be easier to make commensurable comparisons with other studies due to similar survey wording [5].

Research on aging samples faces additional challenges in defining populations. For instance, different researchers may define "aging" (often also termed "older" and "elder") populations with different minimum age requirements (e.g., 50, 55, 60, or 65 years of age at minimum; see [8–10]). As with differences in defining transgender populations, the methodological variations found in IPV research on aging populations may hinder clear cross-study comparisons.

In addition, of particular concern in transgender IPV research among aging populations are time frames regarding whether a participant was transgender identified before, during, or after an IPV relationship occurred. According to the US Transgender Survey – a study of 27,715 transgender people from across the United States and its territories, marking the largest study to date on this population – 82% of transgender people transition their gender identities prior to the age of 35 [11]. Moreover, according to the National Intimate Partner and Sexual Violence Survey (NISVS) – the most recent large, nationally representative study of IPV in the United States, drawing on a sample of 16,507 adults – 84.2% of all IPV survivors (not just transgender survivors) first experience IPV prior to the age of 35. Only 10.3% of survivors first experience IPV between ages 35 and 44, and just 5.5% of survivors first experience IPV at or after age 45 [12]. That is to say, it is likely that the majority of first-time IPV experiences occur when transgender people are younger, and likewise the majority of transgender people transition genders when they are younger as well. The exact timing of whether the gender transition occurs prior to or after IPV victimization may not be clear unless researchers directly inquire about participant self-identity at the time of each abusive relationship. Conversely, asking older transgender samples about lifetime victimization experiences may unintentionally mislabel some abuse as T-IPV at a period in life when a participant identified as cisgender.

5.1.2 Distinguishing Aging T-IPV from Other Violence Types

Beyond hurdles in defining the population appropriately, research on T-IPV among aging populations faces the methodological challenge of adequately distinguishing IPV from other violence types. As noted by Messinger [5], the general field of IPV research struggles with this issue in that it can prove difficult to separate IPV from child abuse and peer victimization. For minors abused by an adult, some survivors may have been persuaded to believe they were in a consensual romantic relationship, blurring the conceptual and methodological distinctions between child abuse and partner violence. In addition, for survivors who have been abused by a casual partner or friend, again the conceptual and methodological line between peer victimization (e.g., bullying) and partner violence becomes blurred [5]. Although not unique to transgender research, it is possible that both issues are exacerbated in studies of T-IPV given the high risk of both child abuse and peer victimization among transgender individuals [11].

Research on aging populations presents still another distinct challenge, in that IPV among older individuals is often subsumed conceptually and in research under other umbrella constructs, potentially masking pertinent findings. For instance, IPV is often considered one type of "elder abuse": neglect, as well as psychological, physical, and sexual abuse committed against an older individual. Because the perpetrator of elder abuse can be not only a partner but also a child, relative, or caregiver, prevalence rates and covariates of elder abuse may not accurately reflect those specifically of IPV among older individuals [9, 10]. Adding to the confusion is that, whereas many researchers use the term "domestic violence" synonymously with IPV (e.g., [13]), others use the term to refer to abuse by and against any family members, such as parents, children, and other relatives. In this vein, "domestic elder abuse" has been used by some to refer to elder abuse perpetrated by a family member but not by non-relative caregivers (e.g., [14]). Confusing distinct areas of research, such as child abuse, sibling abuse, IPV, abuse of older individuals by non-partner relatives, and abuse of older individuals by caretakers, has the potential to mask important differences in prevalence, risk factors, outcomes, and service provision needs. Given this, scholars have called for greater care in differentiating distinct types of violence in research (e.g., [5, 10]).

5.1.3 Culturally Appropriate IPV Measures

A final key challenge in understanding T-IPV among aging populations is designing IPV measures that are tailored to the target population. Overcoming this challenge can entail not assuming all participants are cisgender, incorporating unique aging T-IPV tactics in measure items, and validating such measures with samples drawn from the population of interest.

First, to both increase participant honesty and decrease confusion, it is important that IPV measures recognize that some participants may be transgender. Unfortunately, this recognition is rare [5]. For instance, the preamble paragraph of the female version of the original conflict tactics scale [15] refers to "you and your *husband*/partner," as do IPV questions in the measure (e.g., "Did your (*husband*/partner) ever…"; emphasis added). The equally popular revised conflict tactics scale [16] involved similar item wording (e.g., "My partner explained *his* or *her* side of a disagreement to me"; emphasis added). Such IPV measures assume that all participants identify within the gender binary as either men or women, erasing the existence of nonbinary and genderqueer participants. Movement toward gender-neutral terminology, such as "partner," may reduce cisnormative assumptions in future IPV measures.

Second, IPV measures rarely incorporate tactics unique to T-IPV among aging populations (see [5]). One of the rare exceptions to include unique T-IPV tactics was a study by Roch et al. [17], which included items assessing whether abusers had ever shamed survivors for being transgender, limited the survivor's gender expression such as through restricting gendered clothing access or refusing to use their gender-affirming name, limited the survivor's access to gender-related medical interventions such as surgery or hormone therapies, and threatened to out the survivor's transgender identity to others. An additional exception by James et al. [11] assessed whether abusers had ever shamed survivors for not being transgender enough, as well as whether abusers limited or controlled the survivor's access to medical interventions such as hormone therapies. Beyond these two examples, though, IPV measures tend to exclude abusive tactics that occur specifically in T-IPV relationships, let alone T-IPV among older partners.

Finally, to date, no IPV measure has been validated with a transgender sample [5] nor with an aging sample [9]. As Moradi et al. [18] note, IPV measures validated with one population type might not be suitable for studies on other population types.

In sum, past and future studies of T-IPV among aging populations must contend with these aforementioned methodological challenges, regarding defining the population, adequately distinguishing IPV from other violence types, and creating IPV measures that are culturally specific to and validated with transgender populations. That said, although comparatively smaller, the respective literatures on T-IPV and IPV among older individuals offer insights as to the nature of T-IPV among aging populations, detailed below.

5.2 Prevalence, Tactics, and Impact

Understanding the full scope of T-IPV among aging populations requires examining its prevalence, tactics, and impact on survivors. What becomes readily apparent from this review is that T-IPV and IPV among older individuals are not only common and harmful but also unique in the types of abusive tactics that occur in such relationships, tactics which take advantage of societal discrimination and the marginalized identities of survivors.

5.2.1 Past-Year Victimization Prevalence

Researchers typically ask participants about IPV they experienced during one of two possible time frames: the past year or the participant's lifetime. For older individuals in particular, each time frame is important to consider for different reasons. Past-year IPV victimization prevalence for older samples represents the likelihood of abuse occurring in a typical year during older age, and as such those incidents may be more likely to immediately trigger help-seeking strategies such as reaching out to shelters, police, and mental health counselors. Lifetime IPV victimization prevalence for older samples conversely represents the likelihood that abuse occurred at any point in the lives of older individuals, even abuse that may have occurred decades earlier. While such incidents may be less likely to trigger emergency searches for safety such as by calling the police, former victimization is also important to study in that it may increase risk for future victimization and also can have long-lasting consequences warranting mental health treatment [19].

Regarding past-year prevalence, no publication has yet to report on past-year T-IPV victimization prevalence among older individuals. In the absence of the necessary data, in order to currently estimate prevalence rates of IPV victimization occurring in the past year among older transgender populations, findings on older cisgender populations can be compared with transgender population size estimates. Research on predominantly cisgender samples indicates that past-year IPV victimization risk decreases with age. According to the aforementioned NISVS – the current gold standard in US nationally representative IPV studies – people aged 18 years old are at highest risk of experiencing rape, physical violence or stalking by an intimate partner in the past year (14.8% of women and 9.8% of men in that age group), followed by people aged 25–34 years old (8.7% of women and 8.6% of men in that age group). By comparison to every other age bracket, Americans aged 55 and up are at lowest risk of experiencing at least one of these forms of IPV in the past year (1.4% of women and 1.4% of men in that age group). Notably, while past-year IPV victimization rates are lowest for older individuals, numerically this still equates to a substantial group of survivors. According to weighted estimates using NISVS data, IPV survivors ages 55 and older (1.4% of the sample) represent approximately *1,053,000 Americans* [20].

No published reports have yet to show whether IPV victimization risk (whether past year or lifetime) differs between older transgender and older cisgender people in any nation. Research on samples comprised of people of all ages has also been inconclusive as to whether lifetime victimization risk differs for transgender and cisgender people, with studies drawing competing conclusions that transgender people are at higher, lower, and similar risk relative to cisgender people [4, 5, 21–23]. That said, if one were to begin with the assumption that older transgender and cisgender Americans aged 55 and up are at similar risk of past-year IPV victimization, this would mean that, drawing on NISVS data [20], approximately 1.4% of older transgender Americans experienced non-psychological IPV in the past year. Extrapolating from the best available estimates that 0.6% of Americans identify as transgender [24], this might suggest that 6300 transgender Americans aged 55 and older have experienced non-psychological IPV (i.e., intimate partner stalking, rape, or physical assault) in the past year alone. This figure likely underestimates the number of older transgender Americans to experience IPV in the past year, given that it is based on an analysis that excludes psychological IPV (the most prevalent form of IPV among all Americans according to NISVS) and excludes non-rape sexual IPV (which is more prevalent than intimate partner rape) such as sexual coercion, unwanted sexual contact, and being forced to penetrate the abuser [20].

5.2.2 Lifetime Victimization Prevalence

While a number of major studies have been completed that offer the needed data (e.g., US Transgender Survey; [11]), there are next to no publications reporting the lifetime prevalence of IPV victimization specifically among a sample or subsample of older transgender individuals. The sole exception found that, among a convenience sample of 44 transgender people aged 50 and older who answered a question regarding experiencing unwanted sexual touching, approximately 2% experienced unwanted sexual touching by an intimate partner [8]. Although an important first step, this study excluded most forms of sexual IPV, excluded all nonsexual forms of IPV, and used a smaller and less representative sample than ideal.

While data is sorely lacking on lifetime IPV victimization prevalence specifically for *older* transgender populations, such prevalence rates can be found with samples or subsamples of transgender individuals of *all* ages. In studies distinguishing IPV forms among adults, research has found that 57% of transgender people in their lifetimes experience psychological IPV [4], 35–46% physical IPV [4, 7, 11, 17, 25], and 8–47% sexual IPV [4, 7, 11, 17, 25]. A number of reports of T-IPV prevalence have also offered a single estimate representing the risk of experiencing at least one form of IPV (e.g., [11, 26, 27]). Of these, the previously detailed US Transgender Survey is by far the largest and most accurate study currently available, and analysis of this data concluded that 54% of transgender adults in the United States have experienced at least one form of IPV within their lifetimes [11].

Again, these estimates are based on samples of transgender people of all ages. Because these samples include younger transgender people who have lived fewer years in which IPV could have possibly occurred, the aforementioned lifetime rates almost certainly underestimate the prevalence of lifetime IPV victimization specifically for older transgender individuals.

5.2.3 Tactics

Transgender and cisgender people, as well as older and younger people, experience many similar tactics within each umbrella form of IPV. Psychological abuse often entails verbal insults and embarrassment, threats, monitoring and stalking behaviors, controlling finances, and leveraging children for control. Physical abuse can entail hitting, slapping, punching, pulling hair, burning, throwing objects, and so forth. Sexual abuse can involve nonconsensual sexual contact, threats of and completed rape, and so forth [5, 14, 28, 29].

At the same time, there are additional tactics unique to T-IPV and IPV among older individuals. Regarding unique T-IPV tactics, research indicates that 16–73% of transgender people have had an abuser who utilized a psychological IPV tactic that took advantage of the survivor being transgender [5, 17, 30, 31]. Among others, these unique psychological T-IPV tactics can include the following: threatening to "out" or make public a survivor's transgender identity; accusing a transgender survivor of not being a "real" man, woman, or transgender person; shaming a transgender survivor for being transgender; and restricting a transgender survivor's ability to live life as their identified gender, such as by hiding gendered clothing, controlling access to hormone medications, and refusing to use preferred pronouns and names [5, 17, 32–37]. Regarding physical IPV, some research suggests that T-IPV can also exhibit unique physical abuse tactics, including the use of physical violence against locations on the survivor's body that have symbolic, gendered meaning like breasts and genitals [5, 35]. Likewise, sexual T-IPV can entail unique tactics, such as non-consensually touching parts of a transgender survivor's body that have particularly gendered meaning like genitals and breasts or claiming that "real" women and men prefer rough sexual intercourse as a rationale for raping a transgender survivor [5, 35, 37, 38].

Older IPV survivors may also experience unique tactics. For instance, many older individuals experience increased isolation due to deaths within their social circles and due to their own medical challenges, isolation which abusers in turn may draw upon to reduce detection and to increase a survivor's reliance on the abuser [39, 40]. Financial reliance on abusers may also be exacerbated among older IPV survivors, who may be less able to gain financial independence through a new job due to age discrimination among employers and less recent work experience [40]. In addition, abusers may attempt to limit an older survivor's access to needed medical treatment [41]. It is likely that many of the factors that independently increase the IPV vulnerability of transgender individuals and older individuals are magnified particularly for older transgender people.

5.2.4 Impact

T-IPV can have a series of deleterious effects on survivors. Many T-IPV survivors are forced to miss school or work as a result of abuse (27% of T-IPV survivors; [17]), and many T-IPV survivors experience fear (10–13%; [7]), negative mental health consequences (76%; [17]), and physical injury (16–42%; [7, 17]). In addition, transgender women are more likely to have experienced IPV if they are HIV-positive [42]. Research on predominantly cisgender samples suggests that the cause-and-effect relationship of HIV-positive serostatus with IPV is not always immediately apparent. Whereas sometimes IPV can result in survivors becoming HIV-positive (such as when abusers refuse to use protection during sexual activities), in other instances some abusers may intentionally seek relationships with HIV-positive survivors if the abuser perceives such survivors to feel disempowered, reliant on others, and more easily controlled [5].

Likewise, studies on older IPV survivors have found recent negative mental health and medical health consequences to be associated with past-year IPV victimization [43]. Studies on the broader elder abuse literature, where perpetrators may or may not be intimate partners, suggest survivors may be at an increased risk of depression, fatigue, anxiety, confusion, and psychosomatic outcomes tied to trauma and stress such as ulcers [28].

5.3 Help-Seeking and Help-Giving

Successful interventions with older T-IPV survivors require first recognizing and overcoming the many barriers that too often prevent survivors from reaching help. In addition, once help is sought, survivors may face additional hurdles related to missing, discriminatory, non-tailored, or non-multifaceted help-giving resources. This section reviews these challenges pertaining to help-seeking by and help-giving for T-IPV survivors and older IPV survivors.

5.3.1 Challenges in Help-Seeking

Older T-IPV survivors face a series of challenges in seeking help, including (1) not recognizing IPV, (2) financial and emotional dependency on abusers, and (3) fear. While each of these barriers is not unique to T-IPV [5], they do take on added urgency in T-IPV relationships. First, regarding not recognizing IPV, 25% of T-IPV survivors do not self-identify as survivors of IPV [17]. As is common in IPV with other population types, abusers may blame survivors for angering the abuser and "causing" them to hurt their victims. This can hinder a survivor's ability to view themselves as victims, which in turn may make them feel less deserving of help [5]. For survivors of transgender abusers, abusers may use their transgender identity to portray themselves as incapable of being abusive because they are victims of a transphobic society. For instance, consider the story recounted by a cisgender female survivor about when she confronted her transgender male abuser, who deflected blame by saying, "This is not about you, it's about me. I'm transitioning, not you" ([44], p. 375). Of course, experiencing discrimination in society does not justify being abusive. As one representative of a T-IPV and sexual minority IPV service-providing organization aptly noted, "Frequently we hear batterers say, 'I have a disability so I can't batter,' 'I'm genderqueer so I can't batter,' 'I'm a person of color so I can't batter.' There is no identity that inherently bars people from being batterers" ([45], p. 109). That said, abusers who rationalize abuse and deflect blame onto survivors may make it more difficult for survivors to recognize IPV and, in turn, to seek help with their victimization.

Second, regarding dependency, research indicates that survivors may find leaving an abuser challenging when there exists financial or emotional dependency on abusers. Deciding whether to leave an abuser requires weighing many factors, including whether the survivor can survive financially should they leave. For T-IPV survivors in particular, many come to depend on abusers for financial support to pay for needed medications and treatments regarding gender transitions. Indeed, some abusers may threaten to or actually withdraw financial support specifically for medical interventions of survivors as a means through which to gain control [35]. Older IPV survivors may also be vulnerable to abuser's withdrawing financial support for needed medications related to aging, and older survivors may find financial dependence more difficult to break if they are retired and have not recently been in the job market [46]. Love and affection for abusers is another factor considered when weighing decisions of whether to leave. This emotional dependency can be magnified for T-IPV survivors who perceive their abusers as creating a rare safe space within a transphobic society [35, 47]. For older survivors who have been with their abusers for many years, survivors both may be hesitant to give up on such a long-term emotional investment and may fear that potential sources of help will shame them for not having sought help sooner [48]. Emotional attachment to older abusers with medical issues can also impact IPV survivors' decisions of whether to leave, if they fear that leaving will result in the abuser's medical health further deteriorating [49].

Third and lastly, fear can be a powerful motivator in deterring survivors from seeking help. Beyond the types of fear that are common across survivor population types – fear of harm to the survivor, fear of harm to one's family, and fear of abuser self-harm (see [5]) – T-IPV survivors may experience additional unique fears. Some transgender survivors may fear that seeking help will result in their identity being further stigmatized, just as some survivors of transgender abusers may fear that seeking help will result in their abuser being further stigmatized [5, 44]. As reported in one study, Maria, a sexual minority cisgender woman, feared that seeking help would bring greater discrimination upon her transgender abuser: "I can't tell [my family] the whole truth cause I'm busy convincing them that trans is okay [and that they don't need to be worried about me]. I needed them to understand and believe trans, and that was true of all of my friends, but especially my family because I knew they would think trans people were crazy if they heard that this person was treating me that way" ([44], 375). In addition, many survivors fear that their transgender identity will be outed by abusers, a credible concern given that 13% of transgender people report having had a partner out them [34, 36]. In a world that so often discriminates against transgender people, being outed could have substantial negative effects on survivors, ranging from family and community rejection to fear of an inability to rebuild one's life and to losing housing, jobs, and service at public accommodations (see [5]).

5.3.2 Challenges in Help-Giving

Survivor help-giving resources – such as police officers, IPV survivor agency staff and mental health service providers, and IPV survivor shelters – have the capacity to be invaluable in assisting survivors in coping with victimization, escaping from abuse, and seeking justice. At the same time, older T-IPV survivors often face a host of challenges when they do seek help, challenges pertaining to (1) being denied services, (2) being discriminated against when seeking services, (3) being unable to locate tailored services, and (4) needing a multipronged intervention.

First, many T-IPV survivors are denied services due to being transgender, currently or previously identifying as a man, or currently or previously being biological male. For instance, in the United States, the 2013 Violence Against Women Act (VAWA) Reauthorization barred outright exclusion of transgender people and men in shelters and IPV survivor agencies, but the Reauthorization did offer a key exception: if "sex segregation or sex-specific programming is necessary to the essential operation of a program" [50] and if such segregation is needed to "ensure the victim's health and safety" [51]. Thus, effectively shelters and IPV survivor agencies can deny services to T-IPV survivors for being transgender, for currently or previously identifying as a man, or for currently or previously being biologically male. This has resulted in unfortunate situations, such as when a transgender man is denied access to survivor services despite having identified as a woman at the time of the victimization [52]. While federal guidance restricts determinations about service eligibility to gender identity, not biological sex [51], some agencies may nonetheless ask humiliating screening questions of transgender women about their bodies as a means of determining if they are "real" women, such as when one IPV shelter staff member asked a T-IPV survivor, "What is between your legs?" ([53], 11). Research suggests that admission to IPV survivor shelters can be determined by whether a transgender survivor is deemed feminine enough, drawing on such irrelevant factors as the survivor's physical appearance, voice pitch, whether they have or have not had medical interventions, and whether their often difficult-to-change identity documents like birth certificates and driver's licenses reflect their current name and gender identity [52]. While older IPV survivors may not explicitly be barred from survivor services due to their age, generational differences in whether a marriage should persist even in the face of abuse have been shown to impact not only decision-making by older survivors but also whether help is offered by older peers [49]. In addition, some older IPV survivors report perceiving mainstream IPV survivor services as being unwelcoming due to largely advertising to, being designed for, and servicing younger populations [49].

Second, older T-IPV survivors often face discrimination when seeking help, an experience that not only takes a toll on survivors in and of itself but also may deter future help-seeking. For instance, Amnesty International [54] reports that some police officers have insisted on referring to transgender female IPV survivors as "mister" or have told them to "shut up, faggot" ([54], 84–87). It is perhaps owing to this lack of respect by some officers that one study found T-IPV survivors to be least likely to report to police relative to all other possible sources of help [27]. Transgender people have also reported being called "it" or "he-she" in open court [35]. Regarding IPV survivor shelters and agencies, one study found that 21% of T-IPV survivors had been harassed or disrespected while at such a shelter or agency [55]. Anecdotal evidence suggests that cisgender survivors at shelters may also be discriminatory with regard to T-IPV survivors, as was the case when one transgender survivor overheard another survivor saying she did not know what to tell her children regarding "*what* she [the transgender victim] was" (emphasis added; [52], 9). While not all survivors experience discriminatory responses, the reality that some do may be enough to deter certain survivors from seeking help. For instance, for older T-IPV survivors, seeking help may be coupled with concerns that doing so will result in being involuntarily placed in a nursing home, staffed with caregivers who some survivors fear will be largely transphobic [56]. In addition, IPV among older individuals in particular may be taken less seriously by some service providers, in part out of a perception that older individuals have greater agency and resources with which to deflect and evade abuse [57].

Third, even when IPV agencies, shelters, and other help-giving resources do welcome T-IPV survivors and are not overtly discriminatory, services are rarely tailored to the unique needs and nature of T-IPV. There is a growing use of nondiscrimination admission policies and gender-neutral language in service screening and advertising, which on the one hand may signal to transgender and sexual minority survivors that they are welcome to utilize services [5, 58, 59]. On the other hand, inclusion of transgender people does not necessarily mean the services themselves are tailored to the unique experiences of T-IPV survivors, that is, services may fail to account for unique T-IPV abusive tactics, unique challenges survivors face in seeking help from additional service-providing agencies, and the broader context of transphobia. For example, safety planning protocols at IPV agencies may not always account for the unique emergency bag needs of T-IPV survivors, such as hormone medications [60, 61]. Additionally, mental health service provision may not always directly address the role of transphobia in abuse (see [5]). Furthermore, court-mandated batterer intervention programs, designed to decrease the likelihood of recidivism for abusers, largely omit recognition of T-IPV in their rehabilitative treatments [62]. While a one-size-fits-all approach to service provision may on its surface appear to be nondiscriminatory and welcoming to all survivors of IPV, ultimately IPV is not a monolithic experience. Recognizing the unique ways different communities experience IPV – and infusing those differences into tailored services – may improve both community trust in help-giving resources and the effectiveness of those services.

Fourth and finally, many older T-IPV survivors may need multipronged interventions across multiple agencies, creating an additional barrier to receiving comprehensive assistance. Research hints that polyvictimization – and all the related service needs that entails – is a reality in many older transgender people's lives. For instance, according to the National Transgender Discrimination Survey, a study of 6450 transgender people in the United States, 78% of transgender people have experienced harassment in school, 35% physical assault, 12% sexual assault in school, 57% significant family rejection, and 41% attempted suicide. To place that final number in context, only 1.6% of the broader US population has attempted suicide [55]. According to another study of 2560 older lesbian, gay, bisexual, and transgender adults ages 50 to 95, among older transgender individuals (n = 174), 75.7% had been verbally harassed in their lifetimes, 53% physically threatened, and 26.6% physically assaulted, among other forms of victimization. All told, 91.1% reported experiencing some form of victimization in their lifetimes, and, notably, 77.5% had experienced at least three separate incidents of victimization [46]. Thus, comprehensive help-giving for T-IPV survivors necessitates screening for associated forms of victimization, as well as preparedness to offer referrals for transgender-inclusive service-providing agencies.

5.4 Discussion

Transgender persons experiencing IPV face serious obstacles, and these obstacles are exacerbated by aging. This chapter presented the challenges of researchers and practitioners in understanding the full extent and nature of elder T-IPV, the effects of elder T-IPV, and the barriers to seeking services. Of paramount concern is that there is extremely limited data not only on T-IPV but, in particular, T-IPV among older individuals. Despite this, it is staggering that research estimates that at least half of all transgender people experience some form of IPV in their lifetimes [11]. These high rates of victimization demand culturally responsive interventions targeted at prevention of and delivering services within transgender populations.

In addition, responses to T-IPV must include a careful examination of IPV tactics that are unique to transgender and aging communities. For instance, abusive partners may prevent access to medical interventions [11], such as hormone replacement therapy, or may use access to health insurance to control their partner's behavior [41]. Accessible healthcare within transgender communities may mitigate this tactic, especially for T-IPV survivors who do not have employer-based healthcare or are not yet old enough for Medicare. Moreover, accessible healthcare would increase access to treatment to address the effects of IPV on their physical and mental health. Finally, IPV tactics distinctive to elderly transgender persons, such as leveraging a survivor's limited access to social networks, are important in addressing T-IPV. T-IPV survivors may experience high rates of isolation from friends and family because of their gender identity and IPV victimization, and as they age this isolation may become increasingly severe, as their limited social network may be lost to personal medical complications and the deaths of peers and family members [39]. Elder T-IPV survivors may also be at an increased risk of financial abuse, as they frequently do not have the same economic opportunities that younger T-IPV survivors may have. In the end, many elder T-IPV survivors likely experience the tactics present in elder cisgender IPV *and* T-IPV. To effectively address the needs of elderly T-IPV survivors, more research is needed to create data-driven interventions that inform societal responses.

Several barriers prevent elderly T-IPV survivors from seeking help. Many elder T-IPV survivors may not recognize that they are experiencing IPV, and this may intensify with age and longevity of the relationship (see [5]). When elderly T-IPV survivors do decide to seek help, often social service agencies and IPV shelters are not adequately equipped to shelter elder transgender survivors and can even deny services to T-IPV survivors because of their gender identity [52]. In the event that a shelter can and will offer assistance, they frequently are not trained in working with or do not offer elder T-IPV culturally appropriate services. Turning toward law enforcement for help, as well, may not be a viable option for elder T-IPV survivors, as police historically have been a source of discrimination and, in some cases, humiliation for the transgender community [54]. Future efforts to improve help-seeking access and help-giving services for aging T-IPV must simultaneously address the unique needs of transgender survivors and older survivors. Particular attention should be paid toward continual anti-discrimination training for service providers, the creation of targeted advertising, and tailoring one-size-fits-all services to the unique nature of T-IPV among older individuals.

Finally, crucial to the response to T-IPV among older individuals is increasing not only the quantity but the quality of research centered on this population. Presently, serious methodological issues are present in the T-IPV field, which make it difficult to understand the full extent of the problem. Specifically, research varies in how T-IPV is defined and how to measure for T-IPV in the later stages of life. Other concerns include the timing of the abuse as it relates to the overall life course and the course of gender transitioning. Researchers must work with transgender communities to develop community-based research instruments designed to measure the nature and extent of elder T-IPV. Further, qualitative inquiry is desperately needed to paint a portrait of the lifetime histories of survivors, especially elderly T-IPV survivors. These investigations should disentangle IPV from other forms of interpersonal violence, describe abusers' tactics, and document the response and effects of the abuse. Importantly, this investigation into the components of T-IPV and elder T-IPV should include an intersectional examination of the differences and similarities in the experiences of T-IPV survivors and survivors based on race, ethnicity, class, gender, sexual orientation, ability, citizenship status, urbanicity, and nationality.

5.5 Summary

- It is difficult to determine the amount of elder T-IPV abuse because of a lack of research, but extrapolations from research about elder IPV and T-IPV indicate a serious social and public health problem.
- Survivors of elder T-IPV may experience unique tactics similar to elder cisgender survivors while also experiencing tactics present in T-IPV. Special consideration should be paid to how those combined identities create distinctive abusive tactics present in elder T-IPV, and direct responders should be trained in the identification of and response to elder T-IPV.
- Elder T-IPV survivors experience numerous barriers to seeking help from abuse. When they do seek help, they may be barred from services, face discrimination because of their gender identity and age, encounter ill-fitting services not tailored to their unique experiences, and receive services that fail to screen for and treat T-IPV covariates related to polyvictimization. Education about elder T-IPV is warranted for direct service responders, as is the development of culturally appropriate services.
- To understand elder T-IPV more fully, more research is needed, especially community-based research that works with the transgender community to create best practices regarding responses and interventions.

References

1. Colm TF. Freedom and strategy/trauma and resistance. In: Chen C, Dulani J, Piepzna-Samarasinha LL, editors. The revolution starts at home: confronting partner abuse in activist communities. Brooklyn: South End Press; 2011. p. 174–84.
2. Clements K, Katz M, Marx R. The transgender community health project: descriptive results. San Francisco: Department of Public Health; 1999.
3. Courvant, D., & Cook-Daniels, L. (1998). Trans and intersex survivors of domestic violence: defining terms, barriers, and responsibilities. SurvivorProject.org.

4. Turell SC. A descriptive analysis of same-sex relationship violence for a diverse sample. J Fam Violence. 2000;15(3):281–93.
5. Messinger AM. LGBTQ intimate partner violence: lessons for policy, practice, and research. Oakland: University of California Press; 2017.
6. Gates GJ. How many people are lesbian, gay, bisexual and transgender? Los Angeles: Williams Institute UCLA School of Law; 2011.
7. Pitts M, Smith A, Mitchell A, Patel S. Private lives: a report on the health and wellbeing of GLBTI Australians. Melbourne: Australian Research Centre in Sex, Health and Society, La Trobe University; 2006.
8. Cook-Daniels L, Munson M. Sexual violence, elder abuse, and sexuality of transgender adults, age 50+: results of three surveys. J GLBT Fam Stud. 2010;6(2):142–77.
9. Desmarais SL, Reeves KA. Gray, black, and blue: the state of research and intervention for intimate partner abuse among elders. Behav Sci Law. 2007;25(3):377–91.
10. Roberto KA, McPherson MC, Brossoie N. Intimate partner violence in late life: a review of the empirical literature. Violence Against Women. 2013;19(12):1538–58.
11. James SE, Herman JL, Rankin S, Keisling M, Mottet L, Anafi MA. The report of the 2015 US transgender survey. Washington, DC: National Center for Transgender Equality; 2016.
12. Black MC, Basile KC, Breiding MJ, Smith SG, Walters ML, Merrick MT, Chen J, Stevens MR. The National Intimate Partner and sexual violence survey (NISVS): 2010 summary report. Atlanta: National Center for Injury Prevention and Control, Centers for Disease Control and Prevention; 2011.
13. Cannon C. A survey of domestic violence perpetrator programs in the United States and Canada: findings and implications for policy and intervention. Partner abuse. 2016;7(3):226–76.
14. Brandl B, Horan DL. Domestic violence in later life: an overview for health care providers. Women Health. 2002;35(2–3):41–54.
15. Straus MA. Measuring intrafamily conflict and violence: the conflict tactics (CT) scales. J Marriage Fam. 1979;41:75–88.
16. Straus MA, Hamby SL, Boney-McCoy S, Sugarman DB. The revised conflict tactics scales (CTS2) development and preliminary psychometric data. J Fam Issues. 1996;17(3): 283–316.
17. Roch A, Morton J, Ritchie G. Out of sight, out of mind? Transgender people's experiences of domestic abuse: LGBT Youth Scotland and The Scottish Transgender Alliance; 2010.
18. Moradi B, Mohr JJ, Worthington RL, Fassinger RE. Counseling psychology research on sexual (orientation) minority issues: conceptual and methodological challenges and opportunities. J Couns Psychol. 2009;56(1):5–22.
19. Wallace PH, Roberson C. Family violence: legal, medical, and social perspectives. New York: Routledge; 2016.
20. Breiding MJ, Chen J, Black MC. Intimate partner violence in the United States — 2010. Atlanta: National Center for Injury Prevention and Control, Centers for Disease Control and Prevention; 2014.
21. Dank M, Lachman P, Zweig JM, Yahner J. Dating violence experiences of lesbian, gay, bisexual, and transgender youth. J Youth Adolesc. 2014;43(5):846–57.
22. Landers SJ, Gilsanz P. The health of lesbian, gay, bisexual and transgender (LGBT) persons in Massachusetts: a survey of health issues comparing LGBT persons with their heterosexual and non-transgender counterparts: Commonwealth of Massachusetts, Dept. of Public Health; 2009.
23. Zweig JM, Dank M, Lachman P, Yahner J. Technology, teen dating violence and abuse, and bullying. Washington, DC: Urban Institute; 2013.
24. Flores AR, Herman JL, Gates GJ, Brown T. How many adults identify as transgender in the United States? Los Angeles: Williams Institute UCLA School of Law; 2016.
25. Nemoto T, Bödeker B, Iwamoto M. Social support, exposure to violence and transphobia, and correlates of depression among male-to-female transgender women with a history of sex work. Am J Public Health. 2011;101(10):1980–8.

26. Keuroghlian AS, Reisner SL, White JM, Weiss RD. Substance use and treatment of substance use disorders in a community sample of transgender adults. Drug Alcohol Depend. 2015;152:139–46.
27. Langenderfer-Magruder L, Whitfield DL, Walls NE, Kattari SK, Ramos D. Experiences of intimate partner violence and subsequent police reporting among lesbian, gay, bisexual, transgender, and queer adults in Colorado: comparing rates of cisgender and transgender victimization. J Interpers Violence. 2016;31(5):855–71.
28. Hightower J, Smith MJ, Hightower HC. Hearing the voices of abused older women. J Gerontol Soc Work. 2006;46(3–4):205–27.
29. Seff LR, Beaulaurier RL, Newman FL. Nonphysical abuse: findings in domestic violence against older women study. J Emot Abus. 2008;8(3):355–74.
30. National Coalition of Anti-Violence Programs (NCAVP). Lesbian, gay, bisexual, transgender, queer and HIV-affected intimate partner violence in 2013. New York: Author; 2014.
31. Scottish Transgender Alliance. Transgender experiences in Scotland: research summary. Equality Network. 2008. [Retrieved from www.scottishtrans.org/wp-content/uploads/2013/03/staexperiencessummary03082.pdf].
32. Bornstein DR, Fawcett J, Sullivan M, Senturia KD, Shiu-Thornton S. Understanding the experiences of lesbian, bisexual and trans survivors of domestic violence: a qualitative study. J Homosex. 2006;51(1):159–81.
33. Cook-Daniels L. Intimate partner violence in transgender couples: "power and control" in a specific cultural context. Partner Abuse. 2015;6(1):126–39.
34. Farrell J, Cerise S. Fairs fair: a snapshot of violence and abuse in Sydney LGBT relationships. Sydney: AIDS Council of NSW and the Same Sex Domestic Violence Interagency and Working Group; 2006.
35. Goodmark L. Transgender people, intimate partner abuse, and the legal system. Harv CR-CLL Rev. 2013;48:51–104.
36. Mak WW, Chong ESK, Kwong MMF. Prevalence of same-sex intimate partner violence in Hong Kong. Public Health. 2010;124(3):149–52.
37. Tesch BP, Bekerian DA. Hidden in the margins: a qualitative examination of what professionals in the domestic violence field know about transgender domestic violence. J Gay Lesbian Soc Serv. 2015;27(4):391–411.
38. FORGE. Safety planning with transgender clients FAQ. Author. 2013a. [Retrieved from http://forge-forward.org/wp-content/docs/FAQ-01–2013-safety-planning.pdf].
39. Reeves KA, Desmarais SL, Nicholls TL, Douglas KS. Intimate partner abuse of older men: considerations for the assessment of risk. J Elder Abuse Negl. 2007;19(1–2):7–27.
40. Straka SM, Montminy L. Responding to the needs of older women experiencing domestic violence. Violence Against Women. 2006;12(3):251–67.
41. Sawin EM, Parker B. "If looks would kill then I would be dead": intimate partner abuse and breast cancer in older women. J Gerontol Nurs. 2011;37(7):26–35.
42. Brennan J, Kuhns LM, Johnson AK, Belzer M, Wilson EC, Garofalo R, Adolescent Medicine Trials Network for HIV/AIDS Interventions. Syndemic theory and HIV-related risk among young transgender women: the role of multiple, co-occurring health problems and social marginalization. Am J Public Health. 2012;102(9):1751–7.
43. Mouton CP. Intimate partner violence and health status among older women. Violence Against Women. 2003;9(12):1465–77.
44. Brown N. Stories from outside the frame: intimate partner abuse in sexual-minority women's relationships with transsexual men. Feminism & Psychology. 2007;17(3):373–93.
45. Perez-Darby S. The secret joy of accountability: self-accountability as a building block for change. In: Chen C, Dulani J, Piepzna-Samarasinha LL, editors. The revolution starts at home: confronting partner abuse in activist communities. Brooklyn: South End Press; 2011. p. 100–13.
46. Fredriksen-Goldsen KI, Kim H-J, Emlet CA, Muraco A, Erosheva EA, Hoy-Ellis CP, Goldsen J, Petry H. The aging and health report: disparities and resilience among lesbian, gay, bisexual, and transgender older adults. Seattle: Institute for Multigenerational Health; 2011.

47. Singh AA, McKleroy VS. "Just getting out of bed is a revolutionary act" the resilience of transgender people of color who have survived traumatic life events. Traumatology. 2011;17(2):34–44.
48. Leisey M, Kupstas PK, Cooper A. Domestic violence in the second half of life. J Elder Abuse Negl. 2009;21(2):141–55.
49. Zink T, Regan S, Jacobson CJ Jr, Pabst S. Cohort, period, and aging effects: A qualitative study of older women's reasons for remaining in abusive relationships. *Violence against women.* 2003;*9*(12):1429–41.
50. U.S. Government Printing Office. 113th congress public law 4: violence against women act reauthorization of 2013. Author. 2013. [Retrieved from https://www.gpo.gov/fdsys/pkg/PLAW-113publ4/html/PLAW-113publ4.htm].
51. U.S. Department of Justice. Frequently asked questions: nondiscrimination grant condition in the violence against women reauthorization act of 2013. Author. 2014. [Retrieved from https://www.justice.gov/sites/default/files/ovw/legacy/2014/06/20/faqs-ngc-vawa.pdf].
52. Quinn ME. Open minds open doors: transforming domestic violence programs to include LGBTQ survivors. Boston: The Network/La Red; 2010. [Retrieved from www.ncdsv.org/images/TheNetworkLaRed_OpenMindsOpenDoors_2010.pdf].
53. GLBT Domestic Violence Coalition and Jane Doe Inc. Shelter/housing needs for gay, lesbian, bisexual and transgender (GLBT) victims of domestic violence. 2005. [Retrieved from www.ncdsv.org/images/shelterhousingneedsforglbtvictimsdv.pdf].
54. Amnesty International. Stonewalled: police abuse and misconduct against lesbian, gay, bisexual and transgender people in the US. New York: Author; 2005.
55. Grant JM, Mottet L, Tanis JE, Harrison J, Herman J, Keisling M. Injustice at every turn: a report of the National Transgender Discrimination Survey. National Center for Transgender Equality; 2011.
56. Cook-Daniels L. Coping with abuse inside the family and out: LGBT and/or male victims of elder abuse. In: Elder abuse. New York: Springer International Publishing; 2017. p. 541–53.
57. Brossoie N, Roberto KA. Community professionals' response to intimate partner violence against rural older women. J Elder Abuse Negl. 2015;27(4–5):470–88.
58. Hines DA, Douglas EM. The reported availability of US domestic violence services to victims who vary by age, sexual orientation, and gender. Partner Abuse. 2011;2(1):3–30.
59. Renzetti C. The poverty of services for battered lesbians. J Gay Lesbian Soc Serv. 1996;4(1):61–8.
60. Farley N. Same-sex domestic violence: establishing a safety plan with victims. In: Whitman JS, Boyd CJ, editors. The Therapist's notebook for lesbian, gay, and bisexual clients: homework, handouts, and activities for use in psychotherapy. London: Routledge; 2013. p. 229–33.
61. FORGE. Trans-specific power and control tactics. Author. 2013b. [Retrieved from http://forge-forward.org/wp-content/docs/power-control-tactics-categories_FINAL.pdf].
62. Austin JB, Dankwort J. Standards for batterer programs: a review and analysis. J Interpers Violence. 1999;14(2):152–68.

Recommended Reading

James SE, Herman JL, Rankin S, Keisling M, Mottet L, Anafi MA. The report of the 2015 US transgender survey. Washington, DC: National Center for Transgender Equality; 2016.

Messinger AM. LGBTQ intimate partner violence: lessons for policy, practice, and research. Oakland: University of California Press; 2017.

Zink T, Regan S, Jacobson CJ Jr, Pabst S. Cohort, period, and aging effects: a qualitative study of older women's reasons for remaining in abusive relationships. Violence Against Women. 2003;9(12):1429–41.

Substance Use and Recovery in the Transgender and Gender Nonconforming (TGNC) Older Adult Community

6

Stacy Agosto, Kristin Reitz, Kelly Ducheny, and Tatyana Moaton

While a variety of factors can influence the course of a person's substance use, TGNC older adults face unique stressors that can intensify and deepen their reliance on substances as a coping method. TGNC older adults' substance use can be impacted by a lifetime of minority stress, stigma, and discrimination. The impact of substance use is often pervasive, with both short-term and long-term effects that can touch nearly every aspect of an individual's life: physical health, mental health, social support, relationships, financial, and employment stability [8, 9]. Consider these case vignettes as illustrations of the different ways that problematic substance use and gender identity can influence one another. Names and identifying information have been changed.

> "Shanice" is a 60-year-old transgender woman who came out when she was 18. Shanice dealt with painful transphobia and rejection from her family of origin, triggering decades of substance use as a way to cope with ongoing discrimination, harassment, and stigma. As she neared the age of 40, she stopped her use and had several years in which she was abstinent from all substances. As she got older, chronic pain emerged from previous gender affirmation procedures (silicone implants), and she began to take prescribed opiates, increasing the dosage and frequency as both her pain level and tolerance increased. She began to combine alcohol with her pain medication to self-medicate this chronic pain.

S. Agosto · K. Reitz · K. Ducheny (✉)
Behavioral Health Services, Howard Brown Health Center, Chicago, IL, USA
e-mail: stacya@howardbrown.org; kristinr@howardbrown.org; kellyd@howardbrown.org

T. Moaton
Human Resources, Howard Brown Health Center, Chicago, IL, USA
e-mail: tatyanam@howardbrown.org

M. Houlberg et al. (eds.), *Transgender and Gender Nonconforming Health and Aging*,
https://doi.org/10.1007/978-3-319-95031-0_6

"Thomas" is a 72-year-old transgender man who became aware of his transgender identity as he entered adulthood. At that time, he was married to a man and had just had two children, so coming out seemed impossible. He used alcohol to cope with the pain of hiding his transgender identity. Over time, he began to take steps toward coming out, such as presenting as more masculine by wearing certain clothes and binding his chest. When a stressor would occur that could threaten his process of coming out (marital conflict or a fight with his children), he would turn to the familiar pattern of binge drinking. During an episode of binge drinking, Thomas would throw away his clothes, destroy his binder, and attempt to destroy all of the steps he had taken toward coming out. Afterward, he would experience deep regret and loss and begin to build toward coming out again; this cycle continued for years.

"Rita" is a 75-year-old transgender woman who came out when she turned 65. Rita was aware of her TGNC identity when she was a young child but grew up in a time where coming out was not safe and did not feel feasible. She used various substances throughout her life as a way of numbing and escaping the emotional pain of remaining closeted. As she reached her 60s, Rita began to experiment with periods of sobriety and began to take steps toward coming out. As acceptance in mainstream society for the TGNC and LGBTQ communities grew, coming out seemed more possible. As she became more confident and comfortable in her gender identity, sobriety also seemed more possible.

In 2011, Baby Boomers began turning 65, creating the first generation to openly live as LGBTQ individuals in large numbers [3]. Obtaining accurate statistical data on those self-identifying as LGBTQ and particularly as TGNC (at any age) has historically been difficult, creating a current dearth of research on TGNC older adults. Prior generations of TGNC older adults may have been small in number and may not have been "out" in large enough numbers to be studied. Challenges associated with TGNC data collection include a lack of consistent data, comparable data, and standard/comparable definitions related to sexual orientation and gender identity (SOGI) and small study sample sizes. For the limited research that is available on TGNC older adults, very little of this data has examined rates and types of substance use.

According to SAMHSA [1], alcohol and substance abuse has been cited as a "major concern among transgender people in the United States." In their guide for healthcare providers on the top health issues facing LGBTQ people, SAMHSA states that the most common drugs used by transgender people are marijuana, crack cocaine, and alcohol. SAMHSA also cites some evidence to suggest high rates of methamphetamine and injection drug use. However, most of the studies referenced included samples of transgender people of color under the age of 50 [1].

In their study of LGBTQ older adults, Fredriksen-Goldsen et al. [10] suggest that general substance use declines as LGBTQ older adults age. People aged 80 and over used less than those aged 65–79, who in turn used less than those aged 50–64. While it is encouraging that substance use may decline as LGBTQ and TGNC individuals age, there is still significant concern about the effects of problematic substance use at any age.

A lack of ongoing, scalable, and comparable data relating specifically to the substance use behaviors of TGNC older adults exists; however, several studies have provided insight into the behaviors of related populations and similar age groups. Zelle and Arms [3] stated that, in general, LGBTQ older adults face multiple health disparities, including higher rates of substance abuse compared to heterosexual older adults. One study by Gonzalez et al. [11] provided a significant amount of insight into the substance use behaviors of samples of both transgender men and women, shedding light on the characteristics and circumstances that contribute to substance use in transgender people. The sample of 1210 transgender individuals was mainly composed of white transgender women under the age of 50, but it did include a significant number of transgender people over 50 (10% of the sample). Forty percent of the total participants endorsed either excessive alcohol use, cannabis, or illicit drug use at some point in the 3 months prior to the study.

For transgender women in the Gonzalez et al. [11] study, having completed a lower level of education and reporting gender dysphoria were associated with excessive alcohol use. Transgender women of younger age and lower annual income showed increased odds of marijuana use. For these transgender women having a nonheterosexual orientation, living full time in the affirmed gender and increased internalized stigma were all associated with increased marijuana use. Transgender women who identified as white, lesbian, gay, pansexual, or queer also had increased use of illicit drugs. Transgender men were found to have significantly higher rates of marijuana and illicit drug use than transgender women overall. For transgender men, higher rates of internalized stigma were associated with an increased likelihood of excessive alcohol use, with a nonheterosexual orientation being the main factor associated with increased illicit drug. For transgender men, being partnered, being of younger age, and having a sexual orientation of pansexual or queer were all associated with increased marijuana use [11].

Arayasirikul et al. [12] studied the relationship between sexual orientation and alcohol and drug use in a racially diverse sample of transgender women aged 16–24 living in the San Francisco Bay area. While this study exclusively included a sample of youth, the results may help to inform substance use patterns in the TGNC community. The study found that overall, more than half of the participants reported at least one episode of heavy drinking (consuming five or more drinks in one episode) in the last 6 months. Additionally, 13.5% of participants reported methamphetamine use, 16.6% of participants reported any crack cocaine use, and 20.8% reported any illicit prescription drug use. As in the Gonzalez et al. [11] study, a higher proportion of transgender women self-identifying as gay/lesbian, bisexual, pansexual, or queer reported heavy drinking compared with heterosexual transgender women (61.3% vs 40.7%), and transgender women identifying as other than heterosexual were more likely to report illicit prescription drug use compared with heterosexual transgender women (28% vs 7.7%).

Benotsch et al. [13] found similar rates of illicit prescription drug abuse as were found in the Arayasirikul et al. [12] study. In interviews of 155 transgender, mainly younger African-American participants, Benotsch et al. [13] found that 26.5% of the sample reported nonmedical use of prescription drugs, with analgesics being the most commonly abused drug. This was followed by anxiolytics, stimulants, and sedatives. Nonmedical use of hormones was also common in the sample [13].

There are a number of factors that contribute to substance use that present unique challenges for TGNC older adults. Though there is little research specifically geared toward problematic substance use of TGNC older adults, factors of isolation, stigma and discrimination, minority stress, regret, physical health, lack of affirmative care and chronic pain, and violence appear to play important roles. Where gaps in research exist, the authors' clinical experience has been drawn upon to discuss factors that may impact or contribute to substance use in TGNC older adults and treatment approaches that can support TGNC older adults in their recovery.

It is important to acknowledge that while some TGNC older adults may use substances as a coping tool, it cannot be assumed that every TGNC older adult will or will develop patterns of problematic use. In addition, some TGNC older adults may experience problematic substance use because of circumstances or stressful events unrelated to their gender identity. For example, substance use patterns may have emerged as a youth after the death of a parent or from an unrelated medical procedure, such as a hip replacement or injury.

6.1 Isolation

Substance use among older TGNC individuals can result in the loss of support networks, isolating the individual from their chosen family, family of origin, colleagues, friends, and health-care system supports. For TGNC older adults actively engaged in problematic substance use, the impact on one's social network and support system can be pervasive. Isolation from typical support networks can result in increased worry for TGNC elders about how they will be supported as they age and need more day-to-day support. Rejection by families of origin, spouses or partners, children, and friend and professional networks can intensify isolation and loneliness [4]. This loss is additive, intensifying the interpersonal loss of networks as people age. Isolation and loss of social networks through death or identity disclosure can increase the loneliness of TGNC older adults which can, in turn, lead to higher rates of substance use [4, 14]. TGNC older adults may also experience survivor guilt after losing many TGNC loved ones and peers to community violence, suicide, and early death. TGNC older adults may also experience added feelings of isolation and invisibility within the LGBTQ community. This experience of isolation within the LGBTQ community can be intensified by the community's focus on youth and body image, the lack of opportunity to meet and communicate with other TGNC older adults, and potential judgment of non-binary identities, especially within older adult cohorts that grew up in time periods that may have reinforced more rigid gender roles.

This experience of ongoing and cumulative personal and social loss can weigh heavily on individuals, taxing the coping skills of TGNC older adults and resulting in a higher reliance on substances to numb or distance emotional pain. Active problematic substance use can also become the primary focus in a person's life [9], which can reinforce isolative patterns. This can result in individuals going to great lengths to protect their use, sometimes pushing away their supports in the process. Since substance use is often shrouded in secrecy, it may also fuel isolation and separateness, creating a barrier to living openly or in community with others. Substance use can also intensify and increase as TGNC older adults experience loss at a more rapid rate which, while common for those in their age group, can have particularly challenging impacts for TGNC elders. Conversely, while substance use can have a profound impact on isolation, deepening loneliness can also increase substance use [15]. Substance use can often intensify as individuals experience compounding losses, isolation, and rejection. For example, consider a 68-year-old transgender woman who has recently come out to her family. Her family has not accepted her identity but they continue to have some contact. A family member dies, and she is asked not to come to the funeral as other members of the extended family and community do not know about her transition. This rejection and isolation fuels a period of particularly heavy binge drinking as a way of escaping and numbing the painful emotions that emerge.

Patterns of connection can also influence the role of substance use in a TGNC elder's life, as has been shown for other groups [16]. For example, if a TGNC older adult had historically found safety and connection in bars and bath houses where substance use was prevalent, substance use may be intricately interwoven into how that person creates relationships and finds intimacy, sexual satisfaction, and comfort. It can take intentional effort to disrupt those old patterns and find new and meaningful ways to create connection without the presence of substances.

6.2 Stigma and Discrimination

Research has consistently shown that TGNC people experience intense and pervasive discrimination and stigma in every area of their lives [7]. While new generations are experiencing increased visibility and support, TGNC older adults have weathered decades of oppression, discrimination, loss, mistreatment, and abuse. The decades these older adults have survived contained extreme forms of discrimination including hate speech and action, murder, targeted abuse, invisibility, and denial of housing and employment [7]. The impact of long-term, chronic exposure to trauma, threat, oppression, and stigma [17] can contribute to higher rates of substance use and poorer health outcomes [2] for TGNC older adults. Substance use emerges as a long-term coping strategy to manage stigma and discrimination [5, 6], deepening across time as physical dependence builds and when other coping skills fail to develop.

Having to cope with and navigate persistent stigma, discrimination, and rejection can have a significant impact on overall mental health and can contribute to an elevated risk for depression and suicide among TGNC individuals [14], particularly for TGNC people who have accumulated additive or chronic trauma [17] across their lifespan. In a survey by James et al. [7], TGNC older adults (age 65 and older) experienced rates of serious psychological distress that were four times higher than that same age group in the general US population. The survey also found that 82% "of all respondents had seriously thought about killing themselves at some point in their lives" ([7], p. 114) and that 40% had attempted suicide at some point in their lives, compared with 4.6% of the general US population [7]. Problematic substance use presents an additional layer of risk for suicide [18], with substance use increasing suicidal risk [19] and depression potentially increasing substance use [20].

The presence of such stigma and discrimination can contribute to the utilization of substance use as a coping skill to help manage persistent stressors and mistreatment [21, 22]. Over time and with repetition, substance use can emerge as a TGNC individual's primary coping skill. However, substance use as a coping skill is imperfect, as it can exacerbate the very stressors the person is trying to escape from. Prolonged use is never as effective as the initial use. The feelings that people experience when they use substances, especially in the earlier stages of their use, can be perceived as desirable and helpful in numbing and detaching from emotional distress. With continued use, tolerance increases, and the need to use more, or use in riskier ways, increases as people seek to achieve the same level of intoxication and relief [9, 23]. Coping then becomes more challenging as substance use becomes less effective.

6.3 Minority Stress

Exposure to minority stress can create feelings of resignation, anxiety, and hypervigilance to avoid injury [24, 25]. TGNC people experience chronically high, persistent levels of minority stress [6]. Minority stress is additive [26] and is developed through long-term exposure to discrimination, prejudice, and exclusion that increases the likelihood of psychological distress, physical health problems [24], and use of substances [27]. The cumulative effects of this chronic exposure can also increase a TGNC person's internalized transphobia and feelings of shame, fear, and doubt [6]. The continual experience of discrimination creates an expectation of rejection, with TGNC people developing coping techniques to avoid or manage the anticipated distress of being treated disrespectfully. TGNC people may use substances to preemptively numb themselves to be less impacted by the discrimination or disrespectful treatment they know they will face or to manage mood and distress after it occurs [28]. One recent study exploring TGNC people's experience of expecting rejection reported that over half of participants (17 out of 30) identified the use of drugs and alcohol as a coping strategy to manage the rejection and poor treatment they anticipated [25]. Minority stress is compounded for TGNC people of color given the presence of a second visible minority identity [25, 29].

6.4 Regret

Regret can play an important part in the creation and maintenance of disruptive patterns of substance use. Regret can stem from a lack of affirmative care and support in youth, middle adulthood, and older adulthood. TGNC elders can live with sharp and pervasive regret that surfaces in waves as life events trigger previous trauma and lack of access to affirmative resources, care, and support [30–32]. Just as regret about the negative consequences of use can occur for anyone [33], regret can also surface as long-term substance use alters a TGNC older adult's body and health, potentially interrupting affirmative care.

TGNC elders can describe waves of regret and loss that accompany positive events and transition points in their lives. For example, a TGNC elder client who succeeded in having her gender marker changed on her driver's license at 67 years old described feelings of happiness and accomplishment mixed with regret and loss when thoughts of what her life could have been like had she been able to live her authentic life at a younger age surfaced.

6.5 Physical Health

The potential health implications from substance use are numerous and significant. Those who engage in problematic substance use are at risk for changes in appetite, heart rate, or blood pressure as well as heart attack and stroke in the short term [8] and liver damage. Among the various long-term medical risks are heart or lung disease, HIV, cancer, and hepatitis [8]. Like other older adults, TGNC older adults may be managing one or more chronic health conditions as they age, such as diabetes or high blood pressure [34]. Many such chronic conditions require consistent medical care and medication adherence for optimal health.

The presence of problematic substance use can complicate the management of these conditions [35]. Research has been done with regard to HIV treatment in particular, which indicated that substance use is associated with less adherence to HAART medication [36], which can have a significant impact on physical health. Additional research indicates that problematic substance use can also impact various other aspects of HIV treatment, including access to routine lab care/monitoring, initial engagement in care and continued consistency in engagement, and medication adherence [37]. Although this research specifically addressed HIV treatment, problematic substance use may also potentially impact engagement in the treatment of other chronic medical conditions as well.

The CDC has found in recent years that adults aged 50 and over have experienced an increase in HIV infection rates [38] with that trend expected to continue [39]. Dragon et al.'s [34] research with older adult Medicare beneficiaries showed TGNC people were more likely to be living with HIV than their cisgender peers (11% and 0.4%, respectively). Research from Grant et al. [21] shows that TGNC adults experienced HIV infection at a rate of four times the national average. Though a research gap exists related to the HIV infection rates of TGNC older adults, there has been some research done with other members of the LGBTQ community in relation to older adults, risky sexual behavior, and substance use. Heath et al. [40] found that, for older men who have sex with men (MSM), the "likelihood of engaging in risky sexual activities increases with the use of alcohol and other drugs" (Heath 2012, p. 11). Though the Aging and Health Report indicated that TGNC older adults are less likely to have HIV [41], we can surmise that problematic substance use can put TGNC older adults at risk for engaging in risky sexual behaviors, which can increase risk for HIV and other sexually transmitted infections (STI).

6.6 Lack of TGNC Affirmative Care and Chronic Pain

Transphobia and lack of affirmative care in medical and substance use care settings lead to delayed care [42]. Institutional barriers in care can reduce the likelihood that a TGNC elder would approach a care system [4, 43] to access detoxification service, inpatient/residential care, or sober living housing [2]. This delay in accessing care could, in turn, extend substance use and abuse patterns, increasing the likelihood that TGNC people would avoid accessing care to reduce use or attain sobriety.

In addition to chronic illnesses and injuries that are more frequent as people age, TGNC elders may also be managing chronic pain resulting from gender affirmation surgeries completed decades ago and the long-term health impact of other body modifications (i.e., silicon pumping, breast, or other implants) [44, 45]. While surgeries and procedures have dramatically improved in the United States, the gender-affirming surgeries available to older TGNC adults in the 1960s–2000s may have required more surgical repairs and resulted in poorer outcomes as techniques progressed.

In addition, few TGNC older adults have had consistent access to high-quality affirmative care as they aged, with individuals frequently receiving hormones and silicone pumping outside of regulated and licensed healthcare settings. Additionally, some body modifications destabilize across time, with silicone or cement drifting to other parts of the body, causing ongoing and chronic pain [44, 45]. Chronic pain as a result of these surgeries and procedures could result in opioid misuse. Given the opioid epidemic and the intensely dangerous synthetic opioids that are now available [46], TGNC older adults may be at a high risk of opioid misuse and overdose, as studies have shown that older age and nonmedical use of opioids are linked [47].

The presence of problematic substance use can also impact an individual's ability to meaningfully engage in other interventions, not just engagement in medical care. Interventions such as supportive housing, HIV prevention and/or linkage to care, and case management can all be impacted by active, uncontrolled substance use. For example, a 70-year-old gender-nonconforming person might be living in a senior housing facility with access to case management to support their medical needs. If they are binge drinking heavily, this likely contributes to missing appointments with their case manager, which can put their housing in jeopardy.

6.7 Violence

Studies have shown that TGNC adults face high levels of violence and harassment [48, 49]. In one particular study, it was found that "transgender older adults report significantly higher rates of victimization than non-transgender, regardless of age, income, or education" ([41], p 20). Victimization in this particular study was defined in a spectrum containing verbal assault, threats of violence, property damage, and physical assault [41]. The James et al. [7] study found that "nearly half (48%) of respondents reported that they were denied equal treatment or service, verbally harassed, and/or physically attacked because of being transgender in the last year" ([7], p 199). This same survey also found that "58% of respondents who interacted with a law enforcement officer who thought or knew that they were transgender were verbally harassed, physically or sexually assaulted, or mistreated in another way in the past year" ([7], p 187). TGNC people of color experience such harassment, mistreatment, and violence at even higher rates [7, 21].

Conversely, there is also research that demonstrates that older LGBTQ adults generally report less lifetime victimization and discrimination [10]; this must be examined with the appropriate societal context. For older adults, "concealing their sexual and gender identities seems to have been protective and in fact may have resulted in lower rates of lifetime victimization and discrimination, a function of the realities of the historical time" ([10], pg 11). Although this research was not done directly with the TGNC older adult population, it is possible that some TGNC older adults who have not revealed their identities may experience a similar dynamic.

TGNC adults may face a greater risk of intimate partner violence than those in the greater US adult population, although research has shown inconsistent results (Messinger & Roark, this book). The James et al. [7] study found that the rates of experiencing intimate partner violence within the TGNC community were somewhat increased from the general US adult population, with 35% of TGNC adults experiencing intimate partner violence compared to 30% in the general US adult population (James et al. 2016, p 198) [7]. The Aging and Health report found that TGNC older adults reported "significantly higher rates of verbal and physical abuse than non-transgender older adults" [41]. The presence of substance use may complicate the dynamic of intimate partner violence even further. A recent study of MSM individuals found that those experiencing intimate partner violence are also more likely to engage in substance use [50]. This study did not engage TGNC or older adults specifically, and additional research is needed to determine if TGNC older adults in abusive relationships are more likely to use substances.

Whether experiencing societal violence and harassment or intimate partner violence, substance use can emerge as a coping skill. Testa et al. [51] found that a history of experiencing sexual violence was associated with alcohol abuse in transgender women and men, with transgender women experiencing sexual violence also more likely to report illicit drug use. Experiencing psychological or physical abuse or violence as a result of a TGNC identity has been associated with "higher odds of alcohol, marijuana, or cocaine use, as well as an eight-times higher odds of any drug use, among transgender women" ([52], p 2203). Though this particular study only examined the experience of transgender women, it is possible that TGNC adults in general, including TGNC older adults, may have increased rates of substance use in response to experiencing persistent psychological or physical abuse and violence. Additional research is necessary to explore this relationship.

6.8 Protective Factors and Resilience

While some data and research evaluation is available that describes substance use patterns in TGNC older adult populations, few sources have investigated protective factors that support a TGNC elder to moderate substance use or reduce the likelihood of developing patterns of abuse or dependence. While facing a broad range of challenges in navigating cisgender-focused systems and societal stigma, TGNC older adults embody a tremendous resilience [4, 31, 32] and tenacity that can support coping skill development, survival [4], and recovery. By their endurance across decades of discrimination, TGNC older adults have demonstrated strength in the face of adversity, creativity, and innovation in meeting their individual health needs and protecting their community. They have adapted to dramatic societal changes

[30] and navigated oppressive systems to access resources and create chosen families and communities.

Resiliency can take many forms. A 2011 study identified several resiliency themes including a self-defined identity, an embrace of self-worth, supportive community connection, hopefulness for the future, and an awareness of the existence and impact of societal oppression [53]. The ability of TGNC older adults to serve as a role model for others, to mentor others in the community, and to evolve and improve society through activism and advocacy can fuel resilience and meaning [4, 53, 54].

Mobilizing that resilience as a tool in substance use treatment is pivotal. It is important to understand how substance use may have been a critical part of a TGNC older adult's survival infrastructure, acknowledging and valuing its role while reassessing its current utility as a healthy and productive coping tool. Peer-based support from others in the TGNC community can buffer negative effects of stigma [55]. Treatment cohorts that include other TGNC older adults can reduce isolation and offer interpersonal mirroring that TGNC clients may not often find, thus enhancing the effectiveness of care [4].

6.9 Treatment and Intervention

Approaches to substance abuse treatment have evolved over time as the field has shifted. Traditional models of substance abuse treatment tend to follow a model that focuses primarily on the goal of abstinence [56]. However, research has shown that "one-size-fits-all" approaches to substance abuse treatment do not work for everyone [57]. The continuum of care for substance abuse treatment can include several options, including abstinence either from all substances or just from the primary substance of choice. Other options in this spectrum of care include overall moderation and reduction of substance use, as well as a goal to commit to safer and reduced harm with substance use (e.g., using clean needles). The short-term and long-term goals an individual chooses will vary. This continuum of care allows for a more flexible approach that can meet each individual "where they are at" with their substance use, rather than where they "should" be or where the provider would like them to be.

Harm reduction is an approach to substance abuse treatment that is growing in popularity as it presents an option for care that is client-centered, focused on autonomy, and allows for substance use goals to evolve over time [58]. Harm reduction is a client-centered approach and seeks to have a low-barrier threshold for treatment, nonjudgmentally welcoming individuals at any stage of change [58]. Part of this premise is that change is possible within the context of relationship. Engaging people in treatment, and supporting them to stay engaged in treatment consistently, regardless of their goal for substance use, is the foundation for change. Rather than assume that abstinence is the only option, harm reduction offers the approach that any change is positive and that clients make the decision of what change they would like to work toward [58]. Over time, as insight and motivation for change grow, substance use goals may evolve as individuals begin to examine their substance use in a different light.

Focusing on a client-centered, nonjudgmental approach is vital to engaging TGNC older adults in substance abuse treatment. Particularly as TGNC older adults may be facing loss of independence and support in other part of their lives, giving TGNC older adults the autonomy to make decisions about the direction and goals of their care is empowering and can positively impact engagement and rapport. There are also additional factors and treatment considerations that are important to consider when working with TGNC older adults and with the goal of providing competent and affirming substance use treatment. When providing care to TGNC clients of any age, it's important to "follow the client's lead" in terms of disclosure of identity. This means that providers allow clients to decide how and when to disclose or discuss their identity in all settings that the client encounters. It's possible that the client may be open with some providers and not others. It's important that providers do not force clients to talk about their identity if they are not ready, and providers should take caution not to ask invasive questions about the person's identity that do not serve a purpose other than satisfying the provider's own curiosity.

Substance use treatment can provide its own unique challenges for TGNC older adults seeking care. In inpatient or residential settings, TGNC older adults may feel out of place due to intersecting identities that may not match others' in that treatment setting – including their age and gender identity. Although some treatment centers are working to address this, inpatient and residential settings have traditionally been organized by male and female gender. This has subjected TGNC people to humiliating policies that include being assigned to the unit that matches their state identification or placement in units based on sex assigned at birth. Providers can help by being aware of TGNC-affirming treatment centers in their area or, at the very least, have an understanding of the policies of treatment centers and prepare TGNC clients for what they might expect upon entry.

Research supports group therapy as a helpful method of treatment for substance use [59]. While it provides many benefits for clients, including increasing social connection and combatting the isolation that typically accompanies substance use, it can present unique challenges for TGNC older adults. Some clients have disclosed that it is difficult for them to engage in group therapy, even with other LGBTQ people, because age differences make it difficult to relate. Having the availability of a similar age cohort can make treatment settings most impactful and effective for TGNC older adults [4]. In settings with mainly heterosexual or cisgender people, TGNC older adults may also have difficulty relating due to differences in gender expression. This can be difficult because often issues of sexual orientation and gender identity are germane to a person's substance use [60]. TGNC people need to have a place that they feel comfortable discussing issues of gender identity and sexual orientation in order to make progress in their substance use [61].

Many substance use treatment programs, both inpatient and outpatient, often have a family component where family members are engaged in treatment to some degree. TGNC older adults may define "family" for themselves in a number of ways, including both family of origin as well as chosen family of close friends, partners, and community [14]. For this aspect of treatment, TGNC older adults should be able to define and identify their family in whatever way feels most authentic and supportive. Additionally, it is sometimes assumed that those in the LGBTQ and TGNC community come from fractured families of origin; this is not the case for everyone. Providers cannot assume that every TGNC person comes from a fragmented family of origin and should ask each TGNC person what family means to them and whom they would like to include in this aspect of treatment.

Traditionally, 12-step programs such as Alcoholics Anonymous (AA) or Narcotics Anonymous (NA) are foundational to substance use treatment. While these programs can be enormously helpful to some, some people may not find them relatable. Typically, 12-step programs reference the use of a "higher power," which some (but not all) TGNC clients may find off-putting. The TGNC community has not historically been welcomed by many religious traditions and faiths [62]. Although 12-step programs typically allow people to define a "higher power" for themselves, some LGBT clients may be averse to engaging in a program that has any implication of religiosity at all [27]. This means that providers should be knowledgeable of other resources for TGNC clients who use substances, including nondenominational or secular groups or organizations. SMART Recovery (smartrecovery.org) and Refuge Recovery (refugerecovery.org) are two such organizations that may be of interest to clients who are looking for additional options. SMART Recovery utilizes aspects of cognitive behavioral approaches to enhance motivation for change, while Refuge Recovery utilizes mindfulness and Buddhist principles to support recovery from addiction. People can attend in-person meetings nationwide or participate online.

In addition to 12-step programs, substance use treatment programs also utilize evidence-based interventions. Although not all of these interventions have been normed on TGNC clients, some have been adapted for this population. Seeking Safety is an evidence-based intervention focusing on concurrently treating substance use and post-traumatic stress disorder (PTSD). In their study, Empson et al. [63] reviewed the efficacy of a 12-week Seeking Safety program with a group of HIV-positive transgender women with histories of substance use and experiences of violence. Their study found the treatment to be effective in reducing symptoms of PTSD and drug abuse. This research is promising for the TGNC community.

Similar to anyone making changes to problematic substance use [64], when TGNC older adults are able to achieve sobriety or moderated substance use, waves of self-discovery and emotion are common. When substance use is no longer used as the primary coping skill or tool to manage emotional distress, a range of feelings can surface. This influx of emotional experience can be challenging but can also create an opportunity for the TGNC older adult to learn to cope with and regulate emotions in a healthier way [65]. What seemed impossible before may begin to feel more feasible as people learn to manage emotions in a way that feels healthier and more sustainable.

Conclusion

The goal for this chapter has been to explore the limited research on TGNC older adult substance use, discuss factors that may contribute to or influence the substance use of TGNC older adults, and describe ways to provide competent and affirming substance use care to TGNC older adults. The authors drew upon their clinical experience to discuss factors that may influence and intensify the use of substances in the lives of TGNC older adults and treatment approaches that can support TGNC older adults in their recovery. It is hoped that this information aids in the conceptualization of substance use work with this population, improves the care that is provided to TGNC older adults, and generates ideas for future research.

Through research, improved clinical care, and a commitment to ongoing education, healthcare providers can continue a trajectory of greater health for TGNC older adults. Providers and health team members working with the TGNC community are strongly encouraged to take responsibility for deepening and extending their learning rather than relying on TGNC people for guidance and education [4, 66]. While feedback from TGNC older adult clients and the TGNC community is valuable and absolutely necessary, TGNC people should not be obligated to prepare their care teams to work with them [4]. Professionals providing substance use care should advocate for and work toward improved TGNC and older adult competence within their system of care and within the referral networks they use [67]. Systemically improving the capacity of larger professional networks to provide affirmative care can have a profound and powerful impact on TGNC people [67]. Additionally, referring clients to competent and affirming treatment options, whenever possible, should increase the likelihood that a TGNC older adult will be able to fully engage and participate in treatment, greatly improving their outcomes in substance use treatment [68]. When affirming options don't already exist, providers can advocate for their creation and approach existing networks to develop them. If providers are able to offer affirmative and competent substance use care as TGNC people engage in this process, the result can be transformative and deeply support health and recovery.

References

1. Substance Abuse and Mental Health Services Administration (SAMHSA). Top health issues for LGBT populations information & resource kit. HHS Publication No. (SMA) 12-4684. Rockville: Substance Abuse and Mental Health Services Administration; 2012, Benotsch, Non medical prescription drug use.
2. Carmel TC, Erickson-Schroth L. Mental health and the transgender population. J Psychosoc Nurs Ment Health Serv. 2016;54(12):44–8. https://doi.org/10.3928/02793695-20161208-09.
3. Zelle A, Arms T. Psychosocial effects of health disparities of lesbian, gay, bisexual and transgender older adults. J Psychosoc Nurs. 2015;53(7):25–30.
4. American Psychological Association (APA). Guidelines for psychological practice with transgender and gender nonconforming people. Am Psychol. 2015;70(9):832–64.
5. Bockting W. The impact of stigma on transgender identity development and mental health. In: Kreukels BPC, Steensma TD, de Vries ALC, editors. Gender dysphoria and disorders of sex development. New York: Springer; 2014. p. 319–30.
6. Hendricks ML, Testa RJ. A conceptual framework for clinical work with transgender and gender nonconforming clients: an adaptation of the minority stress model. Prof Psychol Res Pr. 2012;43(5):460–7.
7. James SE, Herman JL, Rankin S, Keisling M, Mottet L, Anafi M. The report of the 2015 U.S. transgender survey. Washington, DC: National Center for Transgender Equality; 2016.

8. NIDA. Health consequences of drug misuse. 2017, March 23. Retrieved from https://www.drugabuse.gov/related-topics/health-consequences-drug-misuse on 2018, April 26.
9. NIDA. Drugs, brains, and behavior: the science of addiction. 2014, July 1. Retrieved from https://www.drugabuse.gov/publications/drugs-brains-behavior-science-addiction on 2018, May 6.
10. Fredriksen-Goldsen KI, Kim H, Shiu C, Goldsen J, Emlet CA. Successful aging among LGBT older adults: physical and mental-health related quality of life by age group. Gerontologist. 2015;55(1):154–68. https://doi.org/10.1093/geront/gnu081. Epub 2014 Sep 11.
11. Gonzalez CA, Gallego JD, Bockting WO. Demographic characteristics, components of sexuality and gender, and minority stress and their associations to excessive alcohol, Cannabis, and illicit (noncannabis) drug use among a large sample of transgender people in the United States. J Prim Prev. 2017;38:419–45. https://doi.org/10.1007/s10935-017-0469-4.
12. Arayasirikul S, Pomart WA, Raymond HF, Wilson EC. Unevenness in health at the intersection of gender and sexuality: sexual minority disparities in alcohol and drug use among transwomen in the San Francisco Bay Area. J Homosex. 2018;65(1):66–79. https://doi.org/10.1080/00918369.2017.1310552.
13. Benotsch EG, Zimmerman E, Cathers L, McNultye S, Piercef J, Heckg T, Perrina PB, Snipes D. Non-medical use of prescription drugs, polysubstance use, and mental health in transgender adults. Drug Alcohol Depend. 2013;132:391–4.
14. Ippolito J, Witten TM. Aging. In: Erickson-Schroth L, editor. Trans bodies, trans selves, a resource for the transgender community. New York: Oxford University Press; 2014. p. 476–500.
15. Wilson C, Moulton B. Loneliness among older adults: a national survey of adults 45+. Prepared by Knowledge Networks and Insight Policy Research; 2010. Washington, DC: AAR Retrieved from: http://assets.aarp.org/rgcenter/general/loneliness_2010.pdf.
16. Gruskin E, Byrne K, Kools S, Altschuler A. Consequences of frequenting the lesbian bar. Women Health. 2007;44(2):103–20.
17. Reisner SL, White Hughto JM, Gamarel KE, Keuroghlian AS, Mizock L, Pachankis J. Discriminatory experiences associated with posttraumatic stress disorder symptoms among transgender adults. J Couns Psychol. 2016;63(5):509–19.
18. Borges G, Walters EE, Kessler RC. Associations of substance use, abuse, and dependence with subsequent suicidal behavior. Am J Epidemiol. 2000;151(8):781–9.
19. Voss WD, Kaufman E, O'Connor SS, Comtois KA, Connor KR, Ries RK. Preventing addiction related suicide: a pilot study. J Subst Abus Treat. 2013;44(5):565–9.
20. Conner KR, Pinquart M, Gamble SA. Meta-analysis of depression and substance use among individuals with alcohol use disorders. J Subst Abus Treat. 2009;37(2):127–37.
21. Grant JM, Mottet LA, Tanis J, Harrison J, Herman JL, Keisling M. Injustice at every turn: a report of the National Transgender Discrimination Survey. Washington, DC: National Center for Transgender Equality and National Gay and Lesbian Task Force; 2011.
22. Reisner SL, Pardo ST, Gamarel KE, Hughto JMW, Pardee DJ, Keo-Meier CL. Substance use to cope with stigma in healthcare among U.S. female-to-male trans masculine adults. LGBT Health. 2015;2(4):324–32.
23. NIDA. The neurobiology of drug addiction. 2007, January 2. Retrieved from https://www.drugabuse.gov/neurobiology-drug-addiction on 2018, May 6.
24. Meyer IH. Prejudice, social stress, and mental health in lesbian, gay and bisexual populations: conceptual issues and research evidence. Psychol Bull. 2003;129:674–97. https://doi.org/10.1037/0033-2909.129.5.674.
25. Rood BA, Reisner SL, Surace FI, Puckett JA, Maroney MR, Pantalone DW. Expecting rejection: understanding the minority stress experience of transgender and gender non-conforming individuals. Transgender Health. 2016;1(1):151–64.
26. Blosnich JR. The intersectionality of minority identities and health. In: Kauth MR, Shipherd JC, editors. Adult transgender care, an interdisciplinary approach to training mental health professionals. New York: Routledge; 2018. p. 30–43.
27. Anderson SC. Substance use disorders in lesbian, gay, bisexual, and transgender clients: assessment and treatment. New York: Columbia University Press; 2009.

28. Mereish EH, O'Cleirigh C, Bradford JB. Interrelationships between LGBT-based victimization, suicide, and substance use problems in a diverse sample of sexual and gender minorities. Psychol Health Med. 2014;19(1):1–13.
29. Chen Y, Tryon GS. Dual minority stress and Asian American gay men's psychological distress. J Community Psychol. 2012;40:539–54.
30. Cook-Daniels L. Understanding transgender elders. In: Harley DA, Teaster PB, editors. Handbook of LGBT elders. New York: Springer; 2016. p. 285–308.
31. Porter KE, Brennan-Ing M, Chang SC, Dickey LM, Singh AA, Bower K, Witten TM. Providing competent and affirming services for transgender and gender nonconforming older adults. Clin Gerontol. 2016;39(5):366–88.
32. Witten TM. It's not all darkness: robustness, resilience, and successful transgender aging. LGBT Health. 2014;1(1):24–33.
33. Blumea AW, Schmalinga KB. [Abstract]. Regret, substance abuse, and readiness to change in a dually diagnosed sample. Addict Behav. 1998;23(5):693–7.
34. Dragon CN, Guerino P, Ewald E, Laffan AM. Transgender Medicare beneficiaries and chronic conditions: exploring fee-for-service claims data. LGBT Health. 2017;4(6):404–11.
35. NIDA. Common comorbidities with substance use disorders. 2018, February 27. Retrieved from https://www.drugabuse.gov/publications/research-reports/common-comorbidities-substance-use-disorders on 2018, May 9.
36. Hinkin CH, Barclay TR, Castellon SA, Levine AJ, Durvasula RS, Marion SD, Myers HF. Drug use and medication adherence among HIV-1 infected individuals. AIDS Behav. 2007;11(2):185–94.
37. Campbell ANC, Tross S, Caslyn DA. Substance use disorders and HIV/AIDS prevention and treatment intervention: research and practice considerations. Soc Work Public Health. 2013;28(0):333–48.
38. CDC. HIV/AIDS surveillance report, vol. 19. Atlanta: US Department of Health and Human Services; 2007.
39. High KP, Brennan-Ing M, Clifford DB, Cohen MH, Currier J, Deeks SG, Deren S, Effros RB, Gebo K, Goronzy JJ, Justice AC. HIV and aging: state of knowledge and areas of critical need for research. A report to the NIH Office of AIDS Research by the HIV and Aging Working Group. J Acquir Immune Defic Syndr (1999). 2012;60(Suppl 1):S1–18.
40. Heath J, Lanoye A, Maisto SA. Behavior among older men who have sex with men: a review and critique of the current literature. AIDS Behav. 2012;16(3):578–89.
41. Fredriksen-Goldsen KI, Kim H-J, Emlet CA, Muraco A, Erosheva EA, Hoy-Ellis CP, Goldsen J, Petry H. The aging and health report: disparities and resilience among lesbian, gay, bisexual, and transgender older adults. Seattle: Institute for Multigenerational Health; 2011.
42. Rachlin K, Green J, Lombardi E. Utilization of health care among female-to-male transgender individuals in the United States. J Homosex. 2008;54(3):243–58.
43. Sage Publications. Improving the lives of transgender older adults. 2012. Retrieved from https://www.sageusa.org/resources/publications.cfm?ID=13 on 2018, April 26.
44. Murariu D, Holland M, Gampper TJ, Campbell CA. Illegal silicone injections create unique reconstructive challenges in transgender patients. Plast Reconstr Surg. 2015;135(5):932e–3e.
45. Wilson E, Rapues J, Jin H, Raymond HF. The use and correlates of illicit silicone or "fillers" in a population-based sample of transwomen, San Francisco, 2013. J Sex Med. 2014;11(7):1717–24. https://doi.org/10.1111/jsm.12558.
46. Rudd RA, Seth P, David F, Scholl L. Increases in drug and opioid-involved overdose deaths — United States, 2010–2015. MMWR Morb Mortal Wkly Rep. 2016;65:1445–52. https://doi.org/10.15585/mmwr.mm655051e1.
47. Yarns BC, Abrams JM, Meeks TW, Sewell DD. The mental health of older LGBT adults. Curr Psychiatry Rep. 2016;18(6):60.
48. Kenagy GP. Transgender health: findings from two needs assessment studies in Philadelphia. Health Soc Work. 2005;30(1):19.
49. Kenagy GP, Bostwick WB. [Abstract]. Health and social service needs of transgender people in Chicago. Int J Transgenderism. 2008;8(2–3):57–66.

50. Houston E, McKirnan DJ. Intimate partner abuse among gay and bisexual men: risk correlates and health outcomes. J Urban Health. 2007;84(5):681–90.
51. Testa RJ, Sciacca LM, Wang F, Hendricks ML, Goldblum P, Bradford J. Effects of violence on transgender people. Prof Psychol Res Pract. 2012;43(5):452–9.
52. Nuttbrock L, Bockting W, Rosenblum A, Hwahng S, Mason M, Macri M, Becker J. Gender abuse, depressive symptoms, and substance use among transgender women: a 3-year prospective study. Am J Public Health. 2014;104(11):2199–206.
53. Singh AA, Hays DG, Watson LS. Strength in the face of adversity: resilience strategies of transgender individuals. J Couns Dev. 2011;89(1) https://doi.org/10.1002/j.1556-6678.2011.tb00057.x.
54. Fuhrmann M, Craffey B. Lessons learned on the path to filial maturity. Charlston: Createspace; 2014.
55. Bockting WO, Miner MH, Swinburne Romine RE, Hamilton A, Coleman E. Stigma, mental health, and resilience in an online sample of the US transgender population. Am J Pub Health. 2013;103(5):943–51.
56. Macmaster SA. Harm reduction: a new perspective on substance abuse services. Soc Work. 2004;49(3):356–63.
57. Marlatt GA, Blume AW, Parks GA. Integrating harm reduction therapy and traditional substance abuse treatment. J Psychoactive Drugs. 2001;33(1):13–21.
58. Little J. Harm reduction in therapy groups: engaging drinkers and drug users in a process of change. J Groups Addict Recover. 2006;1(1):69–93.
59. Center for Substance Abuse Treatment. Substance abuse treatment: group therapy. Treatment Improvement Protocol (TIP) Series, No. 41. HHS Publication No. (SMA) 123991. Rockville: Substance Abuse and Mental Health Services Administration; 2005.
60. Senreich E. Are specialized LGBT program components helpful for gay and bisexual men in substance abuse treatment? Subst Use Misuse. 2010;45(7/8):1077–96.
61. Stevens S. Meeting the substance abuse treatment needs of lesbian, bisexual and transgender women: implications from research to practice. Subst Abus Rehabil. 2012;3(Suppl 1):27.
62. Hopwood RA, Witten TM. Spirituality, faith and religion: the TGNC experience. In: Singh AA, Dickey LM, editors. Affirmative counseling and psychological practice with transgender and gender non-conforming clients. Washington, DC: American Psychological Association; 2017. p. 213–30.
63. Empson S, Cuca YP, Cocohoba J, Dawson-Rose C, Davis K, Machtinger EL. [Abstract]. Seeking safety group therapy for co-occurring substance use disorder and PTSD among transgender women living with HIV: a pilot study. J Psychoactive Drugs. 2017;49(4):344–51.
64. Connors GJ, DiClemente CC, Velasquez MM, Donovan DM. Substance abuse treatment and the stages of change: selecting and planning interventions. New York: Guilford Press; 2013.
65. Quello SB, Brady KT, Sonne SC. Mood disorders and substance use disorder: a complex comorbidity. Sci Pract Perspect. 2005;3(1):13.
66. Hopwood RA, Dickey LM. Mental health services. In: Erickson-Schroth L, editor. Trans bodies, trans selves: a resource for the transgender community. New York: Oxford University Press; 2014. p. 291–305.
67. Ducheny K, Hendricks ML, Keo-Meier CL. TGNC-affirmative interdisciplinary collaborative care. In: Singh AA, Dickey LM, editors. Affirmative counseling and psychological practice with transgender and gender non-conforming clients. Washington, DC: American Psychological Association; 2017.
68. Nuttbrock LA. [Abstract]. Culturally competent substance abuse treatment with transgender persons. J Addict Dis. 2012;31(3):236–41.

Trauma and Aging

7

Loree Cook-Daniels

> I was physically assaulted in [city name withheld] by an unknown cab driver – who kicked me and spit on me and knocked me down – calling me puta and filthy cunt, etc. …I was molested by a co-worker at a luncheon one week later. I had been verbally assaulted at same location by a nurse who humiliated me. My ex-wife was verbally very abusive to me… The sexual assault and molestation resulted in a nervous breakdown/post-traumatic stress – I was unable to work. My ex would get drunk and demand sex, starting with our "wedding night." She required me to do stuff outside, in the pool, on the deck, and sometimes in the kitchen with the children or grandchildren out and about in the next room… My ex liked to try and rip my penis off or cut it off with her nails, and verbally abused me while we had sex [1].

Since Dr. Vincent J. Felitti declared in 2002 that adverse childhood experiences (ACEs) are "the most important determinant of the health and well-being of our nation," [2] there has been an ever-growing body of evidence that childhood trauma accompanies us throughout life, affecting our physical as well as our mental health. This is certainly true of transgender adults, as well, but ACEs make up just a small percentage of the universe of traumatic, discriminatory, and violent experiences that may affect the health and well-being of transgender people as they age. This chapter explores those additional experiences and their health and wellness implications. We end with resilience factors and how service providers can provide trauma-informed care.

7.1 It Starts in Childhood

The ACE study has, to date, involved tens of thousands of participants, each of whom has been asked if they experienced any of the following ten adverse childhood experiences:

L. Cook-Daniels
FORGE, Inc., Milwaukee, WI, USA
LoreeCD@aol.com

M. Houlberg et al. (eds.), *Transgender and Gender Nonconforming Health and Aging*,
https://doi.org/10.1007/978-3-319-95031-0_7

1. A parent, stepparent, or adult living in your home swore at you, insulted you, put you down, or acted in a way that made you afraid that you might be physically hurt.
2. A parent, stepparent, or adult living in your home pushed, grabbed, slapped, threw something at you, or hit you so hard that you had marks or were injured.
3. An adult, relative, family friend, or stranger who was at least 5 years older than you ever touched or fondled your body in a sexual way, made you touch his/her body in a sexual way, or attempted to have any type of sexual intercourse with you.
4. Your mother or stepmother was pushed, grabbed, slapped, had something thrown at her, kicked, bitten, hit with a fist, hit with something hard, repeatedly hit for over at least a few minutes, or ever threatened or hurt by a knife or gun by your father (or stepfather) or mother's boyfriend.
5. A household member was a problem drinker or alcoholic, or a household member used street drugs.
6. A household member was depressed or mentally ill, or a household member attempted suicide.
7. Your parents were ever separated or divorced.
8. A household member went to prison.
9. You often or very often felt that no one in your family loved you or thought you were important or special.
10. You often or very often felt that you didn't have enough to eat, had to wear dirty clothes, and had no one to protect you [3].

The US Centers for Disease Control and Prevention reports that the ACE results show that as the number of ACEs increase, so does the risk for "...alcoholism and alcohol abuse; chronic obstructive pulmonary disease; depression; fetal death; health-related quality of life; illicit drug use; ischemic heart disease; liver disease; poor work performance; financial stress; risk for intimate partner violence; multiple sexual partners; sexually transmitted diseases; smoking; suicide attempts; unintended pregnancies; early initiation of smoking; early initiation of sexual activity; adolescent pregnancy; risk for sexual violence; [and] poor academic achievement" [2].

Briefly, the mechanisms believed to be at work here are these: ACEs lead to disrupted neurodevelopment, which cause social, emotional, and cognitive impairment, in turn leading to symptom management behaviors that are health risks (substance use, risky sex). These risky behaviors in turn lead to disease, disability, social problems, and even early death [2].

Although an estimated 64% of all US adults have experienced one ACE and 40% have experienced two or more [4], many studies have indicated that transgender- or gender-nonconforming children experience even higher rates of childhood emotional maltreatment [5], including physical, sexual, and psychological abuse [6] and "poorer relationships with parents, peer rejection, harassment, and physical and verbal victimization" [6]. If the ACEs questionnaire asked about such common trans-specific childhood traumas as denial of or opposition to a child's identity, being forced to wear clothes or be groomed in a way one found deeply distressing, or being thrown out of the house, transgender individuals' ACE counts would certainly rise even more.

7.2 Adult Violence and Trauma

Unfortunately, childhood is not the only time transgender adults experience trauma. Indeed, many studies have shown that once someone has experienced one type of victimization, they are at increased risk for experiencing even more victimizations [7]. It is important to note that while any one victimization may or may not in any way relate to the transgender individual's gender identity or history, overall transgender older adults experience much more victimization than do their peers. For example, in one large study that compared transgender older adults (aged 50+) to their lesbian, gay, and bisexual age peers, the non-trans LGB older adults had an average of six incidents of lifetime discrimination and victimization. The transgender older adults, in contrast, had almost double that number: 11 lifetime incidents of discrimination and victimization [8]. This study found that the most common types of discrimination and victimization experienced by transgender older adult participants were verbal assaults (76%), being threatened with physical violence (54%), not being hired for job (46%), being denied or provided inferior health care (40%), being denied a promotion (39%), and being hassled by the police (37%) [8]. Transgender elders were also more than twice as likely to have experienced domestic violence in the past year (physical or verbal) than were their LGB peers [9]. One elder transgender woman explained how law enforcement refused to help her when her husband abused her:

> I was physically assaulted by my legal FTM spouse, to the extent that I had to go to the hospital emergency room for treatment. I got a restraining order against his return, but he violated it several weeks later and attempted to rape me. On both occasions the police appeared to think these behaviors were very funny. After the initial assault, one of the responding police officers stated, "Why the hell didn't you just punch his lights out? You must be about twice his size." When I responded, "Then you would have taken me in for assaulting him!" he just shook his head. Since it was clear that [city name withheld] would give me no protection at all, I abandoned my home, along with most of my personal possessions, and used the last of my money to fly back to [city name withheld] where I had friends [1].

A common transgender elder trauma is abandonment. When asking transgender older adults about their experiences of abandonment (using the typical elder abuse definition, "when someone with physical needs is left alone without care by their designated caregiver"), FORGE elicited experiences that did not necessarily meet the definition but clearly were highly traumatic, including these:

> I am [a male-to-female post-operative transsexual] and aged 52. I have a 14-year-old daughter who just said to me one day, "My father died." I have had no contact in years.

> My son and daughter-in-law will not let me see my grandson. They think I will do something to him. I don't even know him now. It breaks my heart not to see him.

> My closest friend of over 30 years finally said, "I just can't handle this." No contact in years.

> My ex-wife was very supportive in the beginning but when physical changes started taking place there was anger. She moved away when I went for surgery. Never seen her or my daughter again [10].

Where transgender individuals are the victims of hate crimes, the impact can be outsized. "Hate crimes are a particularly painful type of event because they inflict not only the pain of the assault itself, but also the pain associated with the social disapproval of the victim's stigmatized social group. The added pain is associated with a symbolic message to the victim that he or she and his or her kind are devalued, debased, and dehumanized in society. Such types of experiences affect the victim's mental health because it damages his or her sense of justice and order" [11]. Another researcher "delineates ways in which violence that is perceived to be related to one's gender identity or expression disproportionately increases distress, compared to violence motivated by other reasons. Such violence leads to internalized transphobia, which can involve negative self-appraisal and rejection of this critical aspect of the person's sense of self, as well as expectations for future rejection and/or victimization. Experiences of violence related to one's gender, alongside these resultant sources of stress, may also lead to concealment of one's trans identity or expression" [12].

Transgender older adults are far more likely to be military veterans (41%) [8] than are the general public (~1%) [13], LGB elders (24.4%) [8], and the transgender population as a whole (20%) [9]. Obviously, military veterans run a relatively high risk of combat-based traumas, but transgender military veterans seem to run a special risk: one study has found that transgender veterans are nearly twice (23% to 12%) as likely to have experienced sexual assault in the military as are non-transgender veterans [14].

7.3 Little-t Traumas

They have been called by many names, including little-t traumas, microaggressions, minority stress, and insidious traumas. They are described as "everyday experiences of disrespect and disparate treatment" [15] or "brief and commonplace daily verbal, behavioral, or environmental indignities, whether intentional or unintentional, that communicate hostile, derogatory, or negative slights and insults toward members of oppressed groups" [16]. They are uniquely damaging: "...stress related to stigma is not assessed solely by its intrinsic characteristics but also by its symbolic meaning within the social context: even a minor event or instance can have symbolic meaning and thus create pain and indignity beyond its seemingly low magnitude" [11]. One 67-year-old transgender woman reported about a visit to her primary physician:

> I had not had a surgery of any kind. The only thing I had done was laser. So when I walked into the doctor's office,...the receptionist started laughing at me. One had to excuse herself and go in the other room because she was laughing so hard [17].

One set of researchers identified twelve categories of trans-specific microaggressions. These include (a) use of transphobic and/or incorrectly gendered terminology, (b) assumption of universal transgender experience, (c) exoticization, (d) discomfort/disapproval of transgender experience, (e) endorsement of gender normative and binary culture or behaviors, (f) denial of existence of transphobia, (g) assumption of sexual pathology/abnormality, (h) physical threat or harassment, (i) denial of individual transphobia, (j) denial of bodily privacy, (k) familial microaggressions, and (l) systemic and environmental microaggressions [16].

A particularly potent trans-related set of little-t traumas revolve around public bathrooms and locker rooms. One observer noted, "...as a matter of tradition and policy, we have built minority stressors for transgender and gender non-conforming people into our very environment due to our reliance on gender segregation in public facilities" [15]. Multiple studies have found very high incidences of bathroom-based problems among transgender people. One reported that 70% of survey respondents reported being denied access, verbally harassed, or physically assaulted in public restrooms; 18% had been denied access altogether, while 68% were verbally harassed and 9% were physically assaulted [15]. FORGE was told of one story involving a transgender elder:

> A very conservatively dressed trans woman was eating, with two friends, a man and a woman, at a local pizza place. When she wanted to use the bathroom (a single use bathroom), she was approached by one of the staff, who loudly told her that she could not use either the women's or the men's room. When her friends asked to see the manager, they were told to leave, which they did. There was no follow-up to the incident [10].

These problems can result in such a high level of fear that people limit their activities, with a British study finding that 38.8% of transgender individuals avoided public restrooms altogether [18]. In Virginia, 11% of transgender people reported that a lack of appropriate restroom facilities had prevented them from seeing a doctor or getting health care [15]. One researcher noted that bathroom-related stress had caused their transgender respondents to reorganize their schedules and change their eating and urinary habits in order to avoid restrooms altogether [19]. Another researcher concluded: "These experiences impacted respondents' education, employment, health, and participation in public life" [15].

Another seldom-acknowledged source of stress for transgender people is public legislative and/or ballot debates over their rights. What happened to LGB people when their rights went to a public vote is telling. One study compared LGB populations living in states that banned marriage equality during the 2004 and 2005 elections with LGB populations living in states that did not go through such public debates. Among LGB people in the banned marriage states, they found psychiatric disorders and comorbidity went up in 11 of their 13 measures. The findings included a 248.2% increase in generalized anxiety disorder, a 41.9% increase in any alcohol use disorder, a 36.6% increase in any mood disorder, and a 36.3% increase in psychiatric comorbidity. The researchers noted that the mood disorders and generalized anxiety disorders were characterized by hopelessness, chronic worry, and hypervigilance [20]. The researchers theorized, "Public campaigns in states debating [anti-gay marriage ballot issues]...have fostered a negative social climate for those with a minority sexual orientation. LGB individuals living in these states confronted increased exposure to stressors, including misleading stereotypes in the media and hostile interactions with neighbors, colleagues, and family members. This exposure to antigay attitudes can lead to greater shame about

LGB identity and more negative feelings about LGB group membership, a construct known as internalized homophobia" [20].

There are no specific studies on how transgender people react to anti-transgender legislative efforts such as the current debates over which bathrooms transgender people should be allowed to use. However, a recent study of transgender and sexual minority women found that the United States post-2016 election environment is having a mental health effect: "[N]early 70 percent of participants reported having 'moderately' or 'much' higher concerns about their safety since the election, while 73 percent reported higher levels of sadness or depression, and 76 percent, of anxiety. …Those who identified as transgender reported significantly higher fears for their safety than those who identified as female" [21].

7.4 Health Results of Trauma

As discussed above, ACE researchers have postulated a sequence of experiences, behaviors, and consequences that link childhood adverse experiences to later-life disability, medical disorders, and even early death. Those who have studied transgender older adults have confirmed some of these connections. The Aging with Pride: National Health, Aging, and Sexuality Study that compared older transgender adults with their LGB peers found that "transgender older adults were at significantly higher risk of poor physical health, disability, depressive symptomatology, and perceived stress compared with non-transgender participants. We found significant indirect effects of gender identity on the health outcomes via fear of accessing health services, lack of physical activity, internalized stigma, victimization, and lack of social support; other mediators included obesity for physical health and disability, identity concealment for perceived stress, and community belonging for depressive symptomatology and perceived stress. Further analyses revealed that risk factors (victimization and stigma) explained the highest proportion of the total effect of gender identity on health outcomes" [8]. Sometimes these connections play out in unexpected ways. One transgender woman explained her decision to engage in sex work (widely regarded as a high-risk behavior) this way:

> I prostitute myself at age 55 because even though I'm a [post-operative transsexual] and passable [as a woman], no one passes 100% of the time. NO ONE. Job discrimination is bad because you're stuck with fellow employees 8 hours a day, 40 hours a week. That much harassment is bad for one's mental health [10].

A renowned minority stress researcher, Ilan H. Meyer, has articulated three main reactions to small-t traumas: (1) identity concealment, (2) internalized stigma, and (3) expectations of rejection [18]. All of these have been demonstrated among transgender older adults, and all may lead to further health disparities. Concealment, for example, "distances the individual from community resources that may otherwise be a source of resilience. Concealment, internalized transphobia, and expectations of future violence, may also exacerbate hesitancy to seek help, which may in turn prolong or intensify distress" [12].

7.4.1 Identity Concealment

If a transgender person has an appearance such that they are not typically "read" as transgender, they may try to minimize both small- and large-t traumas by being hypervigilant about what they say and do. One researcher called it "concealing" (it is also frequently known as "going stealth") and said of it: "Concealing requires constant monitoring of one's interactions and of what one reveals about his or her life to others. Keeping track of what one has said and to whom is very demanding and stressful, and leads to psychological distress. Among the effects of concealing are preoccupation, increased vigilance of stigma discovery, and suspiciousness" [11]. Analysis of a sample of transgender older adults found that concealment was significantly associated with higher degrees of depressive symptomatology and perceived stress [8]. More than half of the adult participants in one large study reported that they had concealed their transgender identity [12].

7.4.2 Internalized Transphobia

Some transgender individuals incorporate negative social beliefs (such as those aired in public debates about transgender rights or parental admonishments that they will never find a partner) into their own self-image, resulting in internalized stigma or internalized transphobia. A study that specifically compared transgender older adults with LGB peers found that the transgender respondents reported higher rates of internalized stigma as well as victimization and that these "were significantly associated with poorer physical health, higher likelihood of disability, and higher degrees of depressive symptomatology and perceived stress" [8].

7.4.3 Expectations of Rejection

Anticipation or fear of violence, discrimination, or rejection can be just as – or even more – debilitating than the incidents themselves. One transgender stress researcher concluded: "Qualitatively, participant narratives were punctuated with a sense of urgency, distress, and resignation. In other words, they shared stories about expecting rejection in ways that suggested that the experiences were intense and often life-threatening (e.g., experiencing fear, anger, and hypervigilance); upsetting and disparaging (e.g., experiencing frustration, sadness, and shame); and an expected part of their existence (e.g., thinking about the possibility of rejection in most contexts and with most people)" [18]. These reactions can lead to further problems. One young adult noted:

> Whenever I get stressed out [about expecting rejection], I let go of my stress by being angry. I tend to lash out. …It always ends up being more harmful right? You always regret that [18].

Transgender individuals in one study coped with expectations of rejection by engaging in avoidance strategies, avoiding certain situations altogether, and developing behavioral routines as a way to avoid becoming a target such as hiding in a restroom stall, keeping earphones on at the gym, and not making eye contact with anyone [18].

One transgender young adult said:

> Any time I'm in the presence of someone who knew me before [transition] – so, past family members, past friends, anybody like that – it's almost like every muscle in my body is in a heightened state of alert and my blood pressure, I can almost feel it pumping. Every word they say, every word they don't say, every flick of their eyes, everything they do is something that I'm focusing on and reading… So, constantly, I'm ready for them to say the wrong pronouns or use the wrong name, or speak to me in some negative way even if they haven't done it or aren't going to. Usually, by the time that situation is over, whether or not anything bad happened, I'll just burst into tears or just decompress emotionally after it's done because I'm so ready to be hurt, expecting to be hurt [18].

Another young adult called it "preemptive stress" and discussed how it impacted their health care:

> So I recently went to a doctor in [home city] for the first time – nothing related to my transition at all, just a medical problem I was having. Literally four or five hours before I went, I just felt really nervous or anxious about going there and just being like, 'What if this happens? What if that happens?' Nothing happened. The doctor was really understanding, but it's just that preemptive stress, I guess [18].

One way avoidance strategies can have a negative health impact is by causing transgender elders to eschew health care. One set of researchers noted this can be self-compounding: "Considering that 40% of the transgender older adults in this study feared accessing health services, both discrimination from health care providers and internalized stigma can exacerbate chronic stress and act as further impediments to accessing needed health care" [8]. Avoidance can even be life-shortening. Here's what one trans elder told FORGE:

> I have decided not to have any life-extending surgery because of past mistreatment by nurses at [the Veterans Administration hospital] [10].

7.5 Aging-Specific Issues

One of the most potent negative impacts on transgender elders is the one that affects all of us: ageism. Radical Age Movement defines it this way: "Ageism refers to discriminatory or prejudiced behavior and attitudes towards people based solely on age. Ageism causes the systematic mistreatment and marginalization of people based on age alone, just as racism and sexism does so based on categories of skin color and gender" [22]. Ageism is so widespread in the United States that it is seldom even recognized as a dangerous stereotype. Moreover, it is a stereotype that appears to be particularly dangerous to those who hold it: "A study by Yale researcher Becca Levy and colleagues followed several hundred older adults for more than two decades. Researchers found that people who had internalized more negative attitudes towards aging were *significantly more likely to suffer impairments and need nursing home care, and died on average 7-1/2 years earlier* than people with less negative attitudes towards aging" [22] (emphasis in original). One of the most pervasive consequences of ageism is that its adherents frequently believe that life will only get worse as they age. One measure of its effect on transgender older adults came in a 2014 study that indicated 65% of respondents believed that their access to health care would be limited as some point in later life and 55% expected to be denied medical coverage completely [23].

Particularly feared is the possibility of needing a nursing home. While this prospect worries many elders, transgender elders (and even younger adults) often have very specific, detailed, and trans-specific fears of what might be in store for them. One 60-year-old told researchers:

> They're going to call me sir and they're gonna treat me like one of the guys and I'm gonna have to complain. And I don't know how effective I'll be, but I expect to fight a lot. I already told my daughter, "Expect me to get kicked out of every nursing home from Maine to Baja and then start in Washington and go to Florida because I'm not gonna put up with it." But I expect it's gonna be a nightmare and the only hope I have is if I have another heart attack that's fatal before I end up having to be in a nursing home [17].

A much younger transgender person who actually worked in the aging field told FORGE:

> …[A]s a trans 35 year old – who is a service provider who has borne witness to incidents of violence and abuse for elders, I'm scared to death about my own future. There is Alzheimer's in my family, and I know there's a good chance it's going to claim me as well. What will happen to me once I can no longer advocate for myself? Will they call me "she"? Will they make fun of my body right in front of me, knowing I won't really understand? Without a significant other, and without children, I fear I'll be left in a nursing home somewhere where no one actually cares about me as a human being. At 35 I've already written a living will…. a Power of Attorney for Personal Care. And honestly? I have more or less decided that I just won't let myself get to that point where I can't take care of myself. I'd rather take matters into my own hands and self-euthanize (that's a nice way to say it, don't you think?) while I am mentally cognizant and physically capable of it. Should the time come when I need to take my own life in order to avoid these horrific experiences, I will [10].

The theme of preferring suicide over being transgender in a nursing home is not uncommon; Minnesota's Transgender Aging Project study quotes at least three trans elders who expressed similar sentiments [17].

Nor are the fears unfounded. A national study soliciting examples of abuse of LGBT people in nursing homes found that 9% of the 853 reported incidents involved "staff refused to refer to transgender resident by preferred name or pronoun" [24]. One advocate told of a transgender resident who was not allowed to eat with the other residents, talk with them, or engage in the communal social and recreational activities [24]. Another informant told FORGE about an incident involving a cross-dresser: "[She] was basically told, 'You can't do that here.' She said she felt she'd been threatened. Don't do it, or you'll be kicked out" [10]. Transgender residents also reported negative treatment from other residents [24].

The under-discussed phenomenon of trauma reemergence in mid- to later- life can also affect transgender older adults. Many trauma survivors are successful in suppressing their memories and/or trauma symptoms for many years through substance use, overwork, devotion to childrearing, or other diversions. Some types of trauma – including, especially, sexual assault – seem particularly prone to being held at bay for long periods of time. In a sexual violence survey FORGE conducted, it was not unusual for transgender sexual violence survivors to first seek emotional help for coping with their sexual assault(s) 10 years or more after the assault(s) took place [25]. One 50-year-old transgender woman felt she still needed help coping with her childhood abuse:

> [Question: What kinds of services would you find useful?] Social support, and therapy to help me develop the missing social skills that are a consequence of my childhood abuse, and my years and years of cognitive dissociation [10].

Intimate partner violence may also play out in a way that only becomes obvious late in the game. One transgender elder reported:

> My life got really, really small, slowly over thirty years, and it took me more than a year to get to where I was comfortable with myself, and six more months before I dealt with any of the abuse – only in the last month has most of the dealing with the abuse happened [10].

Even elders who feel they have "dealt with" or are long past previous abuse may be surprised when a health crisis, life change (such as retirement or moving into congregate living), or death of a loved one suddenly causes the trauma to reemerge and produce painful symptoms. One woman, a survivor of both childhood sexual abuse and several types of abuse perpetrated over decades by her ex-wife, told FORGE:

> I have good coping skills and attitude, and at the same time was able to stow/compartmentalize both abuse situations away from my conscious awareness. It didn't come up seriously until I started volunteering for a group for "stopping abuse in the lesbian, bisexual women's and transgendered communities" – the training I went through kicked it ALL loose. The sexual abuse was only a part of what was going on, with physical and emotional and financial abuse as well [1].

7.6 Resilience

It would be a mistake to develop a picture of transgender elders' lives as being sad and trauma-filled. In fact, transgender people who have survived many decades of derision, myths, and worse are – by definition – survivors who are incredibly resilient and skilled.

Many researchers and theorists have tried to define what makes a person "resilient." An everyday definition is the capacity for overcoming difficult times and experiences [26]. Another simple description is: "The construct of *resilience* has been defined as a set of learned behaviors evolving from an individual's system of beliefs that precedes one's ability to cope" [26]. The LGBT aging researchers in charge of the Aging with Pride study operationalized resilience this way: "The resilience conceptual framework has four primary components: (a) key health indicators, including access to health services and health-related behaviors; (b) risk factors related to marginalization, including internalized stigma, victimization, and identity concealment; (c) protective factors, including social support, social network size, participation in religious and spiritual activities, and community belonging; and (d) health outcomes, including general health, disability, depressive symptomatology, and stress" [8].

A small study ($N = 21$, ages 19–52) specifically designed to investigate the ways in which transgender individuals cope with discrimination, misunderstanding, and prejudice identified five resiliency themes: (1) evolving a self-generated definition of self, (2) embracing self-worth, (3) awareness of oppression, (4) connection with a supportive community, and (5) cultivating hope for the future. Two variant themes [a majority but not all of the participants discussed using these tactics] were social activism and being a positive role model for others [26].

Although many commentators have expressed consternation at the proliferation of terms and even invented pronouns within the transgender community, the resilience study found that this creativity was actually a mark of resiliency: "...all shared that being able to use their own words and terms to define their gender helped them cope with discrimination. Language regarding their gender became a way for participants to actively resist the traditional binary definitions of gender" [26].

Believing "they had the right to live their lives and exist as transgender people" was how the researchers defined "embracing self-worth" [26]. "Despite the transphobia they experienced in the world, participants shared about times in their lives when they concluded that they could not control the world but could instead draw on positive beliefs about themselves to cope with stress. Participants described the idea of believing they were valuable human beings as particularly poignant. Embracing their self-worth not only strengthened a positive sense of self, but also allowed them to 'stand up for themselves' when others would not" [26]. This was also described as having a strong internal "coach" who helped them manage prejudice [26].

Being aware of the concept of oppression helped participants identify and counteract social messages that were not "trans-positive." One participant said:

> The world is really built to not see me. It's the world and not me that is wrong. And I will be seen and known. I am a lot more aware of how the world doesn't want to be out of the "gender box." And I see myself these days being like a shark. Sharks have to constantly move to stay alive and feed themselves. Well, I have to keep being aware and knowing what I know to stay emotionally alive as a trans person [26].

"Participants also overwhelmingly described that a significant aspect of their resilience was building a connection with one or more supportive communities. These communities helped encourage participants when they felt overwhelmed and less resilient to challenges." These communities, which included groups focused on performance, religious or spiritual, feminist, LGBT, and racial ethnic themes, "reflected to them their strengths when they could not do so for themselves" [26] One participant who was connected to a transgender community noted that "Having a community of people like me has saved me after growing up in a world that denies I exist" [26].

Social support, a related concept, may be particularly useful to adults who have experienced trauma. "[S]ocial support creates a sense of safety, which can allow an individual to modify defensive and avoidant coping strategies into ones that provide a sense of control over emotional and cognitive processes, which ultimately decreases self-directed violence. Such a process begins to undermine the learned strategies from childhood/adolescence, which once were adaptive, but are no longer needed when safety and stability are present…." [19]. Interestingly, one of the largest studies of transgender elders found a mixed bag when they asked about social support and community belonging. Transgender elders' social network sizes were larger than those of their LGB age peers, but they reported lower levels of social support and community belonging [8]. Clearly, more study is called for to tease apart these findings.

The only example the researchers gave of a participant expressing hope as a resiliency tactic was a young adult discussing how they helped themselves survive childhood. This dearth of forward-looking resiliency stories may in part reflect the pervasiveness of ageism as discussed above: many people can only imagine life getting worse as they age. This viewpoint should be challenged. One resource that may help an older adult find more hopeful and positive ways of using their lifetime of experience is www.Encore.org, "Second Acts for the Greater Good." This organization describes itself as "a movement of millions of people who are using our passions, skills and decades of experience to make a difference in our communities and the world" [27].

In the 2011 resiliency study by Singh, Hays, and Watson, 85% of the study participants felt that engaging in social activism was a major piece of their resilience package, and nearly as many said they focused on being a positive influence on others. One participant addressed both themes:

> I so get energized by the [kids] I work with because they are identified as "at risk." I try to instill resilience in them, and I try to model my self-talk with them…I try to be positive for them and that helps me be positive for myself. How can I get down about being trans when I see what these youth experience every day? They need me to be strong [26].

It may be worth noting that the researchers concluded that the resilience themes participants discussed were not only individual learned behaviors but involved actively confronting transphobia: "…participants described the essence of their resilience as being the ways they disrupted both societal and internalized transphobia, despite the pervasive discrimination these participants faced" [26].

7.7 Trauma-Informed Care

The Substance Abuse and Mental Health Services Administration (SAMHSA) says a program or approach is trauma-informed when it (1) *realizes* the widespread impact of trauma and understands potential paths for recovery; (2) *recognizes* the signs and symptoms of trauma in clients, families, staff, and others involved with the system; (3) *responds* by fully integrating knowledge about trauma into policies, procedures, and practices; and (4) seeks to actively prevent re-traumatization (emphases in the original) [28]. SAMHSA has also articulated six principles various types of organizations can use to gauge how trauma-informed their approach is:

1. *Safety* – throughout an organization, the staff and people they serve feel physically and psychologically safe; the physical setting must be safe, and interactions should promote a sense of safety.
2. *Trustworthiness and transparency* – organizational operations and decisions are conducted with transparency and the goal of building and maintaining trust among clients, families, and staff.
3. *Peer support* – other individuals who have experienced trauma can serve as key partners in recovery from trauma.
4. *Collaboration and mutuality* – partnering and leveling of power differences between staff and clients and among staff.
5. *Empowerment, voice, and choice* – individual strengths are recognized, built on, and validated, and new skills are developed as needed.
6. *Cultural, historical, and gender issues* - the organization incorporates policies, protocols, and processes that are responsive to the racial, ethnic, and cultural needs of individuals served; there is a responsiveness to gender and consideration for historical trauma [28].

Providing a sense of safety for transgender older adults can be challenging. One trauma expert noted that survivors of prolonged child abuse or neglect can have "trouble reading positive emotions from other people's faces and postures….Unable to recognize caring feelings in the face and posture of others, such a client finds it extremely difficult to feel that anyone is safe or can really be trusted" [29]. Transgender older adults' many experiences of discrimination, violence, and disrespect can also make them cautious with new providers, who will need to earn their trust over time. Practices that are particularly important for trust-building with transgender clients include always using the older adult's preferred name and pronoun; training *all* staff – including, in particular, those who staff telephones and front desks – on how to be respectful to transgender people; carefully avoiding stereotyping by allowing the client to share their own unique story; and ensuring all questions follow the dictum, "Know and Tell Why."

It can be hard for people who have never questioned the gender identity they were assigned to understand how important pronouns are to transgender individuals. It may help to think of pronouns as equivalent to personal names rather than as inconsequential and tiny nouns. Just as it would be considered extremely rude to say to someone you just met, "You look like a Bob to me. I'm going to call you Bob," it can be extremely rude to assign a pronoun to someone based on how you think they look. Providers should make a practice of giving their own pronoun when they introduce themselves and soliciting the pronoun as well as the name of new clients. The pronoun as well as the name should be noted on intake forms and records to ensure that other staff also address clients respectfully.

Many conscientious service providers who obtain training on how to appropriately work with transgender clients fail to extend that training to all of the personnel they work with. This is a mistake. A well-trained professional may never be able to use what they know if transgender people who are seeking services are turned away or turned off by receptionists or other frontline practitioners who (intentionally or not) treat them disrespectfully.

While avoiding stereotyping is a best practice in all service settings, it is particularly important when working with transgender adults who are also trauma survivors. The desire to be "seen" is "especially true of individuals with abuse histories, who have been actively discouraged from asserting their rights and needs, whose personal boundaries have been violated, and who may have been penalized for trying to stand up for themselves" [30]. Allowing people to tell their own story also gives you the opportunity to provide more effective care by ensuring you address what is actually bothering the person rather than treating what you presume their issue is.

Because transgender people are so often subjected to questions that are irrelevant and that distract the service provider from attending to the reason the person is seeking services (e.g., "Have you had the surgery?" "How do you and your partner have sex?"), "know and tell why" – while a helpful practice with all service recipients – is particularly important to use with transgender elders. "Know and tell why" involves thinking about how the answer to a particular question shapes care, ensuring that the question is correctly phrased to clearly solicit the needed information, and telling service recipients in advance why and how the question you are about to ask will help shape their care. Obviously, questions that are not directly relevant to clients' care but are merely asked out of curiosity should be avoided [31].

Since cumulative trauma burden can become overwhelming, especially if an older adult is also coping with other stressors like a new health challenge, grief, or other major changes, service providers may wish to more directly support their client's resilience. If an older adult is showing symptoms of stress, they may benefit from psychoeducation about the aftereffects of trauma and/or by being taught relaxation, mindfulness, or stress management techniques [5].

Advocacy skills may also be called for. A guide for therapists of transgender people advises: "remind clients about their rights and also prepare them for interactions by engaging in role-playing activities" [5]. Another set of transgender trauma researchers go even further, recommending: "[P]ractitioners should explore acting…on behalf of transgender clients in order to ensure they have adequate resources they need for their overall well-being" [19].

Connecting an older trauma survivor to other transgender survivors who can normalize and validate their experiences may be helpful; FORGE sponsors several such forums (see Readings and Resources, below) [5]. Professionals can also support clients' exploring their own internalized transphobia by "evaluat[ing] the nature of clients' inner dialogue in terms of how positively or negatively their internal dialogue affects their well-being...[and] striv[ing] to provide alternative, affirmative messages when counselors encounter clients who are internalizing transphobia" [26].

Finally, assessing and educating about coping styles may also be useful. Early researchers suggested that there are two overarching coping styles: (a) emotion-focused coping and (b) problem-focused coping [32]. Researchers studying coping and psychological distress among genderqueer individuals described these concepts as avoidant and facilitative coping. "Avoidant coping occurs when individuals attempt to prevent an emotional response to the stressor, often by minimizing the problem, trying to disengage oneself from the results of a problem, or using substances. Facilitative coping occurs when an individual seeks psychotherapy, becomes open to learning new skills, attempts to positively adapt, and are [sic] open to other/additional avenues of happiness" [32]. The genderqueer researchers reported that in their respondents, avoidant coping styles were associated with more depression and anxiety than those with higher scores of facilitative coping [32]. Interestingly, they also found a connection between social support and coping styles: "...individuals who reported greater social support...also reported greater use of facilitative coping, and thus experienced less anxiety.... Individuals who reported lower social support...also reported greater use of avoidant coping, and thus experienced greater anxiety...." [32]. Thus, practitioners may want to encourage clients who seem focused on simply ducking their emotions to take more problem-solving approaches and/or seek out more social support.

Take-Home Points

- As a group, transgender older adults have experienced more trauma, discrimination, and abuse throughout their lifespans than non-transgender older adults.
- Some of this trauma is transgender-specific (related to bathrooms, public referenda, and friends and family abandonment) and can include what is often called "microaggressions" or "everyday experiences of disrespect and disparate treatment."
- Experiences of trauma, discrimination, and abuse have myriad, long-lasting negative implications for both mental and physical health.
- Aging-specific traumas may be related to ageism, fear of nursing homes, and trauma reemergence.
- Transgender older adults are by definition resilient survivors. That resilience can be bolstered if they self-generate a definition of self, embrace their self-worth, cultivate an awareness of oppression, connect with a supportive community, and cultivate hope for the future.
- Professionals working with transgender elders should learn about and practice trauma-informed care to improve the effectiveness of their care and to help those elders learn additional resiliency strategies.

References

1. Cook-Daniels L. Abuse and violence directed at transgender elders. Milwaukee: FORGE; n.d. 7 p.
2. U.S. Centers for Disease Control and Prevention. About the CDC-Kaiser ACE study [internet]. Washington DC: Centers for Disease Control and Prevention [cited 2018 Apr 5]. Available from: https://www.cdc.gov/violenceprevention/acestudy/about.htm.
3. U.S. Centers for Disease Control and Prevention. About the CDC-Kaiser ACE study [internet]. Washington DC: Centers for Disease Control and Prevention [cited 2018 Apr 5]. Available from: https://www.cdc.gov/violenceprevention/acestudy/about.htm and Nakazawa DJ. Childhood disrupted: How your biography becomes your biology, and how you can heal. New York: Atria Books; 2015. 279 p.
4. Nakazawa DJ. Childhood disrupted: how your biography becomes your biology, and how you can heal. New York: Atria Books; 2015. 279 p.
5. Richmond K, Burnes TR, Singh AA, Ferrara M. Assessment and treatment of trauma with TGNC clients: a feminist approach. In: Singh AA, Dickey LM, editors. Affirmative counseling and psychological practice with transgender and gender nonconforming clients. Washington, DC: American Psychological Association; 2017. p. 191–212.
6. Roberts AL, Rosario M, Corliss HL, Koenen KC, Austin SB. Childhood gender nonconformity: a risk indicator for childhood abuse and posttraumatic stress in youth. Pediatrics. 2012;129(3):410–7.
7. Cohen EP. Polyvictimization: what it is and why it matters [internet]. Washington DC: American Bar Association; [updated 2013 July 11; cited 2018 Apr 5]. Available from: https://www.americanbar.org/content/dam/aba/administrative/child_law/1A_Cohen_Polyvictimization%20-%20What%20it%20is%20and%20Why%20it%20Matters.authcheckdam.pdf.
8. Fredriksen-Goldsen KI, Cook-Daniels L, Kim HJ, Erosheva EA, Emlet CA, et al. Physical and mental health of transgender older adults: an at-risk and underserved population. The Gerontologist. 54(3):488–500.
9. Services and Advocacy for GLBT Elders (SAGE) and National Center for Transgender Equality (NCTE). Improving the lives of transgender older adults: recommendations for policy and practice. New York; 2012. p. 52.
10. Cook-Daniels L, Munson M. Sexual violence, elder abuse, and sexuality of transgender adults age 50+: results of three surveys. Milwaukee: FORGE; 2008. 37 p.
11. Choi SK, Meyer IH. LGBT aging: a review of research findings, needs, and policy implications. Los Angeles: The Williams Institute; 2016. 50 p.
12. Testa RJ, Sciacca LM, Wang F, Hendricks ML, Goldblum P, Bradford J, et al. Effects of violence on transgender people. Prof Psychol Res Pr. 2012;43(5):452–9.
13. U.S. Department of Veterans Affairs. Profile of veterans: 2016 data from the American community survey [internet]. [updated 2018 Feb; cited 2018 Apr 7]. Available from: https://www.va.gov/vetdata/docs/SpecialReports/Profile_of_Veterans_2016.pdf.
14. Brown GR, Jones KT. Health correlates of criminal justice involvement in 4,793 transgender veterans. LGBT Health. 2015;2(4):1–9.
15. Herman JL. Gendered restrooms and minority stress: the public regulation of gender and its impact on transgender people's lives. J Public Manag Soc Pol. 2013;19:65–80.
16. Nadal KL, Skolnik A, Wong Y. Interpersonal and systemic microaggressions toward transgender people: implications for counseling. J LGBT Issues Couns. 2012;6:55–82.
17. Flunker D, Knochel KA. Minnesota transgender aging project community report: focus on providers. Rainbow Health Initiative: Minnesota; 2017. 27 p.
18. Rood BA, Resiner SL, Surace FI, Puckett JA, Maroney MR, et al. Expecting rejection: understanding the minority stress experiences of transgender and gender-nonconforming individuals. Transgender Health. 2016;1(1):151–64.
19. Burnes TR, Dexter MM, Richmond K, Singh AA, Cherrington A. The experiences of transgender survivors of trauma who undergo social and medical transition. Traumatology. 2016;22(1):75–84.

20. Hatzenbuehler ML, McLaughlin KA, Keyes KM, Hasin DS. The impact of institutional discrimination on psychiatric disorders in lesbian, gay, and bisexual populations: a prospective study. AM J Public Health. 2010;100(3):452–9.
21. Columbia School of Nursing [internet]. First national study published after 2016 presidential election finds gender minorities' sense of safety and well-being impacted. New York: 2017 Nov 1[cited 2018 Apr 4]. Available from: http://nursing.columbia.edu/first-national-survey-published-after-2016-presidential-election-finds-gender-minorities-sense.
22. Radical Age Movement. What is ageism [internet]. Radical Age Movement. [cited 2018 Apr 7]. Available from: https://radicalagemovement.org/what-is-ageism/.
23. Dickey LM, Bower KL. Aging and TGNC identities: working with older adults. In: Singh AA, Dickey LM, editors. Affirmative counseling and psychological practice with transgender and gender nonconforming clients. Washington: American Psychological Association; 2017. p. 161–74.
24. National Senior Citizens Law Center, National Center for Lesbian Rights, National Center for Transgender Equality, Lambda Legal, SAGE, National Gay and Lesbian Task Force. Stories from the field: LGBT older adults in long-term care facilities. Washington, DC; n.d. 35 p.
25. FORGE, unpublished data from Sexual Violence in the Transgender Community Survey, 2004.
26. Singh AA, Hays DG, Watson LS. Strength in the face of adversity: resilience strategies of transgender individuals. J Couns Dev. 2011 Winter;89:20–7.
27. Encore.org. Home page [internet]. San Francisco: Encore.org; [cited 2018 April 7]. Available from: https://encore.org/.
28. Administration for Children and Families. Resource guide to trauma-informed human services [internet]. Washington DC; [cited 2018 Apr 7]. Available from: https://www.acf.hhs.gov/trauma-toolkit#chapter-6.
29. Levine PA. In an unspoken voice: how the body releases trauma and restores goodness. Berkeley: North Atlantic Books; 2010. 369 p.
30. Cloitre M, Cohen LR, Koenen KC. Treating survivors of childhood abuse: psychotherapy for the interrupted life. New York: The Guildford Press; 2006. 338 p.
31. Know and Tell Why FAQ. http://forge-forward.org/wp-content/docs/FAQ-08-2012-know-tell-why.pdf.
32. Budge SL, Rossman HK, Howard KAS. Coping and psychological distress among genderqueer individuals: the moderating effect of social support. J LGBT Issues Couns. 2014;8:95–117.

Recommended Reading and Resources

Transgender Aging Network (TAN). Networks professionals interested in transgender aging and hosts a peer-support listserv for transgender people and their close loved ones aged 50+. Also hosts a collection of publications and training webinars for both elders and service providers. www.FORGE-forward.org/aging.

Trans Survivor Resources. FORGE sponsors multiple networking websites, social media sites, and resource collections for transgender survivors of domestic violence, sexual assault, dating violence, stalking, hate violence, and other traumas. Start here: www.FORGE-forward.org.

Trauma Toolkit. This online "Resource Guide to Trauma-Informed Human Services" was put together by the Administration for Children and Families, the Substance Abuse and Mental Health Services Administrations, the Administration for Community Living, and the Offices of the Assistant Secretary of Health and Assistant Secretary for Planning and Evaluation at the US Department of Health and Human Services. It is "intended to provide an introduction to the topic of trauma, a discussion of why understanding and addressing trauma is important for human services programs, and a 'road map' to find relevant resources". https://www.acf.hhs.gov/trauma-toolkit.

Religion, Spirituality, and Health Behaviors: Intersections with Gender Diversity and Aging

8

Ruben A. Hopwood

This chapter discusses associations between health and religion and spirituality in gender-diverse populations broadly. It is noteworthy for this chapter that there is a paucity of data to fully understand the direct impact of religion and spirituality on gender-diverse populations of any specific age group. Given this, the chapter presents the available literature while also offering expected connections and impact implied by the data to an elder gender-diverse population. For the purpose of this chapter, *religion and spirituality* or *religious and spiritual* will refer jointly to beliefs, actions, and practices of people while seeking whatever they understand as sacred to create meaning, purpose, and/or significance in their lives.

Additionally, *gender diverse* will refer to any gender identity that is nontraditional, including transgender, trans, non-binary, agender, genderqueer, gender expansive, gender nonconforming, etc. It is important to pause here and acknowledge that those we may classify today for convenience of discussion as gender-diverse older adults may have lived for 30+ years in their authentic gender without anyone in their lives being aware of their medical treatment history. They may not identify with or want to be part of an identified gender diverse, transgender, or other gender minority grouping. They may not have disclosed their medical treatment history to any health-care providers, spouses, children, or anyone other than their parents and siblings who may no longer even be alive or in contact with them. They appear and live as any other older adult in society without incidence or perceived difference from any non-transgender person in the society [1]. This group may therefore be invisible by choice, and their concerns and needs may be quite different than those who are known to be part of or who identify as part of a gender-diverse population.

R. A. Hopwood
The Danielsen Institute, Boston University, Medical Department, Fenway Health, Boston, MA, USA
e-mail: rhopwood@bu.edu

M. Houlberg et al. (eds.), *Transgender and Gender Nonconforming Health and Aging*,
https://doi.org/10.1007/978-3-319-95031-0_8

For the purposes of this chapter, *aging* is defined as the process of humans as they grow older in a deleterious sense—complex biological changes over time progressively lead to poorer mental and physical functioning, greater susceptibility to illness and injury, and a greater likelihood the individual will die [2]. Research on aging has often focused on the negative aspects of growing older, including factors leading to increased morbidity and mortality. Research into the positive aspects and factors contributing to optimal aging have been fewer, leaving gaps in knowledge about what makes for optimal aging in different groups [1, 3]. *Optimal aging* herein refers to the capacity to function in life across several physical, mental, and social domains in a way that the individual perceives as satisfactory despite any medical conditions or limitations due to aging or infirmity [4].

Aging can engender negative feelings about oneself due to declines in mental and physical capacity and function [5]. Negative feelings can be mild to severe and may include significant worries about becoming a burden to family, friends, and communities, leading to suicide and suicidal ideation in elder populations in the absence of depressive symptoms [6]. Additionally, gender-variant older adults are often subjected to hostility, sexual abuse, and other elder abuse [7, 8]. Suicidality in aging transgender and non-binary populations appears to be a significant risk that is compounded by the absence of supportive and welcoming communities, safe elder care options, and welcoming religious and spiritual communities [9]. This chapter focuses on the role of religion and spirituality in health and wellbeing in an older gender-diverse population and on how the integration of religion and spirituality by health-care professionals may enhance the wellbeing and optimal aging opportunities for this population.

8.1 Impact of Spirituality and Religion on Health and Wellbeing

The integration of health with religion and spirituality has been the norm and the foundation of health care historically [10]. However, as history changes and societies shift, there is increasing separation of the two, particularly within Westernized health care, in such a way that it may be challenging for health-care professionals to utilize or even recognize the potential for sustained health, resilience, and recovery from illnesses and adversity through engagement with religion and spirituality throughout life. There is clear evidence that the overall effect of religious and spiritual involvement on health and wellbeing in the general population is positive, providing protective and sometimes preventative benefits in hardship and in aging [11]. As the number of older adults increases across the country [12], growth of the elder population amplifies the need to know more about what factors contribute to or detract from quality of life and health across the latter end of the life span [13]. Religion and spirituality are known to both contribute to positive coping and wellbeing and to contribute to distress and illness in the general population [14, 15].

Less is known about the contribution of religious and spiritual practices and communities to the wellbeing of transgender and non-binary elders. There is a paucity of data on religious and spiritual involvement in transgender and non-binary elders [9, 16, 17]. This area of research has scant interest among academic research institutions and near total absence of funding with which to explore the roles and connections to health of religion and spirituality for gender-diverse elders. What is available as a result is limited in generalizability. Nonetheless, this chapter addresses what we may reasonably extrapolate from the data available about the connections between religion, spirituality, and health in aging and in gender-diverse populations and offers suggestions for engaging positive links, beliefs, and practices to enhance optimal aging in this population.

8.2 Stigma, Discrimination, Coping, and Resilience

The field of mental health focuses on understanding and supporting people as they work to achieve a sense of wellbeing. *Wellbeing* herein refers to a positive state of perceived comfort, happiness, and/or health. Wellbeing does not equate to perfect health or wealth. Wellbeing is subjective and may change across situations and ages. A person typically self-defines whether they feel they have a sense of wellbeing. External markers that may indicate whether a person feels they have wellbeing can include the presence or relative absence of anxiety, distress, depression, hopelessness, hope, or a sense of self-determination (e.g., control). Mental health and medical professionals may be active participants in the process of supporting a person to achieve their own optimal wellbeing. However, despite their efforts to enhance wellbeing by accessing health care, people who are given some diagnostic labels (e.g., gender dysphoria, borderline, bipolar, fibromyalgia, eating disorder, substance use, HIV, lung cancer, obesity, etc.) may also experience discrimination due to those same diagnoses [18, 19].

Classifying individuals as pathological when they do not experience or express their gender in conformity to dominant cultural definitions (e.g., gender dysphoria) [20, 21] is profoundly stigmatizing [22]. While this diagnosis may enable access to some gender-affirming health care, the negative reactions to the individuals and to the diagnosis also demonstrate ignorance of natural human biologic and cultural variations [22]. Health-care professionals are in a position to provide substantial individual and social support to either normalize or stigmatize the experiences and needs of gender-diverse people. The role of mental health professionals in stigmatizing or normalizing variance in human behavior and development is not new [23]. There is a need to support people to manage the impact of stigma based on gender identity that differs from social expectations. Compounding the problems from stigma, transgender and non-binary populations face a paucity of health-care access and social policy/legal support to protect their wellbeing. There is an important role for health-care professionals to help alleviate stress and buffer stigma in order to reduce the negative impact and attitudes of the culture on gender-diverse people. Integration of spirituality and religious beliefs and practices into treatment needs to be combined with advocacy on behalf of the individual in treatment and the population at large to increase protections against bias and to reduce social stigma, victimization, and violence based on gender identity [24].

Transgender and non-binary older adults have a significantly higher incidence of physical health problems and depression than the general population. This higher incidence of health problems is strongly correlated to the effects of chronic discrimination in the lives of transgender and non-binary people [24, 25]. The combination of depression with the feeling of being a potential burden to others and inability to get needed supports for survival and health is deadly [6, 24]. Whether the individual feels valued and supported or whether they worry about being a burden to others may indicate level of suicide or early mortality risk [6].The rejection of many gender-diverse people from their families [26, 27] may make the presence of spiritual and religious support communities vital to the person's survival. Encouragement of the individual to explore how they may engage or increase supports may help reduce distress and suicidal thoughts and greatly improve quality of life and wellbeing [28]. Exploration about the individual's religious and spiritual understanding of suicide, self-care, and the role of mutual care of others in a community may further reduce or reframe the perception of being a burden and reduce suicide risk [6].

The absence of health care combined with repeated discrimination and bias results in significant health disparities among gender-diverse populations [29, 30]. The lack of protections against overt discrimination in particular contributes to persistent and recurring experiences of bias and unabated violence toward gender-diverse people that does not decrease as one ages [7, 26, 31]. Continual discrimination and trauma throughout one's life span often results in inability to seek, or fear of seeking, care and supports. This results in poor health and fuels self-defeating coping patterns such as substance use and self-injurious behaviors that may significantly shorten the life span and/or result in suboptimal aging [32–34].

There is limited literature on resilience and coping processes in aging gender-diverse populations [1]; nevertheless, it is reasonable to expect that there may be positive benefits from religion and spirituality available to this population similar to other populations [13, 36]. In other marginalized populations such as sexual identity minorities, religious and spiritual involvement is shown to increase positive coping and resilience in the face of adverse life events [35]. Religious and spiritual beliefs, practices, and community involvement are shown to increase positive relationships, deepen a sense of meaning and purpose in life, and to reduce onset of physical and mental illnesses [35]. Engaging in religious and spiritual practices and participating in a welcoming faith or spiritual community are further shown to enhance recovery from severe mental and physical illness, to protect against development of post-traumatic stress disorder, and to reduce early mortality [11, 31–34, 38].

There may be unique challenges to achieving these same beneficial effects within gender-diverse populations. Rejecting messages and actions from religious and spiritual communities may add to discrimination and distress and increase negative outcomes instead of relieving distress. Rejecting religious and spiritual communities and condemning faith-based beliefs and attitudes may keep transgender and non-binary people out of communities, or they may be rejected from previous places of belonging, increasing isolation and loneliness considerably [26]. Spiritual and religious traditions may also have an impact on whether and what gender-affirming body alterations are permissible. For example, under Jewish *Halakhah* (law), alterations of the body must conform to a set of categories and laws that prohibit self-harm or endangerment, castration, interference with God's image, or unnatural changes to the body [40]. However, there are exceptions to these restrictions that can and do allow surgical gender affirmation that is medically necessary, relieves psychological or physical pain, and is performed under safe medically regulated conditions [40]. Likewise, the prohibition against castration has an exception if the surgery is the best hope of preserving life. Similarly, the prohibition against men or women assuming the dress and socially sanctioned roles and behaviors of the opposite assigned sex do not apply to trans men or trans women receiving appropriate medical care, hormone treatments, and appearing congruent with their gender identity [40]. Other religious traditions may prohibit end-of-life or other important rites of passage, such as the proscription in certain Muslim traditions that forbid burial in a religious ceremony or burial site if the genitals have been altered, thereby compounding the distress the individual experiences [41]. Experiences of rejection and discrimination or affirmation by communities of faith may further impair or empower an individual's coping skills and ability to experience wholeness.

The existential impact of rejection from religious and spiritual communities, which may be experienced as rejection directly from a divine being or eternal condemnation, may result in depression, increased anxiety about death, and suicidal thoughts or actions [16, 42, 43]. Even in the case of religious and spiritual rejection, a substantial number of transgender and non-binary people are resilient. They report finding welcoming and supportive religious and spiritual communities after being rejected by their original communities [44]. The research which does explore the current affiliations of gender-diverse older people reports that many espouse connection to some religious, spiritual, or faith tradition in their lives [17]. Among them, a large group (28.78%) identified with some form of prominent Christian traditions. A small percent of respondents affiliated with other prominent traditions (Judaism, Islam; 7.64%). And another small group (9.88%) identified with non-dominant traditions such as Taoism/Buddhism/Confucianism, Baha'i, Pagan/Celtic, Earth/Sun/Goddess worship, Wiccan, First Nations Traditional, and Alternative Healing Circles.

The largest combined group (53.7%) reported "nonspecific spirituality," "not sure," a mixture of beliefs, none, other, agnostic, or atheistic [17]. Within this large varied group, the majority (21.09%) affiliated with an undefined "nonspecific spirituality" with the next biggest proportion (13.25%) identifying as atheist. Looked at another way, this study shows that nearly three-quarters of the gender-diverse elders identified as currently having some religious, spiritual, or faith community affiliation [17]. While the data pool ($n = 1963$) is too small to generalize with certainty to a global gender-diverse older population, it appears there is continued involvement and, therefore, potential benefits of religion and spirituality in the lives of many gender-diverse people as they age. Additional data lends support to this conclusion and indicates that despite the effects of social stigma, widespread and persistent discrimination, lack of access to health care, and limited overall support for living in one's authentic gender, many gender-diverse people report that they are aging successfully, affiliate with some religion or spirituality, and demonstrate the ability to be resilient [1, 9, 17, 30, 45]. Thus, it is important to examine and understand more about the interaction specifically between transgender and non-binary gender-diverse people and religion and spirituality and how we might integrate these relationships into health care to enhance this support for optimal aging.

8.3 Religion, Spirituality, and Aging

Religion and spirituality emerge in several studies as important to optimal aging in general [13, 17, 46, 47]. Religiousness and spirituality also appear to provide a buffer against anxiety and fear of death by providing a sense of hope and a framework by which to find meaning and purpose in one's life and possible opportunities for continued existence past the current experience [48]. Factors connected to religion and spirituality that contribute to wellbeing in the elderly in particular may arise in part from the tendency of older individuals to increase engagement with spiritual and religious practices such as prayer, meditation, reading of sacred texts, and forgiving past offenses of others [13]. In addition, enhanced social support and increased healthier behaviors are associated with involvement in spiritual and religious communities [39, 49, 50]. These positive effects of community involvement and supports may further reduce stress and isolation common in elder gender-diverse populations and may further increase the likelihood to meet their various needs. Enhancement of supports and meeting of needs may enable a more positive outlook and greater sense of wellbeing for transgender and non-binary older adults [17, 39, 49, 50].

Addressing needs and enabling supports within one's community are important to building resilience in any population. Furthermore, social support for and affirmation of authentic gender serve critical roles in the development of resilience in gender-diverse populations [30]. What distinguishes religious and spiritual supports from general and nonspecific supports is that overall wellbeing appears to be uniquely supported through the explanatory framework that religious and spiritual beliefs, practices, and attitudes provide to create life meaning, provide purpose to existence, and engender a sense of control in late life [47]. A sense of control that is often lost due to the functional declines of aging may be restored through religious and spiritual practices or ritual actions that change situations [5, 47]. The increased sense of control is founded on the ability to "do something" through actions, such as prayer or meditation, which bring about healing, safety, comfort, needed resources, calmness, etc. [5, 51–53]. This sense of control may then help reduce a sense of victimhood, powerlessness, or helplessness. Many religious and spiritual practices are already commonly used within health care and demonstrated to assist people to achieve greater control over their individual wellbeing and health, such as meditation, yoga, centering, grounding, changes of diet, forgiveness, gratitude, etc. [52–56].

In addition to social support, explanatory frameworks, and a sense of control, gender differences themselves play a role in the ways religion and spirituality support optimal aging and resilience. For instance, research has found links between gender, religion, and body image in non-transgender older adults [5]. Overall, higher religiosity (e.g., religious devotion, beliefs, attitudes, or practices) predicts lower anxiety about the aging appearance of the body [5]. For non-transgender men, body satisfaction was predicted by religious wellbeing, existential wellbeing (e.g., the reality, experience, and meaning of existing), and feeling their bodies have sacred qualities or are created in the image of God. For non-transgender women, lower aging-appearance anxiety was predicted by intrinsic (e.g., internal) orientation, religious wellbeing, and existential wellbeing [5]. Moreover, the negative effects from a sense of loss of control that may come with aging are mediated by trusting in a higher power or something larger than the self that is personally accessible through prayer or other action/ritual and can intervene to meet needs and comfort [47].

Non-transgender women and men experience support from religious and spiritual community involvement differently from each other. In studies, non-transgender women tend to experience a greater personal connection to the divine or a higher power with non-transgender men tending to experience a greater connection to the religious or spiritual community [57, 58]. These differences of perceived experience may differentially impact wellbeing and perceptions of mental and general health in non-transgender men and women [58, 59]. Even so, how gender-diverse people with masculine, feminine, and non-binary gender identities may experience body image, sense of control, and response to religious and spiritual explanatory frameworks that support wellbeing is largely unexplored in the literature [26, 42, 60, 61]. There is no information to suggest whether transgender and non-binary people experience connections to spiritual and religious communities, beliefs, practices, the divine, or sacredness similar to non-transgender people based on gender or assigned sex. This warrants caution with regard to assumptions about how gender-diverse individuals may experience or understand their connection to religion and spirituality.

For instance, assuming that a trans-masculine person identifies with a masculine deity may overlook any experience of feeling physiologically separated from the physical representation of maleness depicted within religious imagery and language. That sense of physiologic separation may exacerbate gender dysphoria and lead to spiritual and existential conflicts and separation from the religious and spiritual community instead of connection to it. Inquiry about what religious and spiritual beliefs, practices, symbols, etc., the person identifies with offers understanding and insight into spiritual and existential concerns that may impede wellbeing. Understanding more about the person's religious and spiritual beliefs and practices can significantly increase the capacity of the health-care professional to encourage further exploration to potentially strengthen the individual's coping and meaning-making options.

For example, using the above example, a Christian-affiliated trans-male who feels separated by references and images to a male-bodied Jesus may discover a wider range of religious authorities/voices within this tradition who offer other conceptualizations and images of Jesus, including imagery and references to a transformed *Christ* that are non-gendered and androgynous [62–64]. Discovering other voices within a person's larger religious or spiritual tradition may provide access to radical reframing of internal concepts and provide a greater sense of belonging and self-acceptance with the new ability to see their own lived reality also reflected.

Some gender-diverse people may have a blended experience of religion and spirituality as compared to the general population, mixing together the connections and relevance within their traditions in ways that are seen in both non-transgender men or women's gender-distinctive experiences. In some traditions, a more blended experience is more openly reflected, such as in Hinduism, Jainism, Buddhism, and Southeast Asian traditions. In these traditions there are images and stories of divine and non-divine beings that change gender, express fluid gender, or ambiguous gender/third sex whether related to spiritual or moral character or reincarnation [65, 66]. Supporting and encouraging positive connections an individual has to religion and spirituality require asking open, welcoming, and probing questions focused on understanding from what and where the person draws strength within their traditions and practices. Those existing strengths may then form the ground for enhancing and building effective coping strategies and greater chances of optimal aging. Exploration of religion and spirituality means developing some basic concepts of differences across traditions and how those traditions understand gender diversity.

8.4 Religion, Spirituality, and Gender Diversity

Religious and spiritual views on gender-diverse people vary across and within traditions, locations, and time [67]. In the larger society, transgender and non-binary gender identities continue to be conflated with sexual orientation, adding to confusion for everyone as to how to conceptualize gender-diverse people and their experiences. Furthermore, this confusion is compounded by a prevalent and fundamental ignorance of the natural diversity of biological sex, which ignores the existence of animals—including humans—who do not possess exclusively binary sex or gender and who do at times spontaneously change sex [68]. This ignorance then reinforces and reifies uninformed beliefs about the immutability of sex and gender within the natural world that is then used to spiritually and emotionally harm gender-diverse people by implicit or explicit messages that they are abnormal distortions (e.g., "freaks") of nature or representations of evil [69].

Negative social, religious, and spiritual attitudes reinforced by both passive and active ignorance continue to perpetuate bias and violence against gender-diverse populations, complicating connections to support for these individuals [70, 71]. Illustrative of this bias and harm is the impact of dominant US religious traditions (e.g., Christianity, Judaism, Islam) that have historically interpreted gender-diverse people on a range from problematic to evil personified [62, 72–74]. There are, however, exceptions within the dominant and other religious and spiritual groups that are accepting to various degrees and some that have welcomed or found gender diversity to be a spiritual gift to be celebrated or to be an integral aspect of the healthy functioning of a community [37, 75, 76].

As they work to become resilient, gender-diverse individuals may seek out religious and spiritual communities that are more affirming while rejecting those traditions that rejected them [16, 17, 73, 75, 77]. These religious and spiritual traditions may embrace gender-diverse people along a range from "safe enough" [78] to those that are openly welcoming and supportive of individuals living in their authentic gender regardless of sex assigned at birth [16, 42, 45, 61, 75, 79]. The more openly affirmed the person is within their spiritual and religious community, the greater the support and opportunity to achieve wellbeing and optimal aging [35].

In speaking with older gender-diverse people, many report a renewed interest in religious and spiritual practices and communities that increases as they age. This is not unlike the tendency seen in the general population to become more interested in and involved with religious and spiritual communities and practices as they age [47, 80]. Older gender-diverse individuals in particular show a greater participation than younger gender-diverse or sexual minority populations in religious and spiritual traditions and communities that may, in part, be due to their examining religious and spiritual messages more critically [17, 80]. For example, they may explore double standards within spiritual and theological viewpoints of their traditions, such as teaching that all are loved unconditionally, compared to real-life actions by their traditions that reject multiple people and levy heavy conditions on them for acceptance.

Clinicians can support an individual's insights and use this more critical evaluation of the traditions to encourage externalizing seemingly personalized messages of condemnation as separate from their spirituality. Rejecting the condemnation and hypocrisy may then create opportunities to help reframe and reclaim spiritual connectedness to the sacred, to their faith, and to their communities as much as possible [80]. For helping professionals, it is beneficial to talk about how individuals have internalized the old disparaging messages and pain of rejection, to help separate the messages of a particular tradition or group from individual value or worth, and to help shift the emotional energy of that pain into motivating energy to explore and seek knowledge about what they find meaningful in spite of the dominant messages. This rejection of internalized condemnation supports the person by empowering the building of internalized self-worth. Enabling and encouraging a personal commitment to holding one's own experiences and existence as authoritative or informative support spiritual and religious exploration and development of an internalized sense of wellbeing and self-acceptance that is less vulnerable to external messages of rejection. This may be understood as the distinction between the questions "Who are you?" and "Who do others say you are?"

In this process of exploration of messages from an individual's religious and spiritual traditions, it is important to suspend an investment in the person going to where the clinician may wish they would go. Some will remain in and renew commitments to their religious and spiritual foundations with a more open interpretation of their tradition's sacred writings and doctrine informed by personal study beyond the sanctioned and filtered lessons decided by others [63, 73, 81]. Some will boldly claim divine spiritual acceptance in defiance of exclusionary religious interpretations of who is included and excluded from relationships with the sacred, as defined in that tradition, or with the community [82, 83]. Some will rediscover and enliven ancient traditions such as Earth-based traditions, Pagan, or Wicca and reinterpret them into modern life to find acceptance and meaning and belonging for themselves and other gender-diverse and rejected people [75]. Some will reject all religious and spiritual traditions [77]. What is clear is that gender-diverse people do continue to experience vibrant connections to something sacred beyond themselves, to something divine, and to religious and spiritual beliefs and practices in which they find value, meaning, purpose, and support to endure, to be resilient, and to create meaning and purpose in their lives. Health-care professionals need to engage, explore, and support development of the religious and spiritual practices and community connections of gender-diverse people if health care is to be relevant and effective at all in supporting optimal aging in this population.

8.5 Engaging and Utilizing Religious and Spiritual Connections

There is evidence that mental health treatment that incorporates religion and spirituality may have a positive impact on outcome and initial willingness to engage in treatment and supports [84]. Of special significance to older adults who may have increased prevalence of depression and medical challenges are interventions that intentionally incorporate the individual's spirituality and religious beliefs and practices. This spiritual and religious belief and practice-integrated treatment has been shown to have measurable positive effects on relieving depression and depression related to medical illness and to support overall restoration of functioning [10, 84, 85].

Outcomes are improved when people seek supports sooner rather than later. Knowing a health-care provider will ask about and incorporate one's beliefs and practices into treatment encourages people to seek care sooner [14]. When clinicians are not equipped to incorporate spirituality and religious beliefs and practices into treatment, it creates a primary barrier to accessing care in a timely way, and it disrupts the relationship between the clinician and the individual seeking care [86]. Lack of training of health-care professionals in incorporating spirituality and religious beliefs and practices into treatment may cause the professional to deflect, avoid, or squash the person's desire to talk about their existential concerns. Ignorance on the part of the clinician may also cause harm to the individual by violating their beliefs and values and increasing their stress [86].

The problem does not appear to be with the ability to incorporate practices borrowed from religion and spirituality into mainstream treatment but in the awareness of the background of the practices and in the absence of gaining explicit consent to bring religious or spiritual practices into treatment [86]. Health care already incorporates religious and spiritual practices into care in the use of mindfulness, centering, grounding, and meditative practices within mental health fields in particular [87]. These practices arise largely from Eastern religious traditions, with a few from Christianity, though there appears little awareness or acknowledgement of these connections in the application or in educating providers or patients about these practices.

Recognizing and incorporating these practices, while being ignorant of the connection to a specific spirituality or religion, or intentionally divorcing the connection to religious and spiritual beliefs and practices due to professional or personal anti-religious bias, hinders the potential benefit of the treatment. Ignorance of the religious and spiritual origins of many of these practices eliminates the chance to invite other practices and beliefs of the individual into treatment to strengthen their coping skills. It is vitally important to know the spiritual and religious struggles a person may be coping with prior to introducing a spiritual practice that has been adopted by health care and supposedly stripped of its context.

Context is crucial. Some individuals may express resistance to adopting the practices of another religious or spiritual faith by simply not doing the exercises or "forgetting" to do them. This may then be misinterpreted as treatment resistance to the professional who is unaware of the spiritual tradition out of which the intervention arises and who has not asked whether it does or does not integrate with the person's own religious and spiritual beliefs. For instance, centering—the practice of saying a single word or phrase (e.g., *mantra*) repeatedly to focus the mind in a sort of self-hypnosis to clear the mind—may be seen by some Christians as antithetical to the relational connectedness that requires dialog, or as idolatry based on the words or names used to focus. To others, meditation for calming or insight may be seen as a misguided attempt to reach personal divinity or to elevate oneself outside human existence (transcend the current suffering).

One does not need to know the minute details of each potential religion or spiritual tradition to engage in integrative treatment, however. It is important instead to know that there are traditions and history from which came the practices used in treatment and to get informed consent from the individual to bring these practices into their care. This approach enables the clinician to discuss the practices being recommended with the individual, to explore whether the practices would be helpful, or whether there are similar spiritual and religious practices within their own traditions that can be used instead. For instance, a clinician might discuss the reality that meditation, even though used in therapy, is from Eastern religious traditions. They can then ask the individual if that is comfortable for them or if they use similar traditions that are soothing and help reduce worries and problems and increase a sense of calmness.

Instead of a centering or meditation meant to go singularly inside the self and clear the mind, perhaps the person would want to use *Lectio Divina*, a practice out of Catholicism of reading a small section of scripture, focusing on and praying about the words read, and then reflecting on the meaning, before possibly moving to another small portion of the text to repeat the process. This practice is intended to promote relational communication with God and perspective on one's existence. The outcome would be a comparable alternate practice to a more Eastern tradition practice in which one clears the mind of all thoughts and connection with anything other than the individual self and feels one with everything. They are nuanced distinctions, yet for the individual whose religious and spiritual beliefs and practices they align with or offend, the distinctions are critical. Staying focused on the desired outcome and incorporating the practices, beliefs, and coping options that are already meaningful to the person will have a more powerful and enduring result.

The issue is one of competence in health-care professionals who lack knowledge about the origins and significance of "tools" they may employ indiscriminately with a desire to enhance health. There may also be present an assumption on the part of clinicians that gender-diverse people cannot be spiritual or religious, resulting in failure to consider the presence of spiritual or religious beliefs or practices in the individual's life [88]. In addition to the above suggestions, to assist people to explore the role of religion and spirituality in their lives requires active elimination of personal religious and spiritual discrimination and bias in health care. Access to unbiased, relevant, and competent treatment is essential to wellbeing and can enhance optimal aging in the gender diverse—and any—population. To provide equitable and competent care then, clinicians need to develop and exercise intentional restraint from imposing their own religious and spiritual beliefs and practices on the individual in treatment. This restraint from imposing the clinician's own value system and beliefs on the individual enables the individual in treatment to explore their own beliefs and traditions more openly and authentically without fear of punitive action or of upsetting the clinician. Undoubtedly, there will be challenges for some health-care staff in suspending their personal worldviews in order to provide the most unbiased care and supports possible.

When there are significant staff-to-patient differences of personal experiences and cultural and value-based beliefs (e.g., sexual practices, birth control, abortion, psychotropic medicine, religious beliefs, practices, behaviors, etc.) that impede the ability of the clinician to provide objective, respectful, and sensitive care—regardless of population served—it is essential that the clinician recognize and communicate their personal conflict and offer referrals to other clinical professionals who do not have that conflict of interest and can treat the individual equitably according to that person's needs. Conflicts of interest or impeded ability to provide appropriate and unbiased care are not uncommon in many areas of health care and may be due to many factors. Conflicts of interest that would require responsible transfer to another clinician do not always imply negative attitudes toward the person. Recognizing one's discomfort or bias toward spiritually integrated health care may be more challenging in health-care professions. There are no uniform educational and clinical mentoring opportunities within all clinical health fields for training clinicians to recognize and bracket their personal religious and spiritual beliefs and practices from their treatment actions and choices, though it is recognized as beneficial in clinical training [88]. Applying clinical training learned to maintain other professional boundaries may be generalized onto boundaries where it concerns religion and spirituality without the need to shun integrating religion and spirituality into treatment. All helping professionals will encounter challenges to remaining neutral and keeping clear boundaries at times. Protecting individuals from undue influence or harm in the areas of religion and spirituality are not any different.

For example, a provider may overidentify with the discrimination and bias faced by a client if it is similar to something the clinician has experienced. This may in turn trigger the health-care provider who may get caught in their own internal reactions and processes of reliving their personal emotions, reactions, choices, and regrets or anger to the similar experience. When this happens it stops the clinician's ability to engage in any exploration or lend meaningful supports or guidance to assist the individual because they are temporarily unable to separate their own experiences from the individual's situation. Likewise, clinicians may distance themselves from experiences and information so rigidly that they may minimize or dismiss the concerns of the individual. This stops the process of treatment to protect the clinician and blocks engagement in needed supports for the individual [67]. The latter is the more common experience in health care for gender-diverse people and for people who want to bring their religious and spiritual concerns into treatment. For a substantial percentage of people, their understanding of spirituality and the sacred in their lives is essential to their identity and resilience [86]. Blocking or dismissing the importance of religion and spirituality within treatment therefore blocks and dismisses an individual's core sense of identity and removes a potentially significant source of resilience from being used.

Too often in health care, it is specifically a person's religious and spiritual beliefs, practices, and values that are ignored, avoided, demeaned, redirected, or minimized in spite of the clear evidence that these supports and practices may enhance wellbeing, protect against illness and trauma, and increase resilience [13, 17, 46, 47]. The common resistance within modern health care to fully assess and understand religious and spiritual beliefs and practices as integral to clinical care, equivalent to routine biological, psychological, and social assessments, impairs successful treatment and contributes to increased anxiety and suffering at the end of life by refusal or incompetence to incorporate systems of meaning and value into treatment [48, 89, 90]. Professional resistance to spiritually integrated treatment combined with the high potential for professionals to hold religious and cultural beliefs that also reject gender-diverse individuals [88] increases the likelihood of poor outcomes or avoidance of care altogether [19, 26, 31, 91]. In this cycle, unexamined clinician bias leads to supports being ineffective and even harmful through unintentional or willful rejection of the needs and values of the individual. The more times gender-diverse individuals experience discrimination and rejection in health care, the less they seek health care for otherwise treatable conditions [26]. The effect of avoidance of care is cumulative over time and may lead to older gender-diverse people with complex issues due to lack of treatment over decades of life that then limit wellbeing and increase early mortality in this population [3, 24, 92].

In practice, to avoid or deflect issues around someone's religious and spiritual concerns or the interaction with a person's wellbeing and ability to cope is disrespectful to the individual and conveys a message that their values, beliefs, and practices are unimportant or irrelevant to their health [67]. Avoidance or deflection of spiritual and religious issues may indicate an issue of overt or implicit bias imposed on the individual by the health-care support staff or system without regard to the person's values. Likewise, insisting on a gender-diverse person complying with or espousing religious and spiritual beliefs that are not their own in order to receive needed supports is harmful and inappropriate in any health-care setting [88].

8.6 Assessing for Spiritual and Religious Relevance and Strengths

As part of any work with older gender-diverse adults, a full assessment of mental health, medical and social history, and wellbeing needs to include a spiritual assessment. Assessment of religious and spiritual beliefs and practices needs to include evaluating whether the individual feels supported by or a burden to their religious and spiritual community, family, or other interpersonal relationships. An initial assessment may be as simple as expressing interest and curiosity about whether the individual holds spirituality or religion important. Asking, "Do you have any religious or spiritual beliefs or practices that are important to you?" is a start. Based on the answer, the clinician may want to explore more in-depth. Exploring more may take place over time and may include asking whether the person participates in any spiritual or religious services, practices, rituals, or activities [86].

A more exploratory process would need to be increasingly specific based on answers given, such as asking about attendance at a mosque instead of a church or temple if the person identified an affiliation with Islam and not with Christianity or Judaism. Checking back in with the person to assess whether the questions are being respectful of their traditions and beliefs is part of the process. For some religious or spiritual traditions, it is inappropriate to discuss details of practices with someone outside their tradition or who is not a religious guide or leader [86]. The process builds on the early inquiries across time and may include exploring strengths such as particular practices or beliefs the person finds helpful when they experience challenges. In this process a clinician can signal openly that the person's spirituality and religion are welcome and will be integrated into care. The clinician can also determine whether and to what extent the person integrates spirituality and religious beliefs and practices into their lives and whether there are existing practices that enhance coping and can be built upon if needed. Exploration also needs to include respectful curiosity about whether there are any particular things within their religious or spiritual life that cause them distress or whether they believe there is some connection between their life experiences, the current situation, their gender identity, or struggles that are directly connected to their beliefs or their relationship to their religious and spiritual community [60, 86, 93]. It is essential to both assess for and to remain open to the possibility that religious and spiritual beliefs and practices are important to the individual *and* they do not want to discuss them in the current care or with the particular clinician to whom they are speaking.

Conclusion

In summary, engaging with gender-diverse individuals in an unbiased way that affirms their authentic and espoused gender will aid in the establishment or improvement of supports that can lead to greater wellbeing and optimal aging. Inseparable from an affirming and unbiased approach is the need to assess for and integrate the individual's religious and spiritual beliefs and practices initially and throughout the caring relationship [86]. Integrating religious and spiritual beliefs and practices into health care demands unbiased exploration of systems of meaning, coping skills, and strengths available to the individual. Assessment also includes exploring potentially harmful effects from religious and spiritual messages, practices, and experiences in the person's life [94]. With gender-diverse older adults, there is a particular need to assess for any distress that may be directly due to their gender diversity and conflicts with religious or spiritual beliefs, practices, and end-of-life rites of passage, death and burial rituals, or existential anxiety (e.g., fear of eternal damnation, divine rejection or punishment, etc.).

Understanding the role and influence of religion and spirituality in the gender-diverse elder's life may provide key insights into problematic internalized beliefs or behaviors. There may be direct connections between religious and spiritual beliefs and practices and the individual's experience or expression of their authentic gender [29, 41]. Exploring and understanding specific benefits from their current religious and spiritual practices, community, and organizing beliefs is essential to supporting and increasing resilience [95]. There is a critical necessity of addressing and remedying any harmful effects from hostile and abusive care of gender-diverse older adults [7, 9, 29].

Care that enables resilience and optimal aging must include a commitment to integrating what individuals consider sacred, life-sustaining, and organizing systems of value and meaning for their own lives. Optimal care requires integration of spiritual and religious beliefs and practices. Taking an intentional and open approach to exploring the role of religion and spirituality throughout the entirety of care can improve supports. Understanding and making the most of an individual's existing religious and spiritual practices that support self-care (e.g., strengths) will effectively reduce stress, increase a sense of agency and life control, and enable more optimal aging.

References

1. McFadden SH, Frankowski S, Flick H, Witten TM. Resilience and multiple stigmatized identities: Lessons from transgender persons' reflections on aging. In: Sinnott JD, editor. Positive psychology [Internet]. New York: Springer New York; 2013 [cited 2014 Dec 1]. p. 247–67. Available from: http://link.springer.com/10.1007/978-1-4614-7282-7_16.
2. Comfort A. The biology of senescence [Internet]. New York: Rinehart; 1956 [cited 2018 Jan 28]. 284 p. Available from: http://archive.org/details/biologyofsenesce00comf.
3. Vahia IV, Chattillion E, Kavirajan H, Depp CA. Psychological protective factors across the lifespan: implications for psychiatry. Psychiatr Clin. 2011;34(1):231–48.
4. Brummel-Smith K. Optimal aging, part I: demographics and definitions. Ann Long-Term Care Clin Care Aging [Internet]. 2007 [cited 2018 Jan 27];15(11). Available from: https://www.managedhealthcareconnect.com/article/7994.
5. Homan KJ, Boyatzis CJ. Body image in older adults: links with religion and gender. J Adult Dev. 2009;16(4):230–8.
6. Jahn D, Cukrowicz K, Linton K, Prabhu F. The mediating effect of perceived burdensomeness on the relation between depressive symptoms and suicide ideation in a community sample of older adults. Aging Ment Health. 2011;15(2):214–20.
7. Cook-Daniels L, Munson M. Sexual violence, elder abuse, and sexuality of transgender adults, age 50+: results of three surveys. J GLBT Fam Stud. 2010;6(2):142–77.

8. Cook-Daniels L. Lesbian, gay, bisexual, and transgender aging. In: Kimmel D, Rose T, David S, editors. Lesbian, gay, bisexual, and transgender aging: research and clinical perspectives. New York: Columbia University Press; 2006. p. 20–35.
9. Witten TM. It's not all darkness: robustness, resilience, and successful transgender aging. LGBT Health. 2014;1(1):24–33.
10. Pearce MJ. Addressing religion and spirituality in health care systems. In: Pargament KI, Mahoney A, Shafranske EP, editors. APA handbook of psychology, religion, and spirituality (vol. 2): An applied psychology of religion and spirituality. Washington, DC: American Psychological Association; 2013 [cited 2017 Dec 26]. p. 527–41. (APA handbooks in psychology).
11. Koenig H, McCullough ME, Larson DB. Handbook of religion and health. Oxford/New York: Oxford University Press; 2001.
12. US Census Bureau. The Nation's older population is still growing, Census Bureau reports [Internet]. US Census Bureau; 2017 Jun [cited 2018 Jan 22]. Report No.: CB17-100. Available from: https://www.census.gov/newsroom/press-releases/2017/cb17-100.html.
13. Krause N. Religious involvement in the later years of life. In: Pargament KI, Exline JJ, Jones JW, editors. APA handbook of psychology, religion, and spirituality (vol. 1): Context, theory, and research [Internet]. Washington, DC: American Psychological Association; 2013 [cited 2017 Dec 23]. p. 529–45. (APA handbooks in psychology).
14. Koenig H. Research on religion, spirituality, and mental health: a review. Can J Psychiatr. 2009;54(5):283–91.
15. Pargament K, Magyar-Russell GM, Murray-Swank NA. The sacred and the search for significance: religion as a unique process. J Soc Issues. 2005;61(4):665–87.
16. Hopwood RA, Witten TM. Spirituality, faith, and religion: the TGNC experience. In: Singh AA, Dickey LM, editors. Affirmative counseling and psychological practice with transgender and gender nonconforming clients. Washington, DC: American Psychological Association; 2017. p. 213–30.
17. Porter KE, Ronneberg CR, Witten TM. Religious affiliation and successful aging among transgender older adults: findings from the Trans MetLife Survey. J Relig Spiritual Aging. 2013;25(2):112–38.
18. Mizock L, Mueser KT. Employment, mental health, internalized stigma, and coping with transphobia among transgender individuals. Psychol Sex Orientat Gend Divers. 2014;1(2):146–58.
19. Mizock L, Hopwood RA, Casey H, Duhamel E, Herrick A, Puerto G, et al. The transgender awareness webinar: reducing transphobia among undergraduates and mental health providers. J Gay Lesb Ment Health. 2017;21(4):292–315.
20. American Psychiatric Association. Diagnostic and statistical manual of mental disorders: DSM-5. 5th ed. Arlington: American Psychiatric Association; 2013. p. 947.
21. Inch E. Changing minds: the psycho-pathologization of trans people. Int J Ment Health. 2016;45(3):193–204.
22. Drescher J. Queer diagnoses revisited: the past and future of homosexuality and gender diagnoses in DSM and ICD. Int Rev Psychiatry. 2015;27(5):386–95. Early Online:1–10.
23. Boskey E. Sexuality in the DSM 5. (cover story). Contemp Sex. 2013;47(7):1–5.
24. Fredriksen-Goldsen KI, Cook-Daniels L, Kim H-J, Erosheva EA, Emlet CA, Hoy-Ellis CP, et al. Physical and mental health of transgender older adults: an at-risk and underserved population. The Gerontologist. 2014;54(3):488–500.
25. Testa RJ, Habarth J, Peta J, Balsam K, Bockting W. Development of the gender minority stress and resilience measure. Psychol Sex Orientat Gend Divers. 2015;2(1):65–77.
26. James SE, Herman JL, Rankin S, Keisling M, Mottet L, Anafi M. The report of the 2015 U.S. transgender Survey [Internet]. Washington, DC: National Center for Transgender Equality; 2016 [cited 2016 Dec 9] p. 297. Available from: http://www.transequality.org/sites/default/files/docs/USTS-Full-Report-FINAL.PDF.
27. Klein A, Golub SA. Family rejection as a predictor of suicide attempts and substance misuse among transgender and gender nonconforming adults. LGBT Health. 2016;3(3):193–9.

28. Başar K, Öz G, Karakaya J. Perceived discrimination, social support, and quality of life in gender dysphoria. J Sex Med. 2016;13(7):1133–41.
29. Porter KE, Brennan-Ing M, Chang SC, Dickey LM, Singh AA, Bower KL, et al. Providing competent and affirming services for transgender and gender nonconforming older adults. Clin Gerontol. 2016;21:1–24.
30. Bockting W, Coleman E, Deutsch MB, Guillamon A, Meyer I, Meyer W, et al. Adult development and quality of life of transgender and gender nonconforming people. Curr Opin Endocrinol Diabetes Obes. 2016;23(2):188–97.
31. Rood BA, Reisner SL, Surace FI, Puckett JA, Maroney MR, Pantalone DW. Expecting rejection: understanding the minority stress experiences of transgender and gender-nonconforming individuals. Transgend Health. 2016;1(1):151–64.
32. White Hughto JM, Pachankis JE, Willie TC, Reisner SL. Victimization and depressive symptomology in transgender adults: the mediating role of avoidant coping. J Couns Psychol. 2017;64(1):41–51.
33. Reisner SL, White Hughto JM, Gamarel KE, Keuroghlian AS, Mizock L, Pachankis JE. Discriminatory experiences associated with posttraumatic stress disorder symptoms among transgender adults. J Couns Psychol. 2016;63(5):509–19.
34. Longo J, Walls NE, Wisneski H. Religion and religiosity: protective or harmful factors for sexual minority youth? Ment Health Relig Cult. 2013;16(3):273–90.
35. Rosenkrantz DE, Rostosky SS, Riggle EDB, Cook JR. The positive aspects of intersecting religious/spiritual and LGBTQ identities. Spiritual Clin Pract. 2016;3(2):127–38.
36. Harrison MO, Koenig H, Hays JC, Eme-Akwari AG, Pargament K. The epidemiology of religious coping: a review of recent literature. Int Rev Psychiatry. 2001;13(2):86–93.
37. Brewster ME, Velez BL, Foster A, Esposito J, Robinson MA. Minority stress and the moderating role of religious coping among religious and spiritual sexual minority individuals. J Couns Psychol. 2016;63(1):119–26.
38. Webb M, Charbonneau AM, McCann RA, Gayle KR. Struggling and enduring with God, religious support, and recovery from severe mental illness. J Clin Psychol. 2011;67(12):1161–76.
39. George LK, Larson DB, Koenig H, McCullough ME. Spirituality and health: what we know, what we need to know. J Soc Clin Psychol. 2000;19(1):102–16.
40. Sharzer LA. Transgender Jews and Halakhah. 2017 Jun 7;30. Available from: https://www.rabbinicalassembly.org/sites/default/files/public/halakhah/teshuvot/2011-2020/transgender-halakhah.pdf
41. Teh YK. Mak nyahs (male transsexuals) in Malaysia: The influence of culture and religion on their identity. Int J Transgenderism [Internet]. 2001 Jul [cited 2010 May 16];5(3):97.
42. Brandenstein N. Ultimate transformation: therapeutic and spiritual integration within the transgender experience. Indianapolis: Christian Theological Seminary; 2001.
43. Kennedy JW. The transgender moment. Christ Today. 2008;52(2):54–8.
44. Tabaac A, Witten T. Trans* people and religion/spirituality. In: Goldberg AE, editor. SAGE encyclopedia of LGBTQ studies. 1st ed. Thousand Oaks: SAGE Publications, Inc.; 2016. p. 229–41.
45. Bautista D, Mountain Q, Reynolds HM. Religion and spirituality. In: Erickson-Schroth L, editor. Trans bodies, trans selves: a resource for the transgender community. Oxford/New York: Oxford University Press; 2014. p. 62–79.
46. Abeles R, Ellison C, George L, Idler E, Krause N, Levin J, et al. Fetzer multidimensional measurement of religiousness/spirituality for use in health research: A report of the Fetzer Institute/National Institute on Aging Working Group. John E. Fetzer Institute; 2003 [cited 2011 Jan 23]. Available from: http://www.seminare-ps.net/Rel-Psy/Fetzer_Multidimens_Measurement_Religiousness.pdf.
47. Fiori KL, Hays JC, Meador KG. Spiritual turning points and perceived control over the life course. Int J Aging Hum Dev. 2004;59(4):391–420.
48. Soenke M, Landau MJ, Greenberg J. Sacred armor: religion's role as a buffer against the anxieties of life and the fear of death. In: Pargament KI, Exline JJ, Jones JW, editors. APA

handbook of psychology, religion, and spirituality (vol. 1): Context, theory, and research. Washington, DC: American Psychological Association; 2013 [cited 2017 Dec 23]. p. 105–22. (APA handbooks in psychology).
49. Koenig HG, Pearce MJ, Nelson B, Daher N. Effects of religious versus standard cognitive-behavioral therapy on optimism in persons with major depression and chronic mental illness. Depress Anxiety. 2015;32(11):835–42.
50. Park J, Roh S, Yeo Y. Religiosity, social support, and life satisfaction among elderly Korean immigrants. The Gerontologist. 2012;52(5):641–9.
51. Idler EL. Rituals and practices. In: Pargament KI, Exline JJ, Jones JW, editors. APA handbook of psychology, religion, and spirituality (vol. 1): Context, theory, and research. Washington, DC: American Psychological Association; 2013 [cited 2017 Dec 23]. p. 329–47. (APA handbooks in psychology).
52. Gall TL, Guirguis-Younger M. Religious and spiritual coping: Current theory and research. In: Pargament KI, Exline JJ, Jones JW, editors. APA handbook of psychology, religion, and spirituality (vol. 1): Context, theory, and research. Washington, DC: American Psychological Association; 2013 [cited 2017 Dec 23]. p. 349–64. (APA handbooks in psychology).
53. Ai AL, Bjorck JP, Appel HB, Huang B. Asian American spirituality and religion: Inherent diversity, uniqueness, and long-lasting psychological influences. In: Pargament KI, Exline JJ, Jones JW, editors. APA handbook of psychology, religion, and spirituality (vol. 1): Context, theory, and research. Washington, DC: American Psychological Association; 2013 [cited 2017 Dec 23]. p. 581–98. (APA handbooks in psychology).
54. Wachholtz AB, Austin ET. Contemporary spiritual meditation: Practices and outcomes. In: Pargament KI, Exline JJ, Jones JW, editors. APA handbook of psychology, religion, and spirituality (vol. 1): Context, theory, and research. Washington, DC: American Psychological Association; 2013 [cited 2017 Dec 23]. p. 311–27. (APA handbooks in psychology).
55. McCullough ME, Carter EC. Religion, self-control, and self-regulation: How and why are they related? In: Pargament KI, Exline JJ, Jones JW, editors. APA handbook of psychology, religion, and spirituality (vol. 1): Context, theory, and research. Washington, DC: American Psychological Association; 2013 [cited 2017 Dec 23]. p. 123–38. (APA handbooks in psychology).
56. Ladd KL, Spilka B. Prayer: A review of the empirical literature. In: Pargament KI, Exline JJ, Jones JW, editors. APA handbook of psychology, religion, and spirituality (vol. 1): Context, theory, and research. Washington, DC: American Psychological Association; 2013 [cited 2017 Dec 23]. p. 293–310. (APA handbooks in psychology).
57. Bjorck JP, Maslim AA. The multi-faith religious support scale: validation with a sample of Muslim women. J Muslim Ment Health. 2011;6(1). Available from: http://hdl.handle.net/2027/spo.10381607.0006.105.
58. Lazar A, Bjorck JP. Gender differences in the structure and perception of religious support in a religious Jewish sample. Psychol Relig Spiritual. 2016;8(3):235–43.
59. Reid-Arndt SA, Smith ML, Yoon DP, Johnstone B. Gender differences in spiritual experiences, religious practices, and congregational support for individuals with significant health conditions. J Relig Disabil Health. 2011;15(2):175–96.
60. Plante TG. Addressing problematic spirituality in therapy. In: Spiritually oriented interventions for counseling and psychotherapy. Washington, DC: American Psychological Association; 2011 [cited 2014 Mar 24]. p. 83–106.
61. Wood AW, Conley AH. Loss of religious or spiritual identities among the LGBT population. Couns Values. 2014;59(1):95–111.
62. Mollenkott V. Omnigender: a trans-religious approach. Cleveland: Pilgrim Press; 2001.
63. Wilson NL. Our tribe: queer folks, god, Jesus, and the bible. 1st ed. San Francisco: Harper San Francisco; 1995. p. 292.
64. Loughlin G. Refiguring masculinity in Christ. In: Hayes MA, Porter WJ, Tombs D, editors. Religion and sexuality. London: Bloomsbury Academic; 2016. p. 405–14.
65. Ganguly L. "Who are they?": the third sex in India. Int J Eng Sci Res. 2015;6(8):3.

66. Goldman RP. Transsexualism, gender, and anxiety in traditional India. J Am Orient Soc. 1993;113(3):374.
67. Balkin RS, Watts RE, Ali SR. A conversation about the intersection of faith, sexual orientation, and gender: Jewish, Christian, and Muslim perspectives. J Couns Dev. 2014;92(2):187–93.
68. The extraordinary case of the Guevedoces. BBC News [Internet]. 2015 Sep 20 [cited 2018 May 4]; Available from: http://www.bbc.com/news/magazine-34290981.
69. Roughgarden J. Evolution's rainbow: diversity, gender, and sexuality in nature and people. Berkeley: University of California Press; 2009. p. 474.
70. McQueeney K. "We are God's children, Y'All:" race, gender, and sexuality in lesbian- and gay-affirming congregations. Soc Probl. 2009;56(1):151–73.
71. Worthen MGF. An argument for separate analyses of attitudes toward lesbian, gay, bisexual men, bisexual women, MtF and FtM transgender individuals. Sex Roles. 2013;68(11–12):703–23.
72. Roscoe W. Priests of the goddess: gender transgression in ancient religion. Hist Relig. 1996;35(3):195–230.
73. Tanis J. Trans-gendered: theology, ministry, and communities of faith. Cleveland: Pilgrim Press; 2003.
74. Najmabadi A. Transing and transpassing across sex-gender walls in Iran. Women's Stud Q. 2008;36(3/4):23–42.
75. Kaldera R. Hermaphrodeities: the transgender spirituality workbook. Hubbardston: Asphodel Press; 2009.
76. Slater S, Yarbrough FA. Gender and sexuality in indigenous North America, 1400–1850. Columbia: University of South Carolina Press; 2010. [cited 2018 Feb 11].
77. Hopwood R. Conceptualizations of religion in a sample of female-to-male transsexuals: an interpretative phenomenological analysis [Doctoral dissertation]. Boston: Boston University; 2013.
78. Foster K, Bowland S, Vosler A. All the pain along with all the joy: spiritual resilience in lesbian and gay Christians. Am J Community Psychol. 2015;55(1/2):191–201.
79. Levy DL, Lo JR. Transgender, transsexual, and gender queer individuals with a Christian upbringing: the process of resolving conflict between gender identity and faith. J Relig Spiritual Soc Work Soc Thought. 2013;32(1):60–83.
80. Brennan-Ing M, Seidel L, Larson B, Karpiak SE. "I'm created in God's image, and god don't create junk": religious participation and support among older GLBT adults. J Relig Spiritual Aging. 2013;25(2):70–92.
81. Gomes PJ. The good book: reading the Bible with mind and heart [Internet]. 1st ed. New York, NY US: Avon Books, Inc.; 1996 [cited 2018 May 4]. 400 p.
82. Heller LF. In: Johnson JA, editor. By the grace of god: writings for families, friends and clergy. Wheaton: SSP Publications; 2001. p. 368.
83. Gomes PJ. The scandalous Gospel of Jesus: what's so good about the good news? 1st ed. New York, NY US: HarperCollins; 2007 [cited 2018 May 4]. 264 p.
84. Koenig HG, Pearce MJ, Nelson B, Shaw SF, Robins CJ, Daher NS, et al. Religious vs. conventional cognitive behavioral therapy for major depression in persons with chronic medical illness: a pilot randomized trial. J Nerv Ment Dis. 2015;203(4):243–51.
85. Pargament KI. Spiritually integrated psychotherapy: understanding and addressing the sacred. New York: Guilford Press; 2011. p. 401.
86. Hodge DR. Assessing spirituality and religion in the context of counseling and psychotherapy. In: Pargament KI, Mahoney A, Shafranske EP, editors. APA handbook of psychology, religion, and spirituality (vol. 2): An applied psychology of religion and spirituality. Washington, DC: American Psychological Association; 2013 [cited 2017 Dec 26]. p. 93–123. (APA handbooks in psychology).
87. Bergemann ER, Siegel MW, Belzer MG, Siegel DJ, Feuille M. Mindful awareness, spirituality, and psychotherapy. In: Mahoney A, Shafranske EP, Pargament KI, editors. APA handbook of psychology, religion, and spirituality (vol. 2): An applied psychology of religion and spirituality. Washington, DC: American Psychological Association; 2013 [cited 2017 Dec 26]. p. 207–22. (APA handbooks in psychology).

88. McGeorge C, Carlson T, Toomey R. The intersection of spirituality, religion, sexual orientation, and gender identity in family therapy training: an exploration of students' beliefs and practices. Contemp Fam Ther Int J. 2014;36(4):497–506.
89. Dezutter J, Soenens B, Hutsebaut D. Religiosity and mental health: a further exploration of the relative importance of religious behaviors vs. religious attitudes. Personal Individ Differ. 2006;40(4):807–18.
90. Rizzuto A-M, Shafranske EP. Addressing religion and spirituality in treatment from a psychodynamic perspective. In: Pargament KI, Mahoney A, Shafranske EP, editors. APA handbook of psychology, religion, and spirituality (vol. 2): An applied psychology of religion and spirituality. Washington, DC: American Psychological Association; 2013 [cited 2017 Dec 26]. p. 125–46. (APA handbooks in psychology).
91. Gonsiorek JC, Richards PS, Pargament K, McMinn MR. Ethical challenges and opportunities at the edge: incorporating spirituality and religion into psychotherapy. Prof Psychol Res Pract. 2009;40(4):385–95.
92. Rood BA, Puckett JA, Pantalone DW, Bradford JB. Predictors of suicidal ideation in a statewide sample of transgender individuals. LGBT Health. 2014;2(3):270–5.
93. Plante TG. Thirteen tools from religious-spiritual thought: definitions and philosophical grounding. In: Spiritual practices in psychotherapy: thirteen tools for enhancing psychological health. American Psychological Association: Washington, DC; 2009 [cited 2014 Mar 24]. p. 29–46.
94. Pargament KI, Zinnbauer BJ, Scott AB, Butter EM, Zerowin J, Stanik P. Red flags and religious coping: identifying some religious warning signs among people in crisis. J Clin Psychol. 2003;59(12):1335–48.
95. Pargament K. The bitter and the sweet: an evaluation of the costs and benefits of religiousness. Psychol Inq. 2002;13(3):168–81.

Integrating Intersectionality when Working with Trans Older Adults

9

Anneliese A. Singh, Natalia Truszczynski, Lindsay White, Sand Chang, and Zyer Beatty

As older trans adults continue to age, there are multiple and intersecting identities that influence the experiences they have of their gender identities and expressions [1, 19]. For instance, older trans adults of different racial/ethnic identities can have distinctly different racialized experiences of their gender [7]. Over the last two decades in healthcare provision, scholars and providers have used intersectionality theory to explain some of the differences in multiple social identity intersections that can result in advantages, disadvantages, or a mix of both privilege and oppression experiences [4]. However, although intersectionality has become the new "buzz word" in healthcare provision, there is still little understanding of what this word means – especially as this theory relates to working with older trans adults. In this chapter, we define intersectionality theory, discuss examples of social identity intersections and locations so they can be defined fully, and provide case examples of how healthcare providers can use intersectionality theory to best support the resilience and overall well-being of the older trans adults with whom they work.

9.1 Defining Intersectionality Theory, Social Identities, Privilege, and Oppression

"Intersectionality" references not only the multiple and intersecting social identities that people may have but also the systems of interlocking and overlapping oppressions that occur in society for certain groups [8]. Crenshaw described intersectionality as an important perspective for understanding the unemployment experiences of Black women in her essay titled, "Mapping the Margins." In this essay, Crenshaw

A. A. Singh (✉) · Z. Beatty
Department of Counseling and Human Development Services, University of Georgia, Atlanta, GA, USA

N. Truszczynski · L. White · S. Chang
Department of Health Promotion and Behavior, University of Georgia, Atlanta, GA, USA

M. Houlberg et al. (eds.), *Transgender and Gender Nonconforming Health and Aging*, https://doi.org/10.1007/978-3-319-95031-0_9

urged her fellow legal scholars to consider the ways that their experiences of racism and sexism in employment could not be understood by examining race/ethnicity and gender identity as separate social identities. Other Black feminist scholars, such as Patricia Hill Collins and Lisa Bowleg, introduced discussions of intersectionality into their respective disciplines to also urge their disciplines to avoid an "additive" approach when seeking to understand multiple and intersecting social identities. For example, Bowleg [3] studied the experiences of Black lesbian women, asserting the importance of researchers, practitioners, and advocates refraining from use of an "additive" approach to working with this group, such as examining one identity and then the next identity for this group (e.g., "black + lesbian + woman"). Instead, Bowleg [3] encouraged an integrated, intersectional approach that seeks to understand how each of these identities intersect together and cannot be "pulled apart." In addition, Bowleg advocated that people working with Black lesbian women needed to understand that it was not only the women's multiple identities that intersected but also their experiences of multiple oppressions (e.g., experiences of racism, sexism, and heterosexism) and interlocking societal oppressions they experienced.

To apply intersectionality theory [3, 8] to working with older trans adults, health-care professionals must have a foundational understanding of social identities and how those social identities are related to experiences of privilege and oppression. Social identities refer to social identities older trans adults may have, such as gender identity, racial/ethnic identity, social class, disability, age, religious/spiritual affiliation, and immigration status, among others [7]. Some social identities are assigned societal advantages, while other social identities have imposed oppressions. For example, a White older trans woman with an income level below the poverty line has a racial/ethnic identity that has associated societal advantages that are granted and unearned just because this person is White. However, this person's gender identity, age, and social class are associated with experiences of oppression – meaning that there are societal disadvantages that are linked to these social identities (e.g., inequitable access to resources based on these social identities). As Crenshaw, Hill-Collins, Bowleg, and other intersectionality scholars note, it is the intersections of these diverse and multiple identities that influence health disparities that – when applied to older trans adults –drive societal experiences of privilege and oppression.

Related to various social identities, there are also accompanying societal systems of oppression that exist (e.g., racism, sexism, heterosexism, ableism, classism, xenophobia). A table is provided below that lists a few examples of social identity categories and the accompanying privilege or oppression status. As you read through these social identities, consider your own social identities and where these would fall on the spectrum of privilege and oppression [21]. Reflect on what experiences have been related to your multiple and intersecting identities of privilege and oppression. Then, identify which social identities you may have reflected more or less on and why this might be. Engaging in this personal self-examination of your own social identities can help you understand which of your own identities of privilege and oppression may influence how you view issues that trans older adults present with, as well as how you are viewed and experienced by them as their health-care provider (Table 9.1).

Table 9.1 List of social identities trans older adults may have in relation to privilege and oppression

Social identity	Privilege status	Oppression status
Ability status	Able-bodied	Physical/cognitive/mental disability
Gender	Men	Women, transgender
Sex	Male	Intersex, female
Gender identity	Cisgender	Transgender
Immigration status	White, US citizen	Immigrant, people of color
Race/ethnicity	White, non-Hispanic	People of color
Sexual orientation	Heterosexual	LGBQQ+, polyamorous
Social class	Middle to upper class	Poverty to working class
Religion/ spirituality	Judeo-Christian	Muslim, eastern, pagan, atheist
Education level	Higher education	High school/GED/Non-completion
Language	English as a first language	Non-English speaker
Age	Young and middle adulthood children, adolescents, older adults	
Nationality	White, US citizen, Western European, Canadian	Eastern European, Asian, African, Latino, Middle Eastern

Next, we discuss the social identities in this table briefly – some in tandem with one another – to provide an overview of how trans older adults may experience their own privilege and oppression identities.

9.1.1 Gender Identity and Sexual Orientation Identities

Gender identity and sexual orientation identities have been covered in previous chapters. However, it is worth noting that the intersections that trans older adults experience related to their age, gender, and sexual orientation identities are often unique. For example, trans older adults may feel pressured by those in their lives to generate an "origin story" to explain how it was that they came to be "different" from what society has deemed as normal for a given place and time in regard to their gender and sexual orientation identities. These pressures place additional minority stress on trans older adults, and it is important for health-care providers to note that those who fall into dominant culture norms for sexuality and gender (i.e., heterosexual and cisgender) are not asked to generate these kinds of explanations or justifications [7].

Perhaps no other trans subgroup has faced greater pressure to produce narratives to explain why they are trans than trans older adults. Based on their age cohort, trans older adults may have come to know their gender and sexual orientation identities earlier or later in their lives due to either barriers or facilitators to which they had access (e.g., peer support, mentors, community, education) [19]. Before moving forward with an exploration of gender identity and sexual orientation formation, it is important to acknowledge that narratives about gender and sexuality are simply narratives, not universal truths, and that they often change over time with greater perspective. While there are theories about the development of gender identity and sexual orientation, we are not certain that these even hold true for people who are trans, as we are still lacking critical research and information about what these trajectories "look like." Therefore, we encourage you, as a healthcare provider, to be critical of the very process of seeking etiology when it comes to any aspect of human diversity. When working with older trans clients, the most affirming and respectful stance is to listen and believe clients, even if they do not have an articulate or cohesive way of discussing their gender and sexual orientation identity histories.

Some scientists and researchers have devoted a great deal of time to uncovering biological determinants of sexual orientation and gender identity diversity. Stage models for gender identity development tend to be extremely biased toward a Western perspective and should be applied with careful consideration of cultural variations [7]. The theory most commonly cited in the discussion of gender identity development is Kohlberg's gender constancy model (1966), which posited that children become aware of gender identity by age 3 and achieve a "stable" gender by age 4 or 5. Not all trans people report having a clear sense of gender in accordance with this model; there are trans people who come into awareness about gender later in life or report having gender fluidity rather than stability.

The external environment (sometimes referred to as the "nurture" component in discussions of human development) is a powerful force that may provide or deny access to trans identity or transition. Trans older adults are not only influenced by the social norms of their generation but also by the cultural and historical norms within the field of trans health care. There is no universal experience in terms of social and medical transition, health-care access, and identity development for older adults of being trans [10]. For example, a trans woman who sought gender-affirming medical care from a university gender clinic in the 1960s will have had different experiences than a trans woman who was unaware of her gender identity (i.e., that she was trans) until later in life when she started noticing more media attention centered around trans people. Many factors, such as age, generation, and cohort (e.g., people who started transition in the early 2000s), have significant impacts on how people approached the task of acknowledging their own identity and expressing it to others, if they choose to disclose it at all. The degree to which it is safe to come out or disclose having a marginalized trans identity or sexual orientation depends on geographic location, social norms, and policies (e.g., whether there are legal protections against discrimination) [20].

The process of social and/or medical transitioning (if desired by trans older adults) can sometimes affect their sense of sexuality or sexual orientation. While there is not a general model of sexual orientation development for trans people, one model based on trans masculine spectrum people suggests that sexual orientation may interact with gender identity and ought to take into account the experiences of oppression and development of resilience [9]. Some trans people go through a period of sexual exploration and may come into awareness of attractions toward people they previously were not attracted to, which in turn may shift their conception of sexual orientation [17, 23]. For trans older adults who have been in long-term relationships or marriages prior to transition, this newer experience of sexuality can be vulnerable or threatening to their sense of family or security. Providers should be especially attuned to how shifts in sexual attraction or identity may impact long-standing relationships.

In addition, health-care providers should seek to pay special attention to supporting trans older adults who identify as asexual (those who do not experience sexual attraction to others) and aromantic (people who do not experience romantic attractions to others). Older trans adults with these identities often experience microaggressions related to people assuming they "should" have a queer or straight identity or that they do not develop intimate emotional relationships. It is also important to be open to and respectful of nontraditional relationship patterns when working with trans older adults who identify as polyamorous. Polyamorous trans older adults may experience societal messages that their relational orientation is "not normal" and hear sex-negative viewpoints about being polyamorous (e.g., polyamorous relationships are "just about sex" or "won't last" if there are multiple partners) [6]. No matter what sexual orientation and relational orientation trans older adults have, providers can express value and support for TGNC people's intersecting identities and seek to understand how these intersections influence TGNC people's mental and physical health.

9.1.2 Racial and Ethnic Identities, Immigration, and Language

Just as the well-being of trans older adults is influenced by the degree of support and empowerment they have related to their gender and sexual orientation identities, the experiences they have related to their racial and ethnic identities intersecting with their gender and age can be quite impactful. For instance, trans older adults of color often face even higher levels of mental and health disparities than White trans older adults due to structural racism [14]. In a recent survey of the discrimination experiences of trans people, the rates of discrimination in employment, experiences of suicidality, and housing insecurity were even higher for trans people of color than White trans people [14]. In addition, trans older adults of color may face barriers to accessing healthcare that is both responsive to their race/ethnicity and to their gender. For instance, culturally competent healthcare centers for many trans older adults that focus on queer and trans health may be located in predominantly white neighborhoods with large queer and trans populations. These same services are not often available in areas where many LGBT residents of color live. Because financial stressors and transportation are already significant barriers that trans older adults face when accessing health care, it is even more unlikely like trans older adults of color will be able to access this care [16].

Although there has been little research with trans older adults of color, some research with trans people of color has suggested there are resiliencies that trans people of color in general can experience within their own communities that are important for healthcare providers to know [7]. For example, some scholars have noted the "thick trust" that develops between trans people of color, where a shared set of racial/ethnic and gender identities promotes rapid trust building, rapport, and resource sharing within trans people of color communities [11, 13]. Healthcare providers can use thick trust within older trans people of color communities to implement needed community interventions (e.g., access to name changes, counseling, HIV testing). In doing so, providers can work with popular opinion leaders in the community who can help act as mentors for other trans older adult community members in terms of connecting them with important healthcare resources and supports.

The intersection of race/ethnicity with immigration status and language can also position trans older adults for multiple experiences of privilege and oppression. Trans older adults who have recently immigrated to the United States can experience acculturative stress and may need support understanding the trans-affirming health-care resources in this country. Citizenship status is a major privilege, so those older trans adults who are green card and visa holders, have refugee or asylee status, or are undocumented may not understand how to navigate US health-care systems. In addition to the various migration histories trans older adults have, they may have differential English language learning and access. Therefore, having knowledge of bilingual and multilingual trans-affirming resources is critical.

9.1.3 Social Class and Education Access

Social class refers to the amount of privilege and access to monetary and other financial resource facilitators (e.g., housing, food, healthcare, education) a person may have [2]. There are many ways health-care providers consider social class in their everyday settings, such as whether you have a reduced fee scale, engage in pro bono work, and seek to understand how the lack of access to financial resources influences client and patient care. Whether a trans older adult has access to transportation to your office or community setting, whether they can afford to pay co-pays or even have insurance access, and whether they can pay for necessary components of their medical and social transition (if desired) and other healthcare needs all are influenced by a person's social class. The level of education trans older adults have had access to is also vitally important, as are reading level and ability to access and understand health information. Higher levels of educational attainment can also translate into higher-paying employment and careers for trans older adults.

Applied to the lives of trans older adults, social class and related social identities can be very complex. For example, trans people may have access to financial resources in the middle adulthood years, but as they age, they may experience multiple health-care challenges that deplete these resources. Also, trans older adults may experience barriers in career advancement as they engage in a social and medical transition. They may refrain from seeking promotions and other career advancements because they are preparing for a social and medical transition at work and do not want to jeopardize any support they have by "asking for too much." This may result in trans older adults getting promoted less often. In addition, their legal documents may not "match" their gender identity and gender expression, and/or they can experience conflict and lack of support in their workplaces regarding their gender identity. Some trans older adults may feel more comfortable "starting over" at a new employer after their social and medical transition. Each of these instances will have an influence on their earning potential and social class, which also impacts saving for retirement.

As a result, trans older adults may have to seek support from families who may not have been trans-affirming earlier in their lives. Therefore, you may be helping trans older adults identify how to navigate difficult relationships with family, how to identify and meet self-advocacy needs, and manage grief related to becoming dependent on family members and health-care providers who may or may not be trans-affirming. You also may be working with trans older adults to assess the options they have for financial and other needed supports in order to stabilize their needs for housing, medical care, and social support. However, some older trans adults have access to education and information and have been able to build access to people who have financial resources who care about and support them. So, the intersections of their age, gender, and education identities may have positioned them for resiliencies and resources to "spend" on the financial needs they have.

9.1.4 Religious and Spiritual Identities

For many people, religion and spirituality are important social supports and sources of coping [18]. For trans older adults who identify as religious and/or spiritual, their belief systems can greatly help them in times of challenge. For many people of color communities, religion and spirituality are critical sources of community connections, resources, and coping with societal racism. In a study of the resiliencies of trans people of color surviving trauma, participants shared that their religious and/or spiritual beliefs helped them cope with a wide range of traumatic experiences [22]. Health-care providers should keep in mind that religious and spiritual social identities are incredibly diverse and not limited to Judeo-Christian perspectives (e.g., Hindu, Buddhist, Sikh, Pagan, atheist, agnostic), so healthcare providers can seek to learn about and grow their understanding of belief systems they may not have learned about previously [12].

Providers should also be aware, however, that religion and spirituality have been used to harm trans people throughout their lifetimes (e.g., conversion therapy, being told they are "going to hell"). In addition, many trans people experience rejection from religious/spiritual institutions as they disclose their gender identity to their religious and spiritual communities; trans older adults whose sexual and/or relational orientation are lesbian, gay, bisexual, queer, questioning, polyamorous, and asexual may also experience multiple rejections based on these identities [12]. Therefore, providers should assess not only the personal relevance and needs of religion and spirituality for older trans adults but also the ways in which they have experience harm, grief, or loss.

In addition, healthcare providers can seek to understand and support trans older adults who identify as atheist, agnostic, or nonbelievers, or who use other terms to describe this important social identity [5, 15]. As trans people with non-religious identities enter older adulthood, they may be exposed to or feel "forced" to access health-care providers that are religious in nature (e.g., hospice care, home meal delivery services) and interact with multiple people who question their identity or assume that they "will become religious sooner or later." As a provider, you can consider the religious and spiritual symbols you have in your office, including questions about non-religious identities on your paperwork, and explore the needs and support trans older adults with non-religious social identities they have [5].

9.1.5 Disability Identity

One of the shifting identities that trans older adults face as they age can involve the emergence of a disability identity – whether from a temporary disability or one that becomes an everyday part of their lives. In addition, trans older adults may have been living with various mental, physical, and cognitive disabilities at earlier points in their lives. Therefore, health-care providers should have a thorough understanding of how disability identities can shift and change throughout their lives and the influence they may have on their overall well-being as a trans person. For instance, a trans older adult with multiple privileged identities related to race/ethnicity (e.g., White) and social class (e.g., middle class and above) may face healthcare challenges that change their social class identity rapidly as they are acquiring a disability that may be related to aging (e.g., Parkinson's). Grief and loss can be common issues trans older adults face with an emerging disability identity, and they may be unfamiliar with navigating healthcare systems that serve people living with disabilities (e.g., acquiring wheelchairs, accessing reduced-price medication).

People who have lived with one or more disabilities throughout their lives and then come to identify their trans identity can have multiple needs as they disclose their trans identity to others in their lives. For instance, trans older adults may experience fear that their trans identity will position them to experience even more oppression in society. If they have specialized care providers who are not trans-affirming, there may not be many options to select alternative providers who will affirm their gender identities. In addition, while trans older adults may have been well-connected and supported in local disability communities, there may be less acceptance within these communities when a trans identity is disclosed or someone begins to transition (e.g., a person who is deaf and uses ASL their entire life then identifies as trans and has to "come out" to their entire community).

Also, the need for trans older adults to manage the challenges of a chronic illness or disability can influence the amount of coping they have to manage gender identity microaggressions and other oppressions. This additional layer of minority stress could lead trans older adults to withdraw from social support and be hesitant to access community resources. Within trans communities, there may be a lack of awareness and skills about how to be accepting and adept at supporting trans older adults living with disability. If older adults are neurodiverse, they can also experience challenges in finding housing, further complicating the process of locating accessible housing in already limited trans-affirmative options. In these instances, providers can connect older trans adults living with disabilities with trans-affirming resources and mentors (e.g., blogs, social media) that can serve to help affirm their intersecting identities. It is also critical for providers to advocate for – and possibly develop – needed resources that are affirming of trans older adults.

9.2 Chapter Summary

In this chapter, we described some of the potential identity intersections that trans older adults may have in their lives as these can influence their mental and physical well-being. As providers, we have the opportunity to affirm trans older adults in all of the ways they identify and express their gender identities. We cannot provide trans-affirming care to these older adults without a strong intersectional lens that allows us to understand the whole of their multiple identities that position them for advantages, disadvantages, and/ or a mixture of both. However, we can as providers seek to increase our awareness, knowledge, and skills of these identity intersections for trans older adults, thereby increasing quality of life and overall well-being. We can also take action to address multiple and intersecting inequities and oppression that trans older adults may experience. In doing so, we as providers can reflect on our own intersecting identities of privilege and oppression and how the health-care systems in which we work privilege some identities and oppress others in order to become more effective and trans-affirming advocates.

References

1. Adams M. An intersectional approach to services and care for LGBT elders. Generations. 2016;40(2):94–100.
2. Allmon A, Liu W. Social class transitions and positive psychology. In *Perspectives on the intersection of multiculturalism and positive psychology*. New York: Springer; 2014.
3. Bowleg L. When Black+ lesbian+ woman≠ Black lesbian woman: The methodological challenges of qualitative and quantitative intersectionality research. Sex Roles. 2008;59(5–6): 312–25.
4. Bowleg L. The problem with the phrase women and minorities: intersectionality – an important framework for public health. Am J Public Health. 2012;102(7):1267–73. https://doi.org/10.2105/AJPH.2012.300750.
5. Brewster ME, Robinson MA, Sandil R, Esposito J, Geiger E. Arrantly absent: atheism in psychological science from 2001 to 2012. Couns Psychol. 2014;42(5):628–63.
6. Burnes TR, Singh AA, Witherspoon RGA. Sex positivity and counseling psychology: Introduction to the major contribution. Couns Psychol. 2017;45(4):504–27.
7. Chang SC, Singh AA, Rossman K. Gender and sexual orientation diversity within the TGNC community. In: Singh AA, Dickey LM, editors. *Affirmative counseling and psychological practice with transgender and gender nonconforming clients*. Washington DC: American Psychological Association; 2016.

8. Crenshaw K. Mapping the Margins: Intersectionality, Identity Politics, and Violence against Women of Color. Stanford Law Review. 1991;43(6):1241–99.
9. Dickey LM, Burnes TR, Singh AA. Sexual identity development of female-to-male transsexuals: A grounded theory inquiry. Journal of LGBT Issues in Counseling. 2012;6(2):118–38.
10. Dickey LM, Bower K. Aging and TGNC identities: working with older adults. In: Singh AA, Dickey LM, editors. *Affirmative counseling and psychological practice with transgender and gender nonconforming clients*. Washington, DC: American Psychological Association; 2016.
11. Hwahng SJ, Nuttbrock L. Sex workers, fem queens, and cross-dressers: differential marginalizations and HIV vulnerabilities among three ethnocultural male-to-female transgender communities in New York City. Sex. Res. Soc. Policy. 2007;4(4):36–59. https://doi.org/10.1525/srsp.2007.4.4.36.
12. Hopwood RA, Witten TM. Spirituality, faith, and religion: the TGNC experience. In: Singh AA, Dickey LM, editors. *Affirmative counseling and psychological practice with transgender and gender nonconforming clients*. Washington, DC: American Psychological Association; 2016.
13. Hwahng SJ, Nuttbrock L. Adolescent gender-related abuse, androphilia, and HIV risk among transfeminine people of color. J Homosex. 2014;61(5):691–713.
14. James SE, Herman JL, Rankin S, Keisling M, Mottet L, Anafi M. The report of the 2015 U.S. transgender survey. Washington, DC: National Center for Transgender Equality; 2016.
15. Lee L. Research note: talking about a revolution: terminology for the new field of non-religion studies. J Contemp Relig. 2012;27(1):129–39. https://doi.org/10.1080/13537903.2012.642742.
16. Linscott B, Krinsky L. Engaging underserved populations: outreach to LGBT elders of color. Generations. 2016;40(2):34–7.
17. Meyer I. Prejudice, Social Stress, and Mental Health in Lesbian, Gay, and Bisexual Populations: Conceptual Issues and Research Evidence. Psychological Bulletin. 2003;129(5):674–97.
18. Park CL. Religion as a meaning-making framework in coping with life stress. J Soc Sci. 2005;*61*(4):707–29. https://doi.org/10.1111/j.1540-4560.2005.00428.x.
19. Porter KE, Brennan-Ing M, Chang SC, Dickey LM, Singh AA, Bower K, Witten T. Providing competent and affirming services for transgender and gender nonconforming older adults. Clin Gerontol. 2016;39(5):366–88.
20. Samons SL. When the opposite sex isn't. 2009; New York: Routledge.
21. Singh AA, Hwhang S, Chang S, White B. Affirmative counseling with trans/gender-variant people of color. In: Singh AA, Dickey LM, editors. Trans-affirmative counseling and psychological practice. Washington, DC: American Psychological Association; 2016.
22. Singh AA, McKleroy VS. "Just getting out of bed is a revolutionary act": the resilience of transgender people of color who have survived traumatic life events. Traumatology. 2010;17(2):34–44. https://doi.org/10.1177/1534765610369261.
23. Walinsky D, Whitcomb D. Using the ACA competencies for counseling with transgender clients to increase rural transgender well-being. J LGBT Issues Couns. 2010;4(3/4):160–75. https://doi.org/10.1080/15538605.2010.524840.

10 Evolving Aging Service Networks: Meeting the Demands for Inclusive and Comprehensive Older Transgender Adult Services

Kelly Rice, Claire Niemet, and Katt Ross

10.1 Introduction

The percentage of the US population that is above 50 years old is rapidly increasing as the Baby Boomer generation moves into retirement. By 2030, adults aged 65 years and older will account for approximately 20% of the US population or 88.5 million individuals [27]. The National Gay and Lesbian Task Force Policy Institute estimates there are currently 1.4–3.8 million LGBT Americans over 65 and that this population will expand to approximately 2–7 million by 2030 [18]. This population boom is causing a surge in demand for aging-specific, as well as LGBTQ-competent, services to aid older adults in maintaining their health, wellness, and independence.

There is a limited amount of research that has been conducted about and for aging sexual minority populations, especially for transgender older adults. Sexual orientation and gender identity (beyond the male-female binary) are fields that are rarely included in surveys and studies, which leads to knowledge gaps for service providers, funders, and policymakers. This invisibility of older sexual minority populations is, in part, responsible for increased health disparities, especially for individuals that identify on the transgender spectrum. This chapter will primarily utilize the gender identity terms: transgender, transfeminine, and transmasculine, as the majority of people over the age of 65 tend to identify their gender as male, female, transgender, and transsexual. It is rare that an older adult will identify as gender nonconforming or non-binary. Due to the minimal amount of available transgender

K. Rice (✉) · K. Ross
Social Services, Howard Brown Health Center, Chicago, IL, USA
e-mail: kellyr@howardbrown.org; kattr@howardbrown.org

C. Niemet
Parkinson's Disease and Movement Disorders Program, Rush University Medical Center, Chicago, IL, USA

M. Houlberg et al. (eds.), *Transgender and Gender Nonconforming Health and Aging*,
https://doi.org/10.1007/978-3-319-95031-0_10

adult-specific research, this chapter also utilizes research conducted on the broader older LGBTQ population.

Since 1965, the federal government has funded services for older adults, especially the most economically and socially vulnerable, through the Older Americans Act. State and local organizations provide direct services such as nutrition, homemaker, and transportation services to older adults. These types of services and many more allow older adults to live independently in their homes and help avoid crowding of long-term care facilities. However, as sexual orientation and expanded categories for gender identity are frequently not included or are actively removed from national surveys, the necessary funding needed to address health disparities among LGBTQ older adults may never reach organizations helping older LGBTQ communities.

Geriatric health-care often serves as the entryway for older adults to aging services, and the quality of the experience can influence whether or not an older adult chooses to engage in aging services. If a transgender individual experiences negativity and discrimination within health-care systems, this can lead to a fear of and resistance to approaching and accessing services through aging service networks.

While LGBTQ older adults experience many of the same challenges as the general older adult population, they also experience several unique medical and social support challenges and barriers to care. These barriers to services, gaps in available resources, and lack of competent care lead to negative health outcomes and health-related quality of life [15]. The task of addressing health disparities among the transgender older adult community is daunting but certainly possible. To highlight the extent of health disparities through population-level research studies and for funding to be directed to agencies serving the transgender older adult community, state and national surveys need to include questions about sexual orientation and gender identity. On the interpersonal level, cultural competency training will help community and healthcare personnel understand the unique needs of transgender older adults and how to provide affirming care.

10.2 Brief History of Aging Services in the United States

As part of the Great Society, President Lyndon B. Johnson signed the Older Americans Act (OAA) in 1965 to "promote the well-being of older individuals by providing services and programs designed to help them live independently in their homes and communities [2]." Title III of the OAA authorizes the federal government through the Administration on Aging to distribute funds to state and local government in proportion to the population of older adults 60 years old or older [3]. In turn, state units on aging (SUAs) disperse funds to area agencies on aging (AAA) who prioritize delivering services to older adults with the "greatest economic and social need" [26]. To meet the "greatest economic and social need" definition, an older adult must (a) live below the poverty threshold; (b) possess physical or mental disabilities that pose a risk for institutional placement; or (c) have been impacted by cultural, social, or geographical isolation resulting from language, racial, or ethnic status [3]. AAAs organize, manage, and deliver services to older adults through local government and community-based organizations.

The federal administration on Aging, 56 SUAs, 629 AAAs, almost 20,000 service providers, and 244 Tribal and Native American organizations representing 400 tribes comprise what is called the "Aging Services Network" [2]. Over the past four decades, the OAA has expanded the type and number of services provided under Title III for older adults to include meal and nutrition services (i.e., Meals on Wheels), supportive services and preventive health, family caregiver support services, transportation, and homemaker services [14].

Even after the OAA was signed into law 50 years ago, many older adults in the United States continue to face everyday hardship. In fact, older adults receiving Title III services are more likely to live alone, to live in poverty, and to have difficulty with three or more activities of daily living (ADLs) than individuals in the same age group that do not access Title III services [14]. Given the high rates of isolation, low socioeconomic status, and poor health status, Title III recipients are at higher risk of nursing home admissions [4]. Therefore, the aging services network provides vital services to help older adults with the "greatest social and economic need" remain at home and live independently.

Currently, LGBTQ older adults are not designated as a population of "greatest social and economic need" according to the US Administration for Community Living (ACL), an operating division of the US Department of Health and Human Services (HHS) responsible for providing community support to older adults and people with disabilities to help them stay healthy and independent. However, a 2012 ACL provision clarified that SUAs and AAAs may expand the "greatest social and economic need" definition to other populations experiencing cultural, social, or geographic isolation based on other factors such as sexual orientation or gender identity [1]. The expansion of the definition to explicitly include older transgender adults would allow for funding to be provided for programs and services that address the specific health and wellness needs of older transgender adults.

10.3 Identified Needs and Gaps in Services for Transgender Older Adults

10.3.1 Knowledge Limitations

While researchers have increased their focus on and the inclusion of transgender adults in their studies, it is widely understood that a lack of sufficient evidence, specifically in the areas of service needs, remains. Within the existing aging service and healthcare service provision research, the majority of studies combine the heterogeneous LGBTQ communities into a singular population and do not differentiate gender identity from sexual orientation.

An additional limitation for much of the existing research is the potential for sampling bias to be present. Due to the small size of the US transgender older adult population as a whole, as well as varied levels of individual identification and interaction with public transgender networks and communities, it is clear that study samples are not representative of the older transgender population, essentially rendering the diverse constellation of transgender aging people invisible.

In a 2017 literature review of transgender topic-focused articles, Wanta and Unger [28] identified a total of 2405 transgender health topic journal articles published from 1954 to 2015. Of those articles, only 11 (0.5%) focused on the topic of aging, the smallest subcategory of the articles reviewed. Moreover, of the 11 aging-focused articles, none addressed end-of-life or social service concerns of older transgender adults. Because of this scarcity of research including older transgender adults, it is necessary to utilize surveys that may have smaller than ideal sample sizes and/or to make inferences from studies that include a broader-based sample population.

10.3.2 Intersectionality of Identities and Health Disparities

According to a June 2016 Williams Institute report, approximately 1.4 million or 0.6% of adults in the United States identify as transgender [13]. The population of adults ages 65 and older that identify as transgender is estimated at 217,000 adults or 0.05% of the US adult population. The demographic makeup of the transgender population in the United States is heterogeneous. The intersections of identities, including gender identity, sexual orientation, race, ethnicity, and socioeconomic status impact individuals' perceptions of and interactions with aging service networks and healthcare systems. Unfortunately, it is nearly impossible to access statistics regarding the diversity of the US transgender population due to the lack of collected data.

The majority of all aging adults, including LGBT elders, are expected to be living with chronic conditions by 2040 [6]. According to the US Centers for Disease Control and Prevention [9], approximately 7.7% of adults over the age of 50 are currently experiencing depression, and 15.7% have experienced depression in their lifetime. In contrast, Fredriksen-Goldsen et al. [16] found that the overall rate of depression for older LGBT (not including queer) adults was 31% and 48% for transgender older adults specifically. National data shows that older adults do not frequently use mental health services. Currently, aging adults "account for only 7% to 9% of mental health utilization in hospital, community, and private practice settings" [6]. Consequently, higher rates of depression, along with low rates of mental health-care use, lead to poor health outcomes and further demonstrate the mental health disparities experienced by the aging LGBTQ populations. The risk of isolation is particularly high among LGBTQ older adults, as compared to their heterosexual cisgender peers, with LGBT older adults more likely to live alone (34% vs. 21%), less likely to live with a spouse or partner (48% vs. 70%), and have shrinking support networks over time (40% vs. 27%) [24].

Significant health disparities exist for older transgender adults, as compared to both their heterosexual and LGB cisgender peers. HIV is one health condition that disproportionately impacts LGBTQ adults, including older adults. According to the

Centers for Disease Control and Prevention [10], adults over the age of 50 made up 17% of HIV diagnoses in 2015. The overall diagnosis rate for people ages 50 and above decreased by 10% from 2010 to 2014, but the rate of new HIV infection for men who have sex with men over the age of 55 increased 18% during the same time period. Comparing the HIV rates for adults over 50 by sexual orientation demonstrates where health disparities exist. Gay and bisexual men made up 49% of new HIV diagnoses in 2015 compared to 15% among heterosexual men. Unfortunately, the CDC does not provide statistics for HIV rates for transgender adults over the age of 50. However, the statistics the agency provides for HIV rates within transgender populations confirm that significant health disparities exist, including that 22–28% of transgender women have been diagnosed with HIV and approximately 56% of African-American transgender women have been diagnosed with HIV [11]. In one review of the peer-reviewed literature, HIV rates among transgender women varied from 26% to 47% [28].

10.3.3 Comparisons of Concerns on Aging

SAGE conducted a survey of LGBT adults between the ages of 45 and 75 in 2014. Of the 2376 respondents, 137 (0.06%) identified as a transgender adult. As a part of the survey, participants were provided with a list of issues and were asked to respond with a level of concern on a five-point Likert scale from "Not At All Concerned" to "Extremely Concerned." The results identified alarming contrasts in the levels of concern around aging for LGBT older adults as compared to their heterosexual cisgender peers, as shown in Table 10.1.

The study also explored the differences in the survey responses to the aging issues questions between the transgender and cisgender respondents. Again, alarming contrasts were identified in the responses, demonstrating significant inequities that exist between transgender older adults and their cisgender LGB peers (Table 10.2).

Additionally, the SAGE survey found that one in three (33%) transgender older adults felt that work/volunteer activities would not be open to them if others knew

Table 10.1 Percentage of survey participants responding "very or extremely concerned" for measures by LGBTQ status [24]

Measure	LGBT (%)	Non-LGBT (%)
"Having enough money to live on"	51	36
"Being lonely and growing old alone"	32	19
"Will outlive the money they have saved for retirement"	42	25
"Will have to work well beyond retirement age in order to have enough money to live"	44	26
"Declining physical health"	43	33
"Depending on others for money"	33	18
"Not being able to take care of themselves"	43	34
"Not having someone to take care of them"	30	16

Table 10.2 Percentage of survey participants responding "very or extremely concerned" for measures by gender identity [24]

Measure	Transgender (%)	Cisgender (%)
Being a burden to their loved ones	48	32
Knowing where they will live as they grow older	42	27
Losing their physical attractiveness	31	20
Relationship with medical provider would be adversely affected if sexual orientation/gender identity is known	44	20

about their gender identity and over one in three (38%) were not sure how these opportunities would be affected if their identity was disclosed. One in four (25%) transgender older adults reported experiencing housing discrimination on the basis of gender identity. Two-thirds of transgender older people (65%) felt there would be limited access to health-care as they grow older and more than half (55%) felt they will be denied medical treatment on the basis of their age [24].

10.4 Evolution of Service Networks

The current national aging services network is wholly unprepared to provide quality programs and services for transgender older adults. Most aging service programs are based on a heteronormative model and do not explicitly evaluate nor address the needs of older LGBTQ adults. For those services that are marketed directly to older LGBTQ communities, there are differing levels of meaningful inclusion and centering of transgender people and their specific needs and wants.

10.4.1 Individual Level Concerns and Barriers

Each older transgender person experiences a variety of barriers to care and services on personal, institutional, and systemic levels. Of primary concern is the real or perceived discrimination experienced in health-care settings due to an individual's sexual orientation or gender identity. In one study, 83% of lesbians and gay men reported experiencing rejection or stigma from neighbors and medical providers, and 58% stated they feared coming out and being abused or neglected by those on whom they depend for their safety and well-being [25].

Medical providers working in institutional settings who are unaware of the individualized needs of LGBTQ patients fail to create a safe environment for patients. In addition, providers frequently make heteronormative assumptions about patients' identities, sexuality, and experiences which lead to uninformed and incomplete treatment. Stein and Bonuck [25] found that 30% of respondents were concerned about receiving poor treatment if providers discovered their sexual orientation and 13% avoided or delayed health-care due to concerns about provider reactions to their sexuality.

In another study, 40% of transgender older adults experienced inferior healthcare or have been denied services compared to 11% of gay, bisexual men, lesbian, and bisexual women [16]. In fact, fear of accessing healthcare systems is a mediator between gender identity and adverse health conditions such as depression, disability, and perceived health among transgender older adults [17].

10.4.2 System-Level Concerns and Challenges

In 2010, a nationwide study of a total of 320 AAAs and State Units on Aging (SUAs) was conducted to determine readiness to meet the needs of lesbian, bisexual, and gay older adults, along with transgender older adults [19]. This survey was significant in its design, as it differentiated between gender identity and sexual orientation, in both the survey question design and the analysis of the results.

Approximately 30% of the agencies reported they offer some level of training related to transgender aging, which varied widely from allowing interested staff to attend external trainings to mandating specific training for all staff. A notable training-related finding is that agencies that reported providing transgender-specific training to their staff received three times as many referrals for services for transgender older adults than agencies that had not provided training. However, only 7.2% of the AAAs and SUAs offered services targeted to transgender older adults, and 12.2% completed specific outreach to transgender communities. A surprising 72% of agencies stated they felt transgender older adults would be made welcome if they were to seek services compared to 16% of agencies that stated transgender older adults would not be welcome to engage in services. The results of this study clearly demonstrate the necessity for cultural competency training for staff members, as well as increased targeted efforts by agencies to provide outreach and services to transgender older adults.

10.4.3 Current Transgender Older Adult Focused Programs and Services

Where aging services do exist for transgender older adults, the services are often housed in LGBTQ health centers or community centers and are often developed for the broader LGBTQ community, with varying degrees of service specifically for transgender older adults. While the programs and services are frequently advertised as trans-inclusive, it is unclear without further research if transgender older adults find the services welcoming and whether or not the services meet their needs.

Several agencies and organizations provide services aimed to serve the broader LGBTQ older adult communities. For example, Callen-Lorde Community Health Center in New York has a collaboration with SAGE to provide programs and services to older LGBTQ adults. Fenway Health in Boston works with multiple community partners through the Aging Project. In Chicago, the Center on Halsted operates a LGBTQ senior center, the Center on Addison, dedicated to providing aging programs and services to the LGBTQ population. Adjoined to the Center on Addison are the Town Hall Apartments, which is an LGBTQ-friendly senior housing development. The Town Hall Apartments include 79 subsidized affordable apartments, and supportive services are available on-site for residents [7].

Along with offering clinical medical care and behavioral health services, Howard Brown Health has created and offered group programming and services to help support the adult transgender and gender nonconforming communities in Chicago. The longest-running program is a bimonthly psychosocial support group named "T-Time." The group invites adults over the age of 25 that identify as transgender, gender nonconforming, and intersex to participate. Currently, the age range of group participants spans from 25 to 70 years old and is predominately attended by participants identifying on the transfeminine spectrum.

The group format is casual and discussion-based, addressing topics including safety, medical and surgical navigation, family systems, and advance care planning. The group previously followed a more structured and activity-based model, but feedback from participants indicated the planned programming and activities made the older adults feel infantilized or as though they were in a nursing home setting. The participants were most interested in the companionship and community-building that the group could provide. According to Jahara Carey, T-Time facilitator since 2013, the group provides several benefits to participants, including reducing isolation, providing a space to share experiences and obtain peer support, and allowing for a format to discuss and assist in navigating complex medical and insurance systems that often discriminate in their policies and procedures against the transgender population. To continue to meet the needs and interests of the older transgender adult populations in Chicago, Howard Brown Health is currently in the process of expanding transgender adult-specific programming to additional clinic sites and has begun the first adult trans-masculine-focused group, ENVISION, which launched in April 2018.

10.4.4 Need for Legal Supports and Protections

While there has been an increase in legislation that has passed to advance the rights of the LGBTQ community, there continues to be a lack of sufficient policy to provide protections from the pervasive discrimination that exists, especially at the levels experienced by transgender and gender non-conforming individuals. As such, transgender people are much more likely to age into poverty (annual income less than $10,000) than the general population, 15% vs. 4%, respectively [8].

Access to affordable and culturally competent legal services is advantageous to LGBTQ individuals as they navigate through areas of life like housing, employment, healthcare, and education with few legal protections. Further efforts should be made to ensure that the LGBTQ community is aware of their rights, such as those afforded to them in nursing facilities under the Federal Nursing Home Reform Act (FNHRA) of 1987. FNHRA protects the right to gender-affirming care, including hormone therapy, as well as provides additional protections from verbal and emotional abuse or harassment from both nursing home staff and other residents. Low-income legal clinics as well as LGBTQ-centered legal clinics exist, but in order to meet the needs of the aging transgender population, legal services must specialize to meet the intersecting needs of low-income, older transgender adults.

10.4.5 Informal Peer Systems

Historically, transgender adults have had limited access to validating and affirming support services. Where traditional service delivery systems have failed or have been inaccessible, due to geography or an individual's desire for anonymity, the resourceful transgender community has created their own care structures online. One example of the informal, peer-led support structures is Susan's Place, a website founded in the 1990s, which began as a chat platform for the transgender community. It has evolved and grown and now provides information, resources, and news, with all content created by and for transgender people.

Online communities, like Susan's Place, truly shine in their ability to provide a space for information dissemination and sharing, especially on topics rarely addressed in traditional service delivery settings. For instance, advice can be found on two distinct yet important matters: where to buy shoes or clothing and how to deal with disrespectful colleagues or nosy neighbors. The use of online communication tools allows for peer-to-peer dialogue, fostering a sense of belonging and reducing isolation, while providing a safe setting to explore one's transgender identity while maintaining a level of anonymity, if preferred. The collective efforts of transgender people empowering one another, sharing their practices of care, creating space, and forging support networks to meet their needs exemplify the resiliency of the community. Practitioners in the field must create seats at the tables of their organizations for transgender people to lead the discussions and to have representation in leadership, which will lend power and resources to design services that meet their needs.

10.5 Future of Aging Service Networks

The ability of the aging service networks and related healthcare provider networks to evolve to provide more inclusive and supportive services for transgender and gender nonconforming older adults will depend, primarily, on the degree of willingness to enhance their own systems. Further development of knowledge of the demographics, health status, and needs of the transgender older adult population, as well as intentional active engagement by the aging services network, will be required to provide culturally competent and responsive services.

10.5.1 Count Me In: Threats to Representing Older Transgender Adults

Under the Obama administration, historical laws were passed that expanded the rights and protections of LGBTQ communities. However, in just a little over 1 year, the Trump administration has undermined some of the progress that had been made. For instance, in 2017, the Trump administration removed LGBT identity questions from two major federal surveys conducted through the Administration for Community Living (ACL) and the US Census Bureau. The ACL sponsored National Survey of Older Americans Act Participants (NSOAAP) collects data from older adults who utilize Title III services funded through the Older Americans Act. This particular survey provides information on program usage and identifies where there are gaps in services. Since 2014, the NSOAAP has asked recipients to identify their sexual orientation and gender identity, thus measuring the needs of the LGBT older adult population on a national level. However, the ACL erased the questions about sexual orientation and gender identity because, according to an ACL spokesperson, the LGBT sample size was too small to ensure reliability [20, 23]. After public outcry from 89 organizations and over 13,900 individuals, the ACL reinstated the question asking for the respondents' sexual orientation, but the response of "transgender" remains eliminated as a response choice for the question on gender identity [12]. Data that specifically identifies the needs of older transgender adults is essential to ensure that needs and service gaps are identified and addressed in these communities.

Additionally, the US Census Bureau removed the sexual orientation and gender identity question from the proposed list of new questions on the American Community Survey (ACS), an annual US demographic survey that helps lawmakers determine how to distribute more than 400 billion dollars. Federal agencies such as Housing and Urban Development (HUD) and the Centers for Medicare and Medicaid Services (CMS), along with 75 members of Congress, supported the addition of both questions to the ACS. However, the US Census Bureau deemed there was "no federal data need" to add either question [21]. By not including sexual orientation and gender identity questions in this survey and similar governmental studies, population-level data will not exist, and the vast majority of US LGBTQ communities remain invisible. Even though current research has demonstrated that health and social disparities exist for LGBTQ people, population-level data is necessary to confirm existing research and answer pertinent questions about the LGBTQ community as a whole and within each subgroup. Furthermore, policymakers and government officials rely upon population data to assess how to direct funding to help populations most in need. Without this critical data, resources will not be appropriately directed toward this vulnerable, and often discriminated against, population.

10.5.2 Recommendations to Improve Transgender Representation in Aging Service Networks

To address health disparities among LGBTQ older adults, SAGE, a leading organization advocating on behalf of LGBT older adults, proposes these policy recommendations [5]:

- Congress should designate LGBT older adults as a population with "greatest economic and social need" in the OAA.

- The OAA needs to include sexual orientation and gender identity in pertinent studies such as the NSOAPP.
- The Administration on Aging should continue to support cultural competency training for healthcare service providers and AAAs.
- AAAs and healthcare service providers should use the National Resource Center on LGBT Aging's *Inclusive Services for LGBT Older Adults: A Practical Guide to Creating Welcoming Agencies* to create inviting and inclusive spaces.

10.5.3 Think Local: Building Community Relationships

A responsive and comprehensive aging services network on the local level also needs to be prepared to address the specific health and wellness needs of transgender older adults. As many health conditions, including HIV, disproportionately impact members of the transgender community, local aging agencies need to create partnerships with health and social service community-based organizations (CBOs) who have earned the trust and credibility of the LGBTQ community through years of authentic, culturally competent work [5]. Effective partnerships involving the sharing of knowledge and resources with established and valued trans-friendly CBOs will ensure that transgender older adults have a wide-ranging support network that will meet both health and wellness needs and support a positive health-related quality of life.

10.5.4 A Better Future Starts with You

As cultural anthropologist Margaret Mead once said, "Never doubt that a small group of thoughtful, committed citizens can change the world; indeed, it's the only thing that ever has" [22]. In the current political environment, these words carry even more significance. To address complex issues such as health disparities, social isolation, and low socioeconomic status among transgender older adults, efforts of multiple parties will be needed: transgender older adults; healthcare personnel; social workers; local, state, and federal representatives; LGBTQ agencies; and family and friends. Advocates for LGBTQ health equity will benefit from acting on the following recommendations:

- Find research articles about the LGBTQ older adult population by visiting the National Resource Center on LGBT Aging https://www.lgbtagingcenter.org and the American Society on Aging website http://www.asaging.org.
- Contact local, state, and national representatives with LGBTQ-friendly platforms.
- Connect with local LGBTQ organizations by volunteering, joining committees, and participating in surveys and focus groups.

Take-Home Points

1. Transgender older adults experience significant health disparities and barriers to aging supportive services and programs in comparison to both their cisgender heterosexual and LGB peers.
2. Research and service provision practitioners need to gather data on sexual orientation and gender identity in order to increase knowledge on the demographics and needs of the transgender older adult population.
3. Creative outreach and service delivery must be intersectional, going beyond LGBTQ older adult identities, weaving in race, gender, ability and disability, and other social positions that interact with one's experience of aging.

- Explore national organizations like SAGE https://www.sageusa.org, Human Rights Campaign https://www.hrc.org, the National LGBTQ Task Force http://www.thetaskforce.org. Sign petitions, write editorials, attend rallies.

References

1. Administration for Community Living, U.S. Department of Health and Human Services: Administration on Aging (AoA): Older Americans Act. [Internet]; 2017 [2018 January 19]. Available at https://www.acl.gov/node/650.
2. Administration for Community Living, U.S. Department of Health and Human Services: Administration on Aging (AoA): Administration on Aging. [Internet]; 2017 [cited 2018 January 19]. Available from https://www.acl.gov/node/915.
3. Administration for Community Living, U.S. Department of Health and Human Services: Administration on Aging (AoA): Frequently Asked Questions. [Internet]; 2017 [cited 2018 January 19] Available from https://oa.acl.gov/AoA_Programs/OAA/resources/faqs.aspx.
4. Altshuler N, Schimmel J. Aging in place: do older Americans act title III services reach those most likely to enter nursing homes. Washington, DC: Mathematica Policy Research; 2010. [Internet]; 2010. Available from https://agid.acl.gov/Resources/DataSources/DataFiles/AoA_1_NursingHomes_041311.pdf.
5. Auldridge A, Tamar-Mattis A, Kennedy S, Ames E, Tobin HJ. Improving the lives of transgender older adults. Services and advocacy for GLBT elders and National Center for transgender equality. 2012. Retrieved from https://www.sageusa.org/resources/publications.cfm?ID=13.
6. Bennett JA, Flaherty-Robb MK. Issues affecting the health of older citizens: meeting the challenge. The Online Journal of Issues in Nursing. 2003;8. Retrieved July 26, 2016, from http://www.nursingworld.org/MainMenuCategories/ANAMarketplace/ANAPeriodicals/OJIN/TableofContents/Volume82003/No2May2003/OlderCitizensHealthIssues.html.
7. Celebrating, Supporting and Uniting LGBTQ Older Adult Community [Internet]. Center on Halsted – Chicago's Lesbian, Gay, Bisexual, Transgender and Queer Community Center. Center on Halsted; [cited 2018 Jan 20]. Available from: http://www.centeronhalsted.org/senior.html.
8. Center for American Progress, Map, et al, Paying an Unfair Price: The Financial Penalty for Being Transgender in America. February 2015. Available at http://www.lgbtmap.org/file/paying-an-unfair-price-transgender.pdf.

9. Centers for Disease Control and Prevention and National Association of Chronic Disease Directors. The state of mental health and aging in America issue brief 1: what do the data tell us? Atlanta: National Association of Chronic Disease Directors; 2008.
10. Centers for Disease Control and Prevention. HIV among people aged 50 and older. 2018a, February 12. Available from: https://www.cdc.gov/hiv/group/age/olderamericans/index.html.
11. Centers for Disease Control and Prevention. HIV among transgender people. 2018b, April 23. Available from: https://www.cdc.gov/hiv/group/gender/transgender/index.html.
12. Community Living Administration. Agency information collection activities; submission for OMB review; comment request; revision of a currently approved collection (icr rev; National Survey of Older Americans Act Participants (NSOAPP). [Internet] Federal Register; 2017 June [cited 2018 January 19]. Available from https://www.federalregister.gov/documents/2017/06/22/2017-13030/agency-information-collection-activities-submission-for-omb-review-comment-request-revision-of-a.
13. Flores AR, Herman JL, Gates GJ, Brown TNT. How many adults identify as transgender in the United States? Los Angeles: The Williams Institute; 2016. Available from: https://williamsinstitute.law.ucla.edu/wp-content/uploads/How-Many-Adults-Identify-as-Transgender-in-the-United-States.pdf.
14. Fox-Grage W, Ujvari K. Insight on the issues, the Older Americans Act. Washington, DC: AARP Public Policy Institute. [Internet] 2014 [cited 2018 January 19]. Available from www.aarp.org/content/dam/aarp/research/public_policy_institute/health/2014/the-older-americans-act-AARP-ppi-health.pdf.
15. Fredriksen-Goldsen KI, Emlet CA, Kim H-J, Muraco A, Erosheva EA, Goldsen J, et al. The physical and mental health of lesbian, gay male, and bisexual (LGB) older adults: the role of key health indicators and risk and protective factors. The Gerontologist. 2012;53(4):664–75.
16. Fredriksen-Goldsen KI, Kim HJ, Emlet CA, Muraco A, Erosheva EA, Hoy-Ellis CP, Goldsen J, Petry H. The aging and health report: disparities and resilience among lesbian, gay, bisexual, and transgender older adults. Seattle: Institute for Multigenerational Health; 2011. Retrieved from: http://www.agepride.org/wordpress/wp-content/uploads/2011/05/Full-Report-FINAL-11-16-11.pdf.
17. Fredriksen-Goldsen KI, Cook-Daniels L, Kim HJ, Erosheva EA, Hoy-Ellis CP, Goldsen J, Muraco A. The physical and mental health of transgender older adults: and at-risk and underserved population. The Gerontologist. 2013;54(3):488–500. https://doi.org/10.1093/geront/gnt021.
18. Grant JM. Outing age 2010. 2009. Retrieved from National Gay and Lesbian Task Force Policy Institute website: http://www.thetaskforce.org/downloads/reports/reports/outingage_final.pdf.
19. Knochel KA, Croghan CF, Moone RP, Quam JK. Ready to serve? The aging network and LGB and T older adults [Internet]. 2010 [cited 2018Jan20]. Available from: https://www.lgbtagingcenter.org/resources/pdfs/ReadyToServe.pdf.
20. Loewy K. Erasing LGBT people from federal data collection: a need for vigilance. AJPH. 2017 [cited 2018 January 19]. Available from https://doi.org/10.2105/AJPH.2017.303914.
21. Lo Wang, Hansi. Census bureau caught in political mess over LGBT data. 2017. Retrieved from https://www.npr.org/2017/07/18/536484467/census-bureau-found-no-need-for-lgbt-data-despite-4-agencies-requesting-it.
22. Margaret Mead Quotes. (2018). BrainyQuote.com. Retrieved April 28, 2018, from BrainyQuote.com Available at: https://www.brainyquote.com/quotes/margaret_mead_101283
23. Nash T. Trump Administration has removed questions on sexuality from surveys on aging. ABC News. 2017 [cited 2018 January 19]. Available from https://www.dallasvoice.com/trump-administration-removed-questions-sexuality-surveys-aging-10234245.html.
24. SAGE. Out & Visible: The experiences and attitudes of lesbian, gay, bisexual and transgender older adults, ages 45–75. 2014. Available at https://sageusa.org/resources/outandvisible.cfm. Accessed April, 25, 2018.

25. Stein GL, Bonuck KA. Physician-patient relationships among the lesbian and gay community. J Gay Lesbian Med Assoc. 2001;5:87–93. https://doi.org/10.1023/A:1011648707507.
26. U.S. Government Accountability Office: Older Americans Act: Options to better target need and improve equity. GAO-13-74: Published: November 30, 2012. Publicly released: December 11, 2012 Available at www.gao.gov/products/GAO-13-74. Accessed August 16, 2017.
27. Vincent GK, Velkoff VA. The next four decades: the older population in the United States: 2010 to 2050, current population reports, U.S. Census Bureau. 2010. Retrieved from http://www.census.gov/prod/2010pubs/p25-1138.pdf.
28. Wanta JW, Unger CA. Review of the transgender literature: where do we go from here? Transgender Health. 2017;2(1):119–28.

Recommended Reading

1. Fredriksen-Goldsen KI, Kim HJ, Emlet CA, Muraco A, Erosheva EA, Hoy-Ellis CP, Goldsen J, Petry H. The aging and health report: Disparities and resilience among lesbian, gay, bisexual, and transgender older adults. Seattle: Institute for Multigenerational Health; 2011.
2. Knochel KA, Croghan CF, Moone RP, Quam JK. Ready to serve? The aging network and LGB and T older adults. Washington, DC: National Association of Area Agencies on Aging; 2010. Retrieved from https://www.n4a.org/files/ReadyToServe1.pdf
3. Espinoza R. Out & visible: the experiences and attitudes of lesbian, gay, bisexual and transgender older adults, ages 45–75. [Internet]. SAGE; 2014 [cited 2018 Jan 20]. Available from: https://www.sageusa.org/files/LGBT_OAMarketResearch_Rpt.pdf

Aging in Place, Caregiving, and Long-Term Care for Transgender Adults

11

Jacqueline Boyd

11.1 Introduction

The social, economic, and health disparities that plague transgender individuals throughout the lifespan result in further marginalization in older age. The effects of life-long stigma and discrimination coupled with the challenges of ageism and insufficient training and education of healthcare and aging services providers present unique challenges for transgender older adults [1].

Transgender, gender nonconforming, and non-binary (TGNCNB) older adults have not been as extensively researched as lesbian, gay, and bisexual (LGB) communities. Often transgender older adults have been included in the wider scope of LGBT studies but without the level of specificity and depth to provide a clear and coherent vision of their needs. As addressed elsewhere in this book, it is known that transgender individuals are at increased risk for negative health outcomes due to a variety of factors. Research indicates transgender older adults are a "critically underserved population at heightened risk of physical and mental health disparities often combined with less social and community support" [2]. The increased rates of smoking, substance abuse, chronic illness, and mental illness speak to how further research is essential in truly supporting transgender adults in older age [1].

The aging patterns of transgender older adults have not been as comprehensively researched as other LGB communities [3]. Invisible to a large degree within healthcare and social service systems, transgender older adults have often leveraged that invisibility to protect themselves or their families. In advanced age when cognitive or physical impairment forces a change in the status quo, transgender older adults find themselves encountering new systems and unexpected challenges [4].

Traditional aging models were developed without LGB or TGNC communities in mind. Traditional aging models are here defined as "aging in place" and

J. Boyd (✉)
The Care Plan, Chicago, IL, USA
e-mail: jacqueline@the-care-plan.com

M. Houlberg et al. (eds.), *Transgender and Gender Nonconforming Health and Aging*,
https://doi.org/10.1007/978-3-319-95031-0_11

"long-term care" with a special focus on caregiving, care planning, and best practices. Aging in place refers to the ability to remain in one's home throughout the aging process [5]. Long-term care encompasses the residential options for older adults who cannot live independently due to cognitive or physical impairments. Examples of long-term care include assisted living, continuing care retirement communities, nursing homes, and memory care units [6].

Transgender older adults who are part of the Baby Boom generation have traditionally been trailblazers. Advocating for equal rights in the 1960s and 1970s, surviving the HIV/AIDS crisis of the late 1980s and early 1990s, and establishing policies such as marriage equality in 2013 have been formative in the personal history of many transgender older adults [2]. This chapter aims to explore the traditional aging models available and identify the resiliencies developed by transgender older adults to best address their evolving needs.

11.2 The Aging Experience of Transgender and Gender Nonconforming Adults

The oppressive stigma and socially enforced gender norms that existed for most of recent history have been particularly impactful to TGNC communities. A 2011 report from Services and Advocacy for GLBT Elders (SAGE) and the National Center for Transgender Equality (NCTE) illuminates that transgender older adults face barriers in these general areas: aging services, health-care, health disparities, privacy, violence, community support, limited research and knowledge base, as well as employment and housing discrimination [7].

In little over a century, transgender and gender nonconforming activists have gained tremendous ground in making the world safer for their communities. Often those who have been most marginalized due to factors such as race, class, education, and employment status have led the fight for equality and visibility.

As far back as the 1880s, pioneers like Lucy Hicks Anderson, who was assigned male at birth, began dressing and behaving like a woman during her early school years. Lucy lived her entire adult life as a woman, facing legal prosecution for marrying her second husband, soldier Reuben Anderson. The court system accused Lucy of committing perjury for signing a marriage license marrying a man. Lucy responded saying "I defy any doctor in the world to prove that I am not a woman. I have lived, dressed, acted just what I am, a woman." Lucy served 10 years' probation and again dealt with the legal system years later after having collected money for military spouses [9].

The historical experiences of transgender people reaching older age at this time include two distinct generations. People born in the 1920s to 1940s belong to the Silent Generation. LGB and TGNC individuals of the Silent Generation lived through horrific events like the Holocaust where TGNC people were collected and incarcerated in concentration camps for their perceived perversion [10]. They also have been affected by anti-LGBTQ laws which made employment and housing discrimination legal. Members of the Silent Generation who expressed their gender identity experienced violence from police and peers in record numbers [2].

Unfortunately, the Silent Generation have experienced pathologization for the majority of their lives. The pathologization of transgender communities has been enforced in part by the *Diagnostic and Statistical Manual,* which governs guidelines for diagnosing mental illness. Homosexuality was included in the DSM as a mental disorder until 1973, and it wasn't until 1987 the last vestiges fell away after "sexual orientation disturbance" was officially removed. Transgender and gender nonconforming communities have not yet been relieved of this stigma from mental health institutions. The 5th edition of the DSM continues to pathologize transgender individuals with diagnoses such as gender dysphoria [11].

In contrast Baby Boomers born between 1946 and 1964 came of age in the midst of shifting cultural and social attitudes in the United States. Anti-war fervor and the civil rights movement were broadcast on media, talked about at the dinner table, and the struggles played out in the streets and in the voting booths. Boomers were activated by the promise of social change and equality for marginalized people. They have lived through much of the same discrimination and oppression that the Silent Generation did but have also lived a longer period of their lives when social attitudes have evolved [12]. Sylvia Rivera and Marsha P. Johnson, for example, are credited with instigating the Stonewall Riots, effectively jumpstarting the gay rights movement. Sylvia and Marsha at the time were active in the Greenwich Village area of New York City and following the Stonewall Riots founded an organization called STAR – Street Transvestite Action Revolutionaries. Marsha had survived as a black transwoman in that era by finding work as a performer, model, and sex worker. Marsha dealt with discrimination and violence throughout her lifetime, eventually being found dead at the age of 48 [8].

In 2013 the Metlife Insurance Company and the American Society on Aging (ASA) published a study which found that as a cohort, LGBT Baby Boomers expect dignity and respect from their health-care providers. The same study also found LGBT Baby Boomers feel better prepared for aging than their heterosexual counterparts. However, the lived experience of transgender older adults varies significantly from their LGB peers. As an example, 39% of Baby Boomers who identified as transgender in the study indicated they were "almost or completely out" to their families in contrast to 74% and 76% for gay men and lesbians, respectively. Transgender aging has not been researched with the vigor and support afforded to the LGBT community as a whole. For this reason, data alone cannot provide an accurate picture of the extent and diversity of transgender aging [13].

Transgender older adults of the Silent and Baby Boom generations lived through the Stonewall Riots and the HIV/AIDS epidemic as adults. They've made a way for themselves in times when the greater society dubbed them as mentally ill, unnatural, and a threat. They have served as caregivers, while 50% of their friends died in the 1980s and 1990s to AIDS. They have been mentors and role models to younger generations. Their unique ability to adapt, survive, and thrive deserves further academic attention and discovery.

11.3 Aging in Place

Aging in place models offer older adults and people living with physical impairments the ability to remain in their home environment for the duration of their lives. For transgender people this option provides many advantages to residential placement. Models for aging are constantly in flux as people create new ways to age successfully.

In the last 30 years, LGBT Baby Boomers in particular have developed pathways for quality of life in the home environment for people who choose to age at home. These adaptations include caring for each other, increased social support from LGBT community, and resulting positive health impact. In addition, transgender older adults in particular tend to be skeptical of traditional social service and health-care systems, so they often rely upon informal networks of friends and trusted long-time providers to achieve their goals [12].

The majority of older adults regardless of gender identity plan to age in place, and approximately 90% plan to remain in their homes according to the United States of Aging Survey completed by AARP in 2012 [13]. Aging in place allows people to maintain their independence and home environment while accessing the providers and community resources they have been accustomed to.

11.3.1 Family of Choice

Informal support systems for transgender older adults often are comprised of close friends or chosen family [14]. Chosen family is understood as "people considered family even though not biologically related." [15] Long-time friends, current or former intimate partners, co-workers, community members, and neighbors are just some of the types of relationships that may evolve into chosen family.

The negative and damaging experiences many transgender older adults have experienced when accessing health-care systems leave many to seek support from trusted loved ones rather than external assistance [4]. In older years, family of choice is a critical advantage for many transgender individuals. Research highlights that LGBT older adults in general are more likely to live with friends and receive care from friends than the general population. Specifically, 19% of transgender older adults and lesbians in comparison to 17% of bisexual respondents and 9% of gay men reported needing assistance from friends in the last 6 months [12].

Family of choice can serve many functions in the life of a transgender, gender nonconforming, or non-binary older adult. For people receiving benefits or subsidies to help pay for caregiving support in their homes, family of choice are an appealing choice. The level of comfort and shared knowledge within chosen family provides emotional security for transgender older adults [2]. Listed below are some of the roles family of choice can fulfill in older adult years (Table 11.1).

Even though we see higher rates of chosen family providing care for TGNC older adults, the reality is that many are hesitant to ask for help. TGNC people may feel they have no support system or people in their lives willing to provide

Table 11.1 How can family of choice help TGNC older adults?

Companionship and socialization
Medical advocacy
Household chores
Meal preparation
Financial management
Pet care

Table 11.2 How service providers can decrease isolation for transgender adults

Allow the older adult to express concerns
Make a list of current and future needs
Brainstorm who their friends, romantic partners, and family are able to contribute
Discuss what roles those people could play and how to ask for help
Identify people in their network they feel comfortable with in a caregiving capacity

assistance. They don't want to be a burden. For medical and social service providers, the importance of identifying chosen family who have capacity to provide direct support cannot be overlooked. Many transgender older adults did not imagine living to be the age they are and lack a plan for who will provide care support. Internalized shame around illness, decreased mobility, and advanced age are other challenges which contribute to feelings of social isolation. As such, service providers will benefit from specific care strategies (Table 11.2).

11.3.2 Naturally Occurring Retirement Communities (NORC)

Naturally occurring retirement communities, or NORCs, are developments "not planned or designed for older people, but which over time come to house largely older people" [6000]. Transgender older adults who lived in neighborhoods with higher concentrations of LGBT people for 20 years or more may already be living in a type of NORC. Typically, the NORC community, whether it is an apartment building, a street, or a neighborhood, was formed when younger adults or middle-aged people lived in the same area and then aged in place. Another phenomenon in which NORCs occur are when older adults move to a particular area in significant numbers at a similar time [16]. NORCs originated primarily in urban environments due to the density of senior populations but have expanded to rural areas as well. It is estimated that there are more than 5000 urban NORCs nationwide. "Healthy" NORC communities tend to be characterized as having vibrant older adult communities, easily maneuvered for those with mobility limitations, access to public transportation, and a host of other qualities that make for a senior-friendly environment [17].

The 2006 reauthorization of the Older Americans Act defines a NORC as an area that is "not an institutional care or assisted living setting" where "[1] 40% of the household heads are older individuals [age 60 or over] or [2] a critical mass of older individuals exists, based on local factors, that, taken in total, allow an organization to achieve efficiencies in health and social services to older individuals living in the community" [16].

The NORC structure holds much promise for transgender older adults, particularly in urban settings. One in five transgender people has experienced homelessness in their lifetime [18]. For transgender adults, the process of securing housing can often be tumultuous and emotionally painful. NORCs are an opportunity for communities to support large numbers of older adults within their home environments.

11.3.3 Independent/Solo Aging

Transgender older adults are at a high likelihood of aging alone or without a clear system of support. In addition, transgender older adults are at increased risk of experiencing financial challenges in paying for health-care services [2]. For these and many other reasons, the strategies employed by solo agers or elder orphans can be leveraged to improve the aging process for transgender older adults. Service providers are in the position to actively advocate for their solo-aging clientele. Strategies for successful care encourage providers to take a comprehensive approach and assist the client with planning ahead. In addition to the ten-step guide included here (Table 11.3), providers can work with transgender solo agers to identify and engage sources of support such as chosen family, neighbors, and family of origin to minimize feels of isolation and loneliness.

11.3.4 Intergenerational Housing

Intergenerational housing models offer an opportunity for residents of various ages to cohabitate long term. Participation in intergenerational activities has been shown to have positive impact on older adults and enhance social support networks [20]. For some of the same reasons that older adults wish to remain at home and age in place, intergenerational housing feels like a more natural fit than entering a

Table 11.3 Ten-step guide to caring for an elder orphan

1. Identify all medical issues
2. Identify cognitive and functional abilities
3. Obtain detailed social support information
4. Create a manageable and realistic treatment plan
5. Utilize service delivery to home
6. Make safety and injury prevention a priority; address safety and injury issues
7. Address goals of care and advance directives
8. Understand privacy issues (HIPAA)
9. Assess decision-making capacity and involve the individual as much as possible.
10. Determine if guardianship is needed, and if so, seek it

Carney et al. [19]

retirement community. Older adults report feeling energized by time spent with children, teenagers, and people of younger years.

Intergenerational housing occurs on large and small scales and may be referred to as co-housing as well. Intentional co-housing began in Denmark over 30 years ago in 1972; the phenomenon caught on in Nordic countries first and then spread to other parts of Europe and the United States [21]. Formalized arrangements wherein older residents apply and are offered a lease to live in an intergenerational home have a variety of activities and services at their disposal. Intergenerational housing also happens on a person-to-person level when older adults rent out rooms in their homes to younger adults or students.

There are community-based programs which promote this style of home sharing specifically for LGBT older adults. The renters often receive a subsidized price in exchange for performing light housekeeping or support responsibilities. These programs vary depending on the community, but for transgender older adults, home sharing with younger TGNC people may serve a number of functions. The increased socialization and income of renting out space in their homes can improve quality of life in older years. In Chicago, SAGE affiliate the Center On Halsted developed a successful example of home sharing to serve area LGBT seniors and community members seeking a house [22].

11.3.5 Village Model

The Village Movement has emerged as a consumer-driven peer-support solution to enhance the ability to age in place. The Beacon Hill community of Boston, Massachusetts, established in 2001, envisioned an active community network where volunteers could provide companionship and basic tasks like transportation, shopping, or running errands in addition to maintaining a list of trusted resources. The model is dependent upon community members' desire for a network of this kind, and as those shared needs and goals develop, the Village begins to take shape [23]. While more common in urban areas, villages can be established anywhere and have gained ground internationally in recent years.

Villages can become official nonprofit organizations or partner with other more established villages as a "spoke" to their hub to function without pursuing their own 501c3 status [24]. They operate on a membership model with members paying monthly or annually for access to the Village. Conservative estimates suggest a Village can take 18 months to 3 years to become viable [23].

Due to the relatively recent phenomena of villages and the lack of research on LGBTQ participants, there is little known about the impact on transgender or gender nonconforming older adults within these networks. However, transgender older adults are able to vet their local Village in their years prior to needing to use the services by reaching out while they are still active. Meeting with other members and leadership, attending events and asking specifically about LGBT or TGNC membership will bring to light whether the particular Village is a good fit. To connect with a local Village or learn more about how to start one, the Village To Village

Network is a helpful starting place. Their website can be accessed here: http://www.vtvnetwork.org

Some of the benefits of aging in place include familiarity, a sense of safety, privacy, access to long-standing support systems, minimal change to expenses (except when care requires paid caregiving services), and protection from harassment perpetrated by peers who discriminate against LGBT people [25]. In contrast to the benefits, there are a number of potential negatives to aging in place models for transgender older adults. Specifically the social isolation, fixed income, and lack of informal caregivers can lead to decreased quality of life and inattention to medical and care needs. To summarize, a few of the challenges to aging in place models are depression and anxiety, lack of social support, higher incidence of medical crises, and unexpected fluctuating expenses.

11.4 Caregiving

Securing caregivers in home is one pathway for transgender adults to maintain independence and some protections of an aging in place lifestyle. Caregivers are found in a variety of manners. Informal caregivers such as family of choice can provide invaluable comfort to transgender older adults as discussed earlier in this chapter [26]. An estimated 27% of LGBT adults 50 and older were serving as caregivers. This included 35% providing care to a partner or spouse, 32% caring for a friend, and 7% caring for some other non-related persons such as a neighbor [2]. A separate study conducted by MetLife found 21% of LGBT Baby Boomers were serving as caregivers, of whom 34% were caring for a partner or spouse, 21% were caring for a friend, and 6% were caring for a neighbor or someone else [12].

Formal caregiving systems, while less familiar to the older adult, offer critical assistance with activities of daily living such as bathing, toileting, grooming, and feeding. Formal caregiving services covered in this chapter include independent caregivers, placement agencies, and agencies.

11.4.1 Independent Caregivers

Typically found by the older adult through advertisements, online databases, or personal network inquiries, independent caregivers offer a high degree of flexibility and choice but are accompanied by significant risk for transgender older adults. Independent caregivers often are recommended through a social network, and the older adults may work with them in a very informal manner. The attraction of paying minimum wage combined with the promise of working with just one person are persuasive to many older adults on fixed income.

However, independent caregivers are considered domestic workers. Domestic worker laws vary state by state, and older adults may not be aware of the wages, tax reporting, workers' compensation, and sleep accommodations required by their state. The risk for abuse and neglect on the part of independent caregivers is higher due to the lack of a supervision and accountability process. If independent caregivers are the older adult's preference, it is important to be educated about the governing laws related to domestic workers and ensure proper procedures are followed to protect the older adult [27]. When hiring independent caregivers, it is important for the older adult to understand the risks and in particular their responsibilities as an employer.

11.4.2 Placement Agencies/Registries

Caregiving as a profession has by and large been left to state jurisdiction, so each state is very different in terms of how they license and oversee those licenses. In many states, placement agencies or registries are a hybrid model, wherein the older adult remains the employer but the agency provides the initial background checks and coordinates payment arrangements. These organizations may utilize technology applications to expedite access to caregivers. For those communities which are at high risk for various forms of abuse and neglect, placement agencies or registries offer a median expense caregiving option. To understand if these organizations are available in your state, contact the local department on aging or the state department of public health.

11.4.3 The Agency Model

The caregiving model which presents the least amount of risk to the older adult is the agency model. Traditional agencies are the employer for the caregivers placed in the home. The agency conducts all of the onboarding, including interviews, background checks, and references and ensures all caregivers are bonded and insured. These protections serve transgender older adults particularly well as the added screening and oversight can ease concerns of potential victimization. Increasingly, agencies are recognizing the diverse needs of LGBTQ communities. Education is available that seeks to prepare health-care staff for this diversity. National organizations such as SAGE provide cultural competency training and Chicago's Howard Brown Health offers a 6-hour Health Resources and Services Administration (HRSA)-funded Health Education About LGBT Elders (HEALE) curriculum for multidisciplinary direct care staff, effectively raising awareness of the experiences of LGBTQ people within aging systems [28, 29]. Some agencies are taking on the tasks of training of staff and screening for LGBTQ cultural competency during the onboarding process to more effectively meet the needs of LGBTQ communities.

11.5 Residential Care

While aging in place is the preference for the majority of older adults, many other alternatives exist in the form of residential care. Residential care may also be called facility-based long-term care and refers to the range of older adult housing comprised of independent living, assisted living, skilled care facilities and rehab,

Table 11.4 Types of residential care

Senior apartments
Independent living
Assisted or supportive living
Intergenerational housing
Memory care
Continuing care retirement communities (CCRC)
Skilled nursing facility
LGBT-friendly housing

memory care, identity-affirming housing, and continuing care retirement communities. Residential facilities attempt to provide housing and care for a variety of older adult needs. Often transgender older adults are overlooked within the largely gender normative and heteronormative culture of residential care.

A landmark study found that 40% of transgender older adults have received inferior healthcare or been denied health-care altogether [30, 31]. In contrast, LGB counterparts report experiencing inferior health-care or denial approximately 11% of the time [2]. A staggering 89% of LGBT older adults predicted discrimination from other residents and moreover, 53% predicted discriminatory treatment at the hands of direct care staff. In actuality, survey results reveal 23% of respondents reported harassment from residents and 14% from direct care staff because they identify as LGBT [30]. As such, it is not surprising that many older LGBTQ people go back in the closet when they enter a residential facility due to fear of harassment and discrimination [32]. For transgender older adults, visibility coupled with the intimate nature of the care that occurs in residential facilities, in many cases, places them at increased risk for violence [30].

The catalysts for transitioning into residential care are variable. Some reasons transgender older adults may wish to find senior-focused housing include loneliness, finances, poor diet and nutrition, decreased mobility, inability to function independently, or a lack of appropriate care support. A residential care model also provides a safety net for people aging alone or without children. The benefits of residential care are many, in particular for transgender older adults living at or below the poverty line. The flat rate packages offered by many residential facilities can include utilities, housekeeping, laundry, meals, as well as medical staff on site. Various types of residential care (Table 11.4) are paid for by a variety of mechanisms some of which are dependent on the person's level of income, insurance coverage, age, disability status, and more. Private pay, long-term care insurance, veterans' benefits, Social Security Insurance, and Medicaid are common avenues to cover the costs of residential care.

11.5.1 How to Find TGNC-Affirming Care

For transgender older adults, often living with complex medical and environmental concerns, consistency, and having trusted supports readily available is very valuable. The invisibility of TGNC older adults within health and aging systems can make finding TGNC-affirming care challenging. The vast majorities of retirement

Table 11.5 Steps to find affirming providers

Ask friends and family of choice for recommendations
Contact local LGBTQ organizations and health centers for recommendations
Conduct online research
Interview providers prior to using services
Find out if they serve TGNC clients currently or in the past
Ask what LGBT cultural competency training staff has completed
What anti-discrimination policies are in place
What is the agency policy if incidents of conflict or discrimination that might occur

facilities, medical systems, and caregiving resources do not screen for LGB competency and fewer still TGNC competency. If the transgender older adult wishes to find affirming providers, here are suggested guides (Table 11.5).

11.6 Resilience and Care Planning

In spite of the challenges faced by transgender older adults, survival strategies and resilience tactics have developed over time. For example, transgender women are more likely to live with a spouse or partner in their older age (75+) than any other segment of LGBTQ communities [26]. In the face of a lack of family of origin support, transgender older adults cultivate connections to chosen family. LGBT older adults are more likely than the general population to have made some arrangements for aging that include other people [12]. Documenting powers of attorney and living wills or developing informal caregiving arrangements is an act of self-advocacy which can be leveraged to protect transgender older adults throughout their lives.

LGBTQ communities in general provide more caregiving responsibilities than the general population, and more than 25% of transgender older adults report currently caring for another person [2, 12]. The lived experience of caring for another aging or ill person may equip transgender older adults with enhanced knowledge of systems and resources to aid their own aging process. As public opinion continues to evolve, social services, research, and healthcare institutions have an opportunity to benefit from the increased visibility and inclusion of transgender professionals. The historical employment discrimination against transgender adults has contributed to the distrust and health disparities discussed earlier in this chapter. An important step to enhancing service delivery to transgender and gender nonconforming people should start with hiring from within those communities.

11.6.1 Care Planning

The challenges experienced by LGB and TGNC communities have given rise to valuable strategies for wellness that can be incorporated into a care plan. The adaptability and resilience that are hallmarks of LGBTQ aging should be applied to personalize a plan of care. Care planning for transgender older adults is a vital tool in successful aging. As with any major life transitions, research and preparation equips the individual with knowledge and confidence. Ideally care planning is an ongoing conversation that is rooted in the client's lived experience and stated goals. Working in collaboration with the transgender older adult, it is important to allow ample time for reflection, discussion, and decision-making. For the many older adults who have had negative experiences with social and healthcare providers in the past, it may take time to build trust and an effective relationship.

11.6.2 Tips for Effective Care Planning

Seeking out appropriate resources and proper care planning (Appendix A) can minimize risk and develop critical support for transgender older adults [33]. By thinking outside the box, holding aging service providers accountable for cultural competency, and stepping up to actively advocate for clients, social service, and healthcare providers can play a vital role in the aging process. This list of guidelines (Table 11.6), developed over years of experience working in transgender communities, is an effective means of supporting aging TGNC folks.

Table 11.6 Guidelines for service providers

1. Prioritize the client relationship – Take the time to understand the priorities, personal history, coping skills, fears, and support networks of your client before beginning the care planning process. Focus on the human before addressing the tasks when seeking to build an effective relationship.
2. Start early – Incorporate elements of care planning over time. Checklists, assessments, and attempts to cover many topics in a limited period of time increase stress and contribute to poor decision-making. Present one or two topics at a time in a relaxed fashion to decrease potential client anxiety.
3. Documentation is key – Documentation is required in many social service and health-care settings, but when working with transgender older adults, documentation is also communication. You may be working with clients who have hearing, vision loss, and memory impairment, which requires service providers to adjust their approach. Ensuring the older adult has a large-print copy of what has been discussed, resources and the care plan will help reinforce and retain the gains you've made together.
4. Outline clear goals – From the beginning, be consistent about the reason for and goals of the care plan. Collaborate with the client to identify the goals. Is the care plan necessary to address short-term goals like a surgery or securing housing, or is the goal advanced planning for long-term wellness? Is it a requirement of your agency? Maintain a transparent and straightforward attitude regarding the process.
5. Stay focused – Often transgender older adults are balancing a wide variety of concerns. In the midst of planning, other crises or relevant issues may arise. In order for you both to feel effective, stay focused on the goals you have identified together. Help the client prioritize what needs to happen when in a realistic manner. If the needs exceed your scope, link the client to additional resources to resolve time-sensitive issues.
6. Actively advocate – LGB- and TGNC-friendly aging resources are few and far between, especially in rural communities. There may be a deficit of culturally competent providers to meet your clients' future needs. Ask your local LGBTQ center for trusted recommendations, and reach out to aging service providers to screen for cultural competency prior to adding a provider to the care plan. Don't hesitate to call medical or other social service providers your client receives services from to coordinate care.

Boyd, J. The Care Plan

11.7 Best Practices

It is imperative upon health and aging service providers to incorporate transgender older adults into the fabric of their organizations and practice. To better meet the needs of transgender and gender nonconforming older adults, there are a number of practices health-care providers can integrate into practice. Working within large institutional systems may make connection to TGNC communities challenging. Partner with community health centers who work with LGBT communities to bridge this separation. When hiring new staff, always seek gender-affirming providers, and hire TGNC employees. Develop diverse literature and marketing material that reflects TGNC communities. Perform a comprehensive review and revision of policies and procedures and institute changes where necessary. It is important to ensure the language in your policies isn't exclusionary to gender nonconforming communities and those without family of origin. Removing gender-specific terms and asking preferred name and pronoun on forms are a signifier that your organization has made steps toward inclusion. Establish a clear policy for the reporting of discriminatory actions and how they will be handled by all staff. Increase cultural competency within your organizations through regular staff training and increase knowledge and comfort of cisgender residents by regular events which celebrate diversity and the inclusion of transgender older adults and curate these events to the interest and activity level of participants. Movie screenings, diversity fairs, lectures with featured speakers, and book clubs are further examples of inclusive activities.

11.8 Conclusion

Transgender older adults experience unique challenges within healthcare, aging, and caregiving settings and have been at the forefront of social change for the better part of a century and now find themselves in the position of pioneering once again. Social service and health-care providers have an opportunity to join them in developing effective routes to successful aging. Transgender older adults are claiming aging in new and creative ways; the onus is on social service, health-care, and aging systems to match those efforts.

Appendix A

Guide	Organization	Link
Prepare To Care: A Planning Guide For Caregivers In The LGBT Community	SAGE and AARP	https://issuu.com/lgbtagingcenter/docs/prepare-to-care-guide-lgbt-aarp/4
Create Your Care Plan: An LGBT Person's Guide To Preparing For Medical Procedures	SAGE	https://issuu.com/lgbtagingcenter/docs/sage_care_planning_final_interactiv

Guide	Organization	Link
Prepare To Care: A Planning Guide For Families	AARP	https://www.aarp.org/content/dam/aarp/home-and-family/caregiving/2012-10/PrepareToCare-Guide-FINAL.pdf
Planning With Purpose: Legal Basics for LGBT Elders	National Center for Lesbian Rights	http://www.nclrights.org/wp-content/uploads/2013/04/Resources_Planning_with_Purpose.pdf

References

1. Fredriksen-Goldsen KI, Cook-Daniels L, Kim HJ, Erosheva EA, Hoy-Ellis CP, Goldsen J, Muraco A. The physical and mental health of transgender older adults: an at-risk and underserved population. The Gerontologist. 2013;54(3):488–500. https://doi.org/10.1093/geront/gnt021.
2. Fredriksen-Goldsen KI, Kim HJ, Emlet CA, Muraco A, Erosheva EA, Hoy-Ellis CP, Goldsen J, Petry H. The aging and health report: disparities and resilience among lesbian, gay, bisexual, and transgender older adults. Seattle: Institute for Multigenerational Health; 2011. Retrieved from: http://www.agepride.org/wordpress/wp-content/uploads/2011/05/Full-Report-FINAL-11-16-11.pdf.
3. Cook-Daniels L. Transgender aging: what practitioners should know (book chapter). In: Orel NA, editor. The lives of LGBT older adults: understanding challenges and resilience. Fruhauf: American Psychological Association; 2015.
4. Winter S, Diamond M, Green J, Karasic D, Reed T, Whittle S, Wylie K. Transgender people: health at the margins of society. www.thelancet.com. 2016. 388. Available at: https://ac-els-cdn-com.proxy.uchicago.edu/S0140673616006838/1-s2.0-S0140673616006838-main.pdf?_tid=1adf8158-09fc-11e8-a5b7-00000aacb360&acdnat=1517784082_2fb9e3356cec46c77a17e97a02fb96c0.
5. Fausset CB, Kelly AJ, Rogers WA, Fisk AD. Challenges to aging in place: understanding home maintenance difficulties. J Hous Elder. 2011;25:125–41. https://doi.org/10.1080/02763893.2011.571105.
6. Galambos C, Popescu M, Khalilia MA, Marek KD, Popejoy LL, Stetzer F, Hicks L, Rantz MJ. Comparing aging in place to home health care: impact of nurse care coordination on utilization and costs. Nurs Econ. 2015;33(6). Available at: https://www.ncbi.nlm.nih.gov/pmc/articles/PMC4749163/.
7. Services and Advocacy for GLBT Elders (SAGE) and the National Center for Transgender Equality. Improving the lives of transgender older adults: recommendations for policy and practice. 2012. Retrieved from https://transequality.org/sites/default/files/docs/resources/TransAgingReport_ExecSummary_FINAL.pdf.
8. Martos AJ, Wilson PA, Meyer IH, Prestage G. Lesbian, gay, bisexual, and transgender (LGBT) health services in the United States: origins, evolution, and contemporary landscape. PLoS One. 2017; https://doi.org/10.1371/journal.pone.0180544.
9. Lucy Hicks Anderson. The Legacy Project. 2012. Retrieved from http://www.legacyprojectchicago.org/Lucy_Hicks_Anderson.html.
10. Cuerda-Galindo E, Lopez-Munoz F, Krischel M., Ley A, Niederkrotenthaler T. Study of deaths by suicide of homosexual prisoners in Nazi Sachsenhausen concentration camp. PLoS One. 2017. doi: https://doi.org/10.1371/journal.pone.0176007 Retrieved from https://www.ncbi.nlm.nih.gov/pmc/articles/PMC5398659/?report=classic..
11. Drescher J. Out of DSM: depathologizing homosexuality. Behav Sci: Open Access J Psychol Cognition. (2015). https://doi.org/10.3390/bs5040565. Retrieved from https://www.ncbi.nlm.nih.gov/pmc/articles/PMC4695779/.

12. American Society on Aging, MetLife. "Still Out, Still Aging": The MetLife Study of lesbian, gay, bisexual and transgender baby boomers. 2013. Retrieved from: https://www.metlife.com/assets/cao/mmi/publications/studies/2010/mmi-still-out-still-aging.pdf.
13. Association for the Advancement of Retired Persons (AARP). The United States of aging survey. 2012. Retrieved from https://www.aarp.org/content/dam/aarp/livable-communities/learn/research/the-united-states-of-aging-survey-2012-aarp.pdf.
14. de Vries B. LGBT aging: research and policy directions. Pub Policy Aging Rep. 2011;21(3):34–5. Available at: https://www.sageusa.org/files/Public%20Policy%20and%20Aging%20Report.pdf.
15. Van Wagenena A, Driskell J, Bradford J. I'm still raring to go: successful aging among lesbian, gay, bisexual and transgender older adults. J Aging Stud. 2013;27(1):1–14. https://doi.org/10.1016/j.jaging.2012.09.001.Retrievedfrom. https://www.ncbi.nlm.nih.gov/pubmed/23273552
16. Hunt, M.E. and Gunter-Hunt, G. 1985. Naturally occurring retirement communities. Journal of Housing for the Elderly, 3(3):3–22.
17. Greenfield EA, Scharlach A, Lehning AJ, Davitt JK. A conceptual framework for examining the promise of the NORC program and village models to promote aging in place. J Aging Stud. 2012;26(3):273–84. https://doi.org/10.1016/j.jaging.2012.01.003.
18. Masotti PJ, Fick R, Johnson-Masotti A, MacLeod S. Healthy naturally occurring retirement communities: a low-cost approach to facilitating healthy aging. Am J Public Health. 2006; https://doi.org/10.2105/AJPH.2005.068262.
19. Quintana NS, Rosenthal J, Krehely J. On the streets: the federal response to gay and transgender homeless youth. 2010 Center for American Progress. Retrieved from https://www.americanprogress.org/wp-content/uploads/issues/2010/06/pdf/lgbtyouthhomelessness.pdf.
20. Carney MT, Fujiwara J, Emmert Jr. BE, Liberman TA, Paris B. Elder orphans hiding in plain sight: a growing vulnerable population. Curr Gerontol Geriat Res. 2016. https://doi.org/10.1155/2016/4723250. Retrieved from https://www.researchgate.net/publication/309393502_Elder_Orphans_Hiding_in_Plain_Sight_A_Growing_Vulnerable_Population.
21. Park AL. Do intergenerational activities do any good for older adults' Well-being? A brief review. J Gerontoly Geriatric Res. 2014; https://doi.org/10.4172/2167-7182.1000181.
22. Lietaert M. The growth of co-housing in europe. The Co-Housing Association of America. 2007. Retrieved from http://www.cohousing.org/node/1537.
23. Tamarkin D. The Center on Halsted's homesharing program. Time Out Chicago. 2011. Retrieved from https://www.sageusa.org/newsevents/news.cfm?ID=49 .
24. Gupta V. Assessing the village model and the village to village network in advocating aging in place for older americans. Submitted to the Department of Urban Studies and Planning in partial fulfillment of the requirements for the degree of Master in City Planning at the Massachusetts Institute of Technology. 2012.
25. Johnson C. Why community based senior villages are growing in the us. www.shareable.net. 2017. Retrieved from https://www.shareable.net/blog/why-community-based-senior-villages-are-growing-in-the-us.
26. Wiles JL, Leibing A, Guberman N, Reeve J, Allen RES. The meaning of "aging in place" to older people. The Gerontologist. 2012;52(3):357–366. https://doi.org/10.1093/geront/gnr098. Retrieved from https://academic.oup.com/gerontologist/article/52/3/357/580905.
27. Croghan CF, Moone RP, Olson AM. Friends, family and caregiving among midlife and older lesbian, gay, bisexual, and transgender adults. J Homosex. 2014; https://doi.org/10.1080/00918369.2013.835238.
28. Paying minimum wage and overtime to home care workers: a guide to consumers and their families to the fair labor standards act. Wage and Hour Division of the United States Department of Labor. 2016. Retrieved from https://www.dol.gov/whd/homecare/homecare_guide.pdf.
29. SAGECare http://sageusa.care/.

30. Health Education About LGBT Elders (HEALE) Howard Brown Health https://howard-brown.org/era/education/curriculum/.
31. National Senior Citizens Law Center in collaboration with Lambda Legal, National Center for Lesbian Rights, National Center for Transgender Equality, National Gay and Lesbian Task Force and Services & Advocacy for GLBT Elders (SAGE). LGBT older adults in long-term care facilities: stories from the field. 2011.
32. Grant JM, Mottet LA, Tanis J, Harrison JH, Herman JL, Keisling M. Injustice at every turn: a report of the national transgender discrimination survey. National Center for Transgender Equality and the National Gay and Lesbian Task Force. Retrived from http://www.thetask-force.org/static_html/downloads/reports/reports/ntds_full.pdf .
32a. Stein GL, Beckerman NL, Sherman PA. Lesbian and gay elders and long-term care: identifying the unique psychosocial perspectives and challenges. J Gerontol Soc Work. 2010;53(5):421–35.
33. Gonzales G, Henning-Smith C. Barriers to care among transgender and gender nonconforming adults. The Milbank Quarterly. 2017. https://doi.org/10.1111/1468-0009.12297 . Retrieved from http://onlinelibrary.wiley.com/doi/10.1111/1468-0009.12297/full .

End of Life: Honor and Celebration of TGNC Individuals

12

Hector Torres, Greg Storms, and Vanessa Sheridan

At the age of 75, after a long life of battling against a heterosexist world, Axel, a trans feminine individual, finally feels she can stop fighting. Soon, there will be no more teaching others about how to treat her fairly and with dignity. She will be finished with having to explain who she is. She will no longer have to make herself visible in front of those who try to ignore her or forcefully deny her identity. She looks in the mirror and smiles at the wrinkles and white hair that signify she has made it to being an older adult.

As she reflects upon her life, she recalls how far she has come since her childhood. She remembers the pain and the happiness. Even though she wishes more of her biological family would be supportive, at the end she feels she has been loved, and her family of choice has been there for her. She knows she will be missed by the other seniors at the LGBTQ center and that if there is consciousness where she is headed, she will miss her friends, too. Axel's body is letting her know it is time to close any pending accounts and start saying her goodbyes. She is unsure of what comes next, yet feels proud of how she has lived her life. She does not know how much longer she has before she departs, but she will start preparing. She will leave her legal documents and farewells in place. She hopes those around her will celebrate her in life once she departs. She also worries about how she will be presented at her memorial.

She is appreciative of her caregivers yet is pleased by the thought of not having to depend on others anymore. She has learned to be vulnerable and accept help, yet it has not always been easy. Kindness from others used to be a scarce commodity. Some caretakers have been compassionate, while others have unintentionally hurt

H. Torres (✉) · G. Storms · V. Sheridan
Center on Halsted, Chicago, IL, USA
e-mail: Htorres@centeronhalsted.org; Gstorms@centeronhalsted.org; vsheridan@centeronhalsted.org

M. Houlberg et al. (eds.), *Transgender and Gender Nonconforming Health and Aging*,
https://doi.org/10.1007/978-3-319-95031-0_12

her. She had often ignored microaggressions in order to keep her environment safe and to not be perceived as confrontational. She knows some of the caretakers don't intend harm, and the pain they do cause feels less intense because she knows that pain comes from ignorance, not malevolence. However, she would have really liked to have a care provider who could have seen her as who she is and who could have been affirming of her identity. She hopes her end-of-life memorial is an opportunity for others to remember, honor, and celebrate her journey. Above all, she hopes she is represented as she is truly is and knows herself to be.

12.1 Transgender and Gender Nonconforming Older Adults and the Process of Facing Death

It has been said that growing old is not for sissies. That may or may not be true, but for many TGNC older adults like Axel, growing old and the prospect of facing the end of life can certainly introduce its share of challenges as well as opportunities.

It is expected that the transgender and gender nonconforming (TGNC) older adult population will continue to grow in the United States and so will the disparities that this population will face [1]. In general, older adults typically face financial, health, and social challenges. Yet, compared to their heterosexual counterparts, TGNC older adults will be more likely to have greater challenges in all of those areas [2]. TGNC older adults are more likely to live alone, have no children, be victims of abuse, and lack access to a competent health care provider [3]. Discrimination, hostile treatment, microaggressions, lack of affirmative care, and other common challenges that TGNC individuals routinely face throughout their lives may become even more prominent as the person ages.

TGNC older adults often experience greater isolation in part because they are less likely to be able to count on their biological families for support and care. Therefore, they have an increased need to rely on systems of care. To depend on the kindness of others can be a frightening thought, perhaps especially when finding kindness has been the exception throughout one's life. It is not surprising that, in a recent study, a majority of LGBTQ individuals reported their concern about a lack of access to LGBTQ-specific services for seniors [4].

Care provider discrimination and a lack of competence regarding TGNC individuals are problematic issues that have been widely documented [3, 4]. Consequently, many TGNC older adults find themselves forced to either avoid receiving necessary services or be vulnerable to discrimination, ill treatment, and abuse from service providers—who are supposed to help, not harm, them.

In addition to the obvious challenges that discrimination and these chronic abusive experiences can pose, it is deplorable that, as a consequence of having to constantly face and cope with discrimination, TGNC older adults may be distracted—and sometimes even prohibited—from focusing on the developmental process customary to individuals in the same age group. The opportunity to successfully face age-related developmental challenges can positively contribute to an individual's overall well-being.

According to Erikson's stages of psychosocial development [5], an older adult has gone through a process of generativity wherein the focus has been to contribute to society and help guide future generations. Now, as the end of life is nearing, they are entering a process of retrospection where they reflect back over their life and accomplishments. Individuals who see their lives as productive are able to develop a sense of integrity about their personal journey. However, those who do not see themselves as productive or successful may develop feelings of despair or worthlessness. TGNC older adults, in particular, may have difficulty engaging in such retrospection. For this reason, care providers can be helpful in assisting TGNC older adults to be involved in reflection, recognize their strengths and survival skills, and frame their experiences as warriors who have survived in a heterosexist world. Regardless of the present challenges, a sense of integrity can potentially be reached by recognizing that simply living as themselves in a world that put so many obstacles in front of them is, in fact, a success.

Furthermore, Erikson explained that during advanced age, individuals may need to rely on others for their care. Consequently, the TGNC older adult might revisit an earlier psychological crisis such as "trust vs. mistrust" [6]. Trust is a fragile thing. Because of the unique needs and gender status of a TGNC older adult, care providers must work diligently to build their TGNC competence, so they can provide care with sensitivity, dignity, and proficiency. Given that the TGNC community spans all cultures, ethnicities, and religions, provider sensitivities include making sure that the client feels safe to be open about their identities, including (but not limited to) their gender identity. When addressing topics such as end of life and death, care providers must consider a complex set of traditions and beliefs as well as social and familial support systems.

End-of-life care includes a variety of services and may involve multiple settings and care providers. TGNC older adults who receive this type of care often worry about every new provider and the possibility of facing awkward or discriminatory interactions. Building a safe, open, and affirming environment is essential to creating trust, building rapport, and providing culturally competent care to TGNC older adults. This is especially important when addressing a subject as emotional as preparing for the inevitability of death. These are areas where care providers can be of great support and play a very significant role.

Preparing to die means preparing to confront the absolute unknown: the end. As individuals reflect on their death, they will usually think about leaving their life in order. This may include legal concerns around estates and inheritances. Also, many worry about managing their interpersonal relationships and bringing closure to them. Others feel the need to go into deeper exploration of their spirituality and/or religion. Nevertheless, as death becomes more evident, individuals tend to go through a grief process.

Elizabeth Kübler-Ross, a pioneer in the study of death, proposed the most cited and commonly referenced model of stages of grief. The Kübler-Ross model describes five stages through which individuals navigate when they become aware that death is approaching [7]. This model gives a good idea of some of the emotions and challenges of facing the certainty of death. The process of grief may start long before certainty of death, as an individual notices loss of capacity and abilities. As death becomes more imminent, this process intensifies. Accepting death is not an easy or linear process; therefore, these stages may not happen in sequential order. The five stages of grief proposed by Kübler-Ross are denial, rage, bartering, depression, and acceptance.

In the denial stage, the person attempts to avoid thinking and denies that the end is near. This may manifest as not having time to plan or talk about it or even attempting to make plans that go beyond life expectancy. This stage is often temporary, as individuals are forced to confront reality when they experience limitations in their health. During the denial stage, the person may question the accuracy of their perception, the reality of their situation, or the intentions of others. Consequently, individuals may isolate and often feel guilty.

The next stage of the grief process is rage. This emotion is often expressed as a sense of unfairness about what the person is experiencing. The rage comes from the inability to change the reality of impending death. The person may be realizing that "This is stronger than me, and there is no way I can change it." Although rage and anger are common expressions of this stage, individuals may also express their feelings through other means such as self-destructive behaviors and a lack of self-care.

The next stage is bartering. In this stage, individuals attempt to negotiate with death to buy more time. This stage may be expressed through rationalization and an attempt to find a logical solution. On the other hand, wishful thinking and attempts to make changes in lifestyles may be proposed as a way to barter for an extension. During the bartering stage, individuals may raise questions to which the answers are unattainable, as if this could somehow earn them more time. Common questions include: "Why do some suffer more than others?" "Why does injustice exist?" "What happens next?" The person may seek assistance from religious/spiritual leaders, family, friends, or care staff. Ultimately, there are many questions without answers, and the most adequate way to move forward is with resolution. Individuals may feel despair at the lack of answers. One solution is to focus, instead, on what has been gained in life that cannot be lost. Their own memories of their journey, the lessons learned, the achievements made, the love received, and the love given are things that cannot be taken away. It is in this space where peace can be found and celebration can start—but before people can reach that place of peace and acceptance, they may first need to visit the stage of depression.

Once the individual realizes that bartering does not change the reality of impending death and that it *will* happen, then this person may go into a stage of depression. During this period, the person starts admitting their inability to change what is to come. Many individuals have great difficulty moving past the pain and sadness of this stage. When someone revisits their past with nostalgia, they often just want someone to listen to them. A trauma-informed and strength-based approach can help caregivers support individuals through this stage. Active engagement, asking questions, reflecting, mirroring, paraphrasing, and demonstrating the appropriate feedback and emotions are good ways to let this individual know that you are accompanying them in their memory-based journey. Other methods to help individuals move toward acceptance may include helping them to express their emotions, validating their reality, helping them to regulate their emotions, and asking questions to help bring added perspective to the situation.

The length of time needed in each stage of grief can vary by individual, yet if someone is stuck and unable to move beyond the depression stage, they can benefit from more in-depth behavioral health support. Care providers do not need to supply all the answers, yet they should be able to offer support in making connections or referrals to others who have the right training and who can be most helpful.

These life processes have a significant impact on older adults and can be particularly intense for TGNC people as they age. The time needed to experience and process their grief has been limited or taken away from many TGNC individuals by society's imposition of oppression. The transgender person may have had to spend countless hours learning about who they really are, how to express their identity in an oppressive world, and how to deal with other barriers to wholeness. For these reasons, TGNC individuals at the end of their life may feel it is unfair that their life ends so soon. It may feel premature that, after so much work, they must now say goodbye. A TGNC individual who is caught up in this scenario may deny their limited time, experience rage about how unfair this has been, barter for more time, and become depressed at the reality of the fast-approaching end of life. Supporting these individuals may mean validating each of the stages, empathizing with them, and helping them gain perspective by acknowledging their personal accomplishments, particularly when society has created conditions that make success feel as though it is only achieved against all odds. This process has led the individual to the beginning of the final stage of grief.

The last stage is acceptance, and it is about finding a positive way to look at the inevitability of the end of life. During the process of acceptance of death, "Life flashes before your eyes." It is practically unavoidable that individuals would engage in reflection about the meaning and purpose of their personal journey. The more the reality of death can be accepted, the easier is for individuals to (1) fully immerse themselves in such existential exploration and (2) hopefully be able to embrace their journey toward the end.

12.1.1 Life Review

One activity that can support this process is a "life review." A life review is a reflective process in which memories are pieced together and meaning is found in those experiences. This activity can be completed independently, but it is most useful when there is someone else to help with the process, such as a support staff member or therapist. Also, it may be very empowering to share the findings with a close group, such as a support group. TGNC older adults may benefit from not only piecing together memories but also connecting them to identity development models and their various stages. For example, an individual could identify times prior to developing a personal, social, or community identity [8] or instances that contribute to the development of pride and a synthesis of their identity [9]. This exercise can help individuals gain a positive insight into their own identity-shaping process.

It can also help them to recognize accomplishments and milestones that they might have not identified before. At the end, the process of accepting impending death can be a process of great insight that leads to personal growth, individual satisfaction, and internal peace.

During the acceptance stage, individuals may be interested in finding closure in their interpersonal relationships, including connections with individuals who may have become distant or who may have strayed. As the approach of death has been accepted, they acknowledge that they have a limited opportunity to resolve any unresolved issues. They tend to seek reconciliation and find peace through resolutions of conflict that now may seem less important than before. Mending broken relationships can bring gratification, yet the process is unpredictable, and there is no guarantee that the relationships can be mended. Care providers should support the individual in whichever decision they make and prepare them to recognize that there are things they cannot control and that some people may never change.

Reaching the final stage of acceptance can help the individual become open to useful conversations that are necessary in preparation for death, including planning a ritual or ceremony such as a memorial event. It is understandable that individuals may have a hard time thinking about their memorial service, and some people may go through similar emotions as the stages of grief when thinking about such an event. For example, individuals may want to deny the importance of planning a memorial. They may become angry at the logistics, try to negotiate not having to think about the situation, and become depressed about who will or will not be there. Hopefully, they can finally accept the reality of the situation and engage in the process. Although it may be initially difficult, becoming involved in the planning of their own memorial event can be an empowering, rewarding, and uplifting experience. In the case of TGNC individuals, there are added layers of concerns connected to their gender identities and societal oppression. In the following section, we will offer an overview of memorial practices and some of the particular challenges faced by TGNC individuals.

12.2 Memorials as Site of Oppression

Every society at every moment in known history—and in much of prehistory—has created at least one socially sanctioned ritual to commemorate the lives and deaths of its constituents. Cultural universals are relatively rare. In the instances where they do exist, the particular forms these rituals take on can differ by sociocultural and temporal contexts. Death and its commemoration are no different. What ultimately ties these diverse cultural practices together, however, apart from their focus on death, are the ways in which both individual and communal constructions of identity can become deeply intertwined with the cultural practices themselves.

Each memorial practice is, in a sense, a production of the departed individual's identity. Importantly, this happens without the active participation of that individual. The fractal nature of this process comes from the many, and often competing, sources involved in the process of creating a "final" story for the deceased individual. From the stories that are told of their life by those mourning to the presentation of the body prior to its burial or incineration, every element of memorial practices creates a new retelling of the dead person's life. In this retelling, some perspectives become dominant and others less so. Often, these more dominant perspectives are offered at the cost of the deceased's self-identification. This happens far too often for sexual and gender minorities, in which the narratives told may actively deny the self-determined identities of those who have passed on.

LGBTQ people have long experienced memorials and end-of-life celebrations as instances of symbolic violence committed against them. It is still not uncommon for more culturally mainstream memorials to erase same-sex partnerships and/or gender fluidity, unfairly punish the deceased with accusations of immorality, or deny community identification through exclusionary acts, e.g., refusing to allow fellow members of the LGBTQ communities to attend/participate in the memorial or wake. This has been particularly true of TGNC persons, whose gender diverse identities are often obscured or outright erased in the tales recounted during these "celebratory" moments. This denial of subjectivity and gender-based authenticity is "a psychic act of violence, foreclosing upon the subject whose gender identity is misread. To be a subject is to be recognized in a social field in which gender matters" [10].

Conventional end-of-life memorial practices, traditions, and rituals may work well for many people when their journey reaches its conclusion. However, and while some of the experiences that TGNC older adults face at the end of life may be similar to those experienced by cisgender people, other situations may be very different. For some TGNC persons, conventional processes and practices may not be fitting, appropriate, or desired. By default, TGNC persons have unique life experiences and a correspondingly different frame of reference for themselves than a cisgender individual will have. It is purely a function of the TGNC person's identity and their personal reality. The end of life should optimally be a meaningful reflection of that reality and understanding.

When a TGNC older adult approaches their life's end, they may have a unique set of questions, such as "Will I be celebrated and/or honored for who I truly am when I die? What will people think or say about me at the end of my life and beyond? Will my gender identity be acknowledged and respected, or will it be ignored, swept under the rug, or even vilified?" Questions such as these are indicators of the significance of a TGNC person's identity and the experiences they encounter while they travel through life. That identity and those experiences will have obviously helped to shape their thinking and their corresponding self-awareness.

As we have already learned, identity construction continues, in a social sense, beyond death. Because this is true, many TGNC older adults have concerns—and rightfully so, given the general antipathy that our society holds toward the transgender community—about whether their transgender identity will be recognized, affirmed, and remembered at the end of life and after their death. The end-of-life experience for a transgender person creates an opportunity to honor, respect, and celebrate who they are—or, following their death, who they were. It can allow those who remain behind to validate the truth of the TGNC older adult's identity, recognize their experiences, and honor the impact that resulted from the manifestation of that identity during the TGNC person's lifetime.

Nevertheless, many transgender persons have concerns about whether others will be respectful or will reject their TGNC identity and/or their gender fluidity. TGNC older adults tend to seek acknowledgement and affirmation of their TGNC identity from caregivers and family members. Sometimes, though, family members and caregivers may refuse to accept the reality of a TGNC person's core identity and have no interest in honoring or appreciating it. Such attitudes and behaviors can create a great deal of unnecessary pain, which is a heartbreaking experience to be imposed on anyone at the end of their life. Cisgender persons are rarely, if ever, forced to deal with this type of unjust situation.

> For transgender people, the lack of recognition of their chosen gender identity, or the humiliation of having to explain that they are transgender, [can be] salient issues. One service provider told of a transgender woman who had lived all her life as a woman, but had never had sex reassignment surgery. She now had dementia and lived in an aged care facility run by a religious charity. Staff there forced her to live as a man. Other transgender people who have not had sex reassignment surgery, or who are left with incontinence after the surgery, have to explain their situation to care providers in order to get appropriate products. One service provider reflected on the very high levels of education, advocacy and training, and personal support, needed to ensure transgender clients received appropriate services, even from transfriendly agencies [11].

12.2.1 Working with Families and Caregivers

Older TGNC adults may have to worry about whether they will need to teach their families or caregivers about TGNC identities, forms of expression, and specific health/medical needs. There are many reports of barriers to health-care service access due to discrimination, inappropriate care, and lack of knowledge among health-care workers about legal rights at the end of life. For some cisgender care providers, this may be the first time in their lives they have ever been confronted with a gender diverse person's existence or particular needs. Since this is a new scenario for them, they may need to be educated about the realities of a TGNC identity, expression, and health needs. The burden of providing such education often falls, unfairly, on the shoulders of the TGNC older adult. Since the gender diverse person may already be in poor or failing health, having to be an educator can be both physically and emotionally difficult, especially for someone who is nearing the end of their life's journey.

Yet another unique aspect of the end of life for TGNC older adults may involve concerns about how they will be presented after their death. For example, if their body is to lie in an open coffin for a memorial, how will that body be dressed and groomed? Also, how will they be identified and spoken about? What gender-based language will be used and applied in such situations? Again, these are potentially problematic areas with which most cisgender persons are never burdened.

Sometimes, TGNC older adults may be forced to deal with a "disenfranchised grief" situation. This can occur when same-sex partners are not legitimized by service providers and/or family members. Also, friends—and sometimes even former partners—may not be respected or recognized as significant members of a "family of choice." As might be expected, this type of situation can create all sorts of potential difficulties and raw emotions. "All of the above problems can lead to isolation, late presentation for treatment which results in the need for crisis management, and complicate the experience of end-of-life care" [11].

End of life for TGNC older adults may hold a particular set of concerns that most cisgender persons never have to think about. However, the end of a TGNC life can also be a time of satisfying reflection, introspection, retrospection, sharing, and appreciation for lessons learned along the way. Additionally, it can be a time of genuine celebration and respect for a life that may have been out of the mainstream but has been lived in a special, unique way that allowed the individual to be their authentic self.

12.3 Memorials as Opportunities to Celebrate Identity and Form Community

Despite the ways that memorials have so often been used as sites of erasure, they have also been adapted and adopted in affirming ways. With regard to LGBTQ people, the queering of memorial practices allows for a new respect to be found for the dead in a world that has largely cast them aside as disposable at best and despicable at worst. Practices that not only affirm but also celebrate trans identities create a space for building community. As Walt Odets notes in relation to individuals who have died from HIV-related complications, "When social ritual is not too conventionalized–which is to say that it remains connected in some way to the subjective experience of the participants–it can be immensely important in helping to confirm individual happiness, or assisting survival of what might otherwise be unendurable, private misery" [12]. Beyond individual happiness, however, these "not too conventionalized" memorials allow for traditionally marginalized peoples to come together and find communal happiness as well.

By creating new cultural practices that center on queer identity, the symbolic violence inflicted upon the dead by unsympathetic or unknowledgeable persons can be alleviated, at least to some extent. People who are planning and facilitating the memorial rites (morticians, religious leaders, family members) may both intentionally and unintentionally misgender and/or commit harm through the eternal reminders of obituaries and gravestones. By queering the funerary space, a celebration of the deceased's life is able to truly take place, as well as a real opportunity for grieving for the memorial attendees.

12.3.1 Queering the Funeral

The act of queering the funeral allows the process of creating subjectivity, thereby supporting the deceased person's narrative and lived experience while affirming both the individual and the community [13]. With regard to the individual, memorial events can provide a space for a lasting image of a person to be continually generated in the minds of others. There is a reason why such time and effort are given to ensuring that a body is presentable in open-casket funerals. These final images of the body and the communal consumption of images and narratives permeating the events help to ensure a malleable but durable recollection of the individual. A body that visibly shows respect for self-identification—and not necessarily the desires of those who remain—leaves a more authentic and honorable final image for those in attendance. It also creates an opportunity in which both transgender older adults and younger folks in attendance are able to see their identities validated in a fundamental way.

In addition to the visual presentation of the body, the actual site of burial also matters. The burial of an individual near their family, of course, indicates kinship and family identification. Conversely, the distancing of physical bodies from each other in death represents, both literally and metaphorically, a distancing of family relations. Like many other queer individuals, TGNC people have often faced the challenge of family estrangement both before and after death. The families of origin of many TGNC folks have disavowed them in death as in life by preventing their burial near that of other "blood kin."

While this has led to numerous unique difficulties for many TGNC people, as with other sexual and gender minorities, it has sometimes also led to spaces of cultural and psychological innovation. Choosing to be buried near one's family of choice, as opposed to one's family of origin, can be a deeply empowering and motivating decision that extends beyond the individual and forges queer kinship in seemingly eternal ways. The ceremonies themselves can provide for community to be built in shared moments of deeply intertwined emotion. The power of grief can limit social interactions in surprisingly useful ways [14, 15]. It can also bring people together.

We see this, for example, here in the United States with the insistence on remembering and saying the names of people who lost their lives to violence. This is especially important in communities of color and LGBTQ communities. In a context where so many TGNC women of color are fatal victims of violence, and in which these victims are often left unrecognized, the movement to #SayHerName provides myriad functions: to honor and remember the deceased, to bring about awareness and justice on a larger social level, and to build a visible and more powerful community of TGNC folks and allies. These are reasons why the annual Transgender Day of Remembrance, held each November 20th, has become such a significant occasion within the TGNC community, providing a space for both respectfully honoring individuals and simultaneously building community.

12.4 Recommendations of Key Elements for TGNC Memorial Planning

We believe it is time to create new end-of-life traditions in honor of TGNC individuals—traditions that do not carry the historical baggage of oppression and invisibility. Here we would like to propose that memorials for TGNC individuals not only be considered opportunities for closure and saying goodbye but that such memorials also become a platform for community building, advocacy, celebration, and tribute. For those reasons, this chapter will conclude with the following recommendations to be considered when planning a memorial event for a TGNC individual:

- Help the individual to make as many decisions as possible prior to the event, so that those decisions are consistent in terms of how the person wants to be represented. This could include preselecting decorations, music, the list of guests, program information, etc. For example, help the individual preselect photos and items to be displayed, so that they are remembered as they would like to be. They might want to create a PowerPoint presentation, video, or memory board. In addition, this would include a plan for announcements in social media or other forms of media.
- Suggest considering art performances such as poems, a singer, or an instrument playing, as these are meaningful ways to celebrate a person's life journey. The TGNC individual may want to highlight specific times/events of their life through some form of artistic expression.
- Connect with local LGBTQ agencies and explore the possibility of their involvement. The presence of community leaders can help heighten the importance of taking this opportunity to build community and honor those who were part of the struggle.
- Help the TGNC person think about the physical location of their memorial service. Remind them about the importance of choosing a place that can be easily accessible to their support network. It would be ideal if the venue utilized is one that has clear nondiscrimination policies, messaging, signage, and affirming practices.
- Clarify, and consider putting in writing, the role of family of origin and family of choice in the programming and the overall event.
- If desired, include a spiritual element of choice that resonates for the TGNC person.
- Consider an activity to honor the TGNC person, such as releasing balloons, marching on the street, or giving those present the opportunity to share thoughts about this person. Activities like this can create long-lasting memories in those who participate.
- Throughout the process, bring up key words such as courage, authenticity, advocate, hero, and warrior. The atmosphere should be one of honoring and paying tribute to this individual.

In the end, there are endless considerations and opportunities when planning a memorial for a TGNC individual. Yet, it is of great importance to make no assumptions, communicate effectively with this individual whenever possible, and seriously take into consideration the sociohistorical elements and challenges that call for these celebrations to be different. Being able to support a TGNC individual in their preparation for the end of life is an honor and a privilege.

References

1. Hughes AK, Harold RD, Boyer JM. Awareness of LGBT aging issues among aging services network providers. J Gerontol Soc Work. 2011;54(7):659–77.
2. Rath T, Harter JK, Harter J. Wellbeing: the five essential elements: Gallup Press; 2010.
3. Lambda Legal. When health care isn't caring: lambda Legal's survey of discrimination against LGBT people and people with HIV. New York: Lambda Legal; 2010.
4. Houghton A. Maintaining dignity: understanding and responding to the challenges facing older LGBT Americans. Washington, DC: AARP Research; 2018. https://doi.org/10.26419/res.00217.001.
5. Crain W. Theories of development: concepts and applications. 6th ed. Upper Saddle River: Pearson Education, Inc.; 2011. ISBN 978-0-205-81046-8
6. Erikson EH, Erikson JM. The life cycle completed (extended version): WW Norton & Company; 1998.
7. Kübler-Ross E. On death and dying: what the dying have to teach doctors, nurses, clergy and their own families: Taylor & Francis; 2009.
8. D'Augelli AR. Identity development and sexual orientation: Toward a model of lesbian, gay, and bisexual development. In E. J. Trickett, R. J. Watts, & D. Birman (Eds.), The Jossey-Bass social and behavioral science series. Human diversity: Perspectives on people in context (pp. 312–333). 1994; San Francisco, CA, US: Jossey-Bass.
9. Cass VC. Homosexuality identity formation: a theoretical model. J Homosex. 1979;4(3):219–35.
10. Cavanagh SL. Queering bathrooms: gender, sexuality, and the hygienic imagination. Toronto: University of Toronto Press; 2001.
11. Auger JA. Passing through: end-of-life decisions of lesbians and gay men. J Palliat Care. 2004;20(3):221.
12. Odets W. In the shadow of the epidemic: being HIV-negative in the age of AIDS. Durham: Duke University Press; 1995.
13. Ellis C, Flaherty M. Investigating subjectivity: research on lived experience, vol. 139: Sage; 1992.
14. Scheper-Hughes, N. Death without weeping: The violence of everyday life in Brazil. Oakland: University of California Press; 1993.
15. Scheper-Hughes N. Violence and the politics of remorse. In: Biehl J, Good B, Kleinman A, editors. Subjectivity: ethnographic investigations. Oakland: University of California Press; 2007. p. 179–234.

Transitioning and Generational Cohort: Retirement

13

D. L. Wilke

13.1 Introduction

Other chapters in this book will cover the science behind transgenderism. Others still will cover specific issues related to substances, violence, spirituality, etc. But this chapter is focused on connection and the aging process. Apart from our very young years, there is probably not a more vulnerable time in our own histories than when we become elders. Developmental losses are the norm for most aging persons, but for this unique population, the impact of those losses can feel singularly painful and isolating. So much more the reason that we help each other find a way to become or stay connected as we grow older.

This will be an exercise in gathering experiential golden nuggets of not just my current and past client stories but of those gleaned from responses to a short survey sent out across the country to a variety of agencies and organizations that serve the transgender and gender nonconforming populations. These places included SAGE (Advocacy & Services for LGBT Elders) in New York City Midtown and Chicago, PHS (Program in Human Sexuality, University of Minnesota), Trans Lounge (LGBT Center Los Angeles, CA), Chicago Gender Society, Chi Chapter, and T-FEM Chicago, IL, and a variety of online and in-person support networks in Michigan and Indiana.

My private practice of 20 years has nested itself in three different bedroom communities of Chicago, Illinois. Former clients, as well as current, were kind enough to complete the following survey (Table 13.1). What is added to these are the many stories that have been shared with me through the years. My early consultant was

This chapter does not follow the academic style or educational rigor of the previous chapters. Rather, it is a social survey and personal narrative by a professional working with the transgender community in and around the Chicagoland area for over 20 years in private practice.

D. L. Wilke
Compassionate, Counseling, Shorewood, IL, USA

M. Houlberg et al. (eds.), *Transgender and Gender Nonconforming Health and Aging*,
https://doi.org/10.1007/978-3-319-95031-0_13

Table 13.1 How we connect as transitioning or gender nonconforming elders survey results ($N = 34$)

Who most likely partners you in activities related to gender transition (gender nonconformance)?	*N*	%
Spouse	9	19.57
Friend made after transition	3	6.52
Friend known before transition	7	15.22
Friend made during transition AT a trans-related activity	12	26.09
Friend made during transition but NOT AT a trans-related activity	12	26.09
No one	3	6.52
Are you retired?		
Yes	19	55.88
No	15	44.12
If so, how long have you been retired?		
≤1 year	3	15.79
1–3 years.	1	5.26
3–5 years.	3	15.79
≥5 years.	11	57.89
If not, how long until you plan to retire?		
≤1 year.	0	0.00
1–3 years.	1	6.67
3–5 years.	1	6.67
≥5 years.	11	73.33
How many trans-related activities do you attend per week?		
<1	3	10.00
1	18	60.00
1–3	6	20.00
≥3	3	10.00
How many of these include other retirees?		
<1	6	26.09
1	8	34.78
1–3	5	21.74
≥3	4	17.39
Do you live in a retirement community or a similarly designated housing area?		
Yes	0	0.00
No	34	100.00
Are there any trans-related activities where you live?		
Yes	21	61.76
No	12	35.29
Unknown	1	2.94
Are there any retiree activities where you live?		
Yes	16	47.06
No	14	41.18
Unknown	4	11.76

Note: Survey by D.L. Wilke. Table shows quantitative results only; % represents valid percent right: Our clients are our very best teachers. I will never be able to repay them for all that they have taught me about what it means to live in the margin of society as a gender nonconforming individual. I hope you find their words on these pages as golden and compelling as I have found them through the years.

13.2 Survey Data

In looking at the low return rate of the surveys disseminated nationally, it is clear that our techno-inclined culture would have surely been more likely to respond to an online survey than the one offered via email requesting a scan and return through the same or faxed or worse yet snail mail. Despite this survey being one which queried the elders of the transgender and gender nonconforming of our gender-variant tribe, they still preferred online responding over the methods that were offered.

While studying the responses to the first question on the survey about who partnered folks in activities related to transition or their gender nonconformance, I was not surprised to see that nearly one-third of respondents had a spouse or partner leave them, considering the age group that was polled. It has been my experience as a gender therapist (with 20 years in private practice and having served over 375 persons to transition to whatever level clients felt comfortable) to see the rate of a wife filing for divorce related to this matter fall into one of the following categories: those married more than 30 years, only one couple; those married 20 to 30 years, most wives stayed, a few left; those married 10 to 20 years, most left, a few stayed; and those married less than 10 years, none stayed.

It was interesting to see how the numbers for "Friends made *during* transition," whether at or *not* at a trans-related activity, were tied. Of our 34 respondents, 19 were already retired and 15 were not yet. Again, our numbers were tied at 11 years relative to how long people had either *been* retired or *until* they would retire. Most people reported attending only one trans-related activity per week, and a slight majority reported that these activities included other retirees.

None of our 34 respondents reported living in a retirement community or similarly designated housing area. A curious response was the finding that 21 of the 34 respondents reported that there *were* trans-related activities where they live. The lengthier essay responses of the people who did not have the luxury of living in an area that offered such activities or companionship spoke of the isolation they experienced feeling cutoff from a sense of TGNC community. In the last of the short answer questions, only by a difference of one did the score find in favor of people having retiree activities where they live. Four of the 34 did not know if there were any retiree activities where they lived, whereas only 1 of the 34 was unsure if there were any trans-related activities where they live.

It was also interesting to look at the variety of answers to the essay questions. The answers were as broad in spectrum as the rainbow itself. The first response (see Appendix A) made a very salient point. Younger people transitioning, or living a more non-binary life, today enter a more informed and welcoming society than did the Baby Boomers generation who make up most of the retirement age persons in the TGNC population.

13.3 Discussion

In 1999, I was asked by my second transgender client to please start a support group for persons like herself. She began to cry and begged me saying, "Please Deb, I am forty-two years old and I have never met anyone like me in my whole life." She had driven five and one-half hours just for her session with me and was willing to repeat the journey to come meet someone like herself.

I gave it considerable thought. I figured I had an out when I considered turning the responsibility over to existing agencies in Chicago, so I could refer her, and others who might ask, over to them. No one had heard of such a thing. It was official. I was on the hook to begin the first professionally facilitated support group for TG/TS persons in Illinois. I began calling a list of 15 churches in the area to host our group. Fourteen told me to seek elsewhere. One said that "This would be a fantastic outreach ministry for our church." The minister on the other end of that line was an atheist. Eighteen years later, the group continues through member-led facilitation.

Through the years, I have noticed groups like this one waning as younger blood seems to have lesser need to associate with those older than themselves. They have their own young people's support and social networks magnificently run by very talented staff. In fact, when I first began my practice in 1998, those coming to me in search of themselves and eventual transition were feminizing males ranging in age from 40 to 75 years old and now are predominantly masculinizing females ranging in age from 11 to 17 years of age. [Those coming to me on the younger end often define themselves as non-binary. It would be a mistake to confuse this term with non-important or non-visible or nonessential to our world. Just because they do not sign on for our strongly held binary exclusionism construct, it doesn't make our belief true or theirs incorrect, no matter how much the English teacher within us struggles to use plural pronouns when referencing an individual.]

I think it is for this reason that there were many more respondents to the survey who were feminizing males than masculinizing females. And although the transmasculine experience is represented in the responses you read here, clearly the transfeminine responses outnumber them significantly largely due to the aging factor. What I have noted in my own practice is that the GNC transmasculine female has had an easier time going stealth melting into the male world than the converse.

One of our first efforts as a support group, which was called *Transitions from the Inside Out*, was to call out the chief of police in the town where we met for still having on their lawbooks a 1965 law prohibiting cross-dressing in public. When I called the chief, who had been on the force over 20 years, he told me he didn't believe there was such a law. He had never heard of it while still a young officer walking the beat. I asked him to research it. He found it and acknowledged it did in fact still exist. I asked him to remove it because it was unnerving to my group's members, understandably. He told me it wasn't that simple. First, we had to write a formal letter of request petitioning the town to remove the law, then the town's lawyers would have to review the request, and then the town council would have to vote on it. It took 9 months to abolish the law, setting the hearts of our members at ease.

Just as no two clients have ever been alike, their responses have been equally varied regarding their perception of how their transition, or life as a gender nonconforming individual, has gone. Some have experienced their TGNC life as less than hoped for, while for some it has been the highlight of their existence. The same holds true for experiences in TGNC-related activities. Many tell of just how plain fun their connections to others have been at these activities, a time to let their "girly persona out" and "have a good time," while others found these connections to be "crucial to their well-being." For some, it gave them "opportunity to make dramatic changes" to their exteriors, while for others, it allowed them to have their interiors "be given expression for the first time."

To truly appreciate how meaningful this can be, we have only to flip open the pages of any introduction to psychology textbook to read about the social motive in young children, or the importance of healthy attachment to others, or further still the deeply needed quiet certainty of one's own self-satisfaction with feeling accepted, loved, and true to oneself. The last of these is difficult to experience if you have forever felt trapped in some sort of costume that never bore your name on the tag inside.

One of the most memorable moments in my session room was when a young adult was trying to explain to her father why she felt it necessary to gender transition. I believe the father was trying to come from a loving and understanding place while addressing his feminizing son with the question, "Why do you feel you need to do this? Can't you find a different way to make peace with your life?"

The youth respectfully responded with words I will never forget. "Dad, it's like you told me you loved me when you sent me off to school and all you asked of me was to wear this bear costume and to never, ever take it off no matter what. And Dad, I have tried. I have really tried to live inside it, even though it was itchy, even though people made fun of me for it, even though I knew it never fit right. I tried. I really tried, Dad, because I loved you. I didn't want to disappoint you. But I can't do it anymore Dad. The costume is coming off. Do you understand, Dad? It's coming off. It's time to just be me."

This young person's father broke down and cried and asked for his child's forgiveness. He didn't realize this is what he had asked of his child. Finally, the father knelt in front of his daughter and whispered, "You have my blessing and my full support."

Now, I wish I could tell you every client had this kind of happy ending. Sadly, they do not. And because they do not, I think therefore some of the remarks in the essay questions reveal lives of pain and isolation. And even when opportunities present themselves in older years, some TGNC people will decline the chance to attend or become involved on any level in activities specifically targeted for them, choosing rather to remain in what they know best, lives of withdrawal and isolation.

You can read this for yourself in some of the comments made in the essay responses (Appendix A).

It is an interesting human phenomenon that it almost doesn't matter the initial circumstance or event each person will create from their own personal story. So, some folks who had it difficult and lonely, feeling wounded and deprived in terms of gender expression, may end up being very involved in TGNC activities, advocacy, and even outreach programs.

One such person comes to mind. This individual had an internal knowing about gender at an early age as our human sexuality textbooks tell us is common. I reference it as the awareness of the gendered self. Despite clients so often wishing me to tell them which gender they are, whether they are transgender, whether they should transition, etc., I cannot possibly know these things. Its knowing is so deeply personal and dwells only within the person themselves. It is the client who must tell me who they are.

One such client then spoke of this early awareness. When feeling brave, he would dare to cross-dress in female attire as a child. The client reported not feeling any sexual gratification from this behavior but rather a correctness, a "rightness." While still a teenager, tragedy struck when both of his parents were killed in an automobile accident. This young man believed in his heart, like so many of us are tempted to do, that this loss was a punishment from God for his cross-dressing behavior.

When this client shared this story with me, he told me, "This is the first time I have ever told anyone this story." I have always considered my session room a safe place for my clients and their disclosures sacred testimony. As he spoke, it was clear to me that he was lifting off his heart a burden he had carried for a very long time. After he laid it on the session room floor, he reported feeling better, lighter. As he was leaving the room, he wept in my arms saying, "Can you believe this is the first time I have spoken of this in over fifty years?"

That same individual braved telling not only me but a spouse of many years, family, and friends. But it didn't stop there. That transwoman went on to follow her journey through physical transition and almost more importantly blossomed into a tremendous advocate for the TGNC community helping others to tell their story and find peace for themselves. Not everyone will respond the same way to beginning circumstances or events in their lives. Each of us write our own script.

One of the things I try to stress with all my clients is their ownership of the "blue pencil," that which all editors use to mark manuscripts for that which they want edited out and that which they want kept or tweaked. I remind clients they are not only the authors of their stories but the editors as well. They get to decide what stays and what goes. They are not their histories. They are not what people tell them they are or were. And, they are definitely greater than the sum of their parts. One respondent said it best, "I get out once a month and that suits me. I enjoy the trans part of my life, but its just a part of me, and I am okay with that."

The focus of this chapter is connection, however, and I want to stress some of the comments made in the essay questions here. One such individual gave a lengthy response to the first essay, which offered a broad explanation of how she remains connected to others in the TGNC community. I appreciate how she first acknowledges that "Transition is a journey, first of discovery, then of progression." She speaks of attending different groups in different states for support across a spectrum of friends who are very similar to her own story and those very different as well. She ends with "There are many challenges to overcome. It's so important to have those around you to love you and support (you) on this journey." Indeed.

I also value her comment on staying close to transgender friends through the medium of Skype. Social media was something I had left out of the survey. I can only imagine I did so because I do my best to avoid these. Well, it's relatively easy because I don't understand how to work many things on the computer or smartphones, nor do I have the time to devote to such things. I'm not sure if that makes me sound stupid or industrious, probably a little of both. Still, the value of connecting through the computer and social media is incalculable. People of almost any age can attest to their significant connections using these means. It afforded them a window to the world with the introduction of the World Wide Web. They could look up anything, connect with almost anyone anywhere, play infinite games, and have a private vehicle that could whisk them away from any otherwise painful here and now. They could create an avatar, multiple avatars; change genders, body types, and abilities; explore curiosities; build armies, farms, and cities; and travel to new galaxies all from the comfort of their own bedrooms.

Another piece I have consistently found interesting in the TGNC population (particularly transwomen), and this was mentioned in the first essay response as well, is that there seems to be this cycle so many of them go through and that is the URGE, SPLURGE, and PURGE cycle of buying clothes, accessories, wigs, etc. This seemed to be true for the cross-dresser and for the early days and years of the transitioning individual. I encourage them all to invest in larger storage containers instead of being faithful donors to resale stores.

It's not that I don't understand the stages of this cycle. It's just that I understand poverty better. For some of these folks, particularly those who opt to transition, money will become a large issue. And even for those who are enjoying cross-dressing much to the distress of their spouses, divorces can be pricey, too. I encourage all of them simply to save their stuff and save their money. If they live long enough, most clothes do come back in style. It's a thing. It's a cycle in fashion.

13.4 Retirement

For many TGNC people, retirement unlocks the key to the freedom to truly expressing one's gendered self in a way that the workplace would not have tolerated. I've been writing letters for HRT (hormone replacement therapy) and GCS (gender confirmation surgery) for years, and despite my respect for WPATH's (World Professional Association for Transgender Health) Standards of Care methodology, I will never ask of a client that they cross-dress in the workplace if they feel it would be unsafe to do so or if their pension would be on the line for doing so. The RLT (real-life test), in my mind, can occur in other places and count just as much than if I asked the impossible, unreasonable, or dangerous of my client. I won't do it. I will follow SOC as the guidelines they were meant to be, not laws etched into stone. It will do my aging client no earthly good to become penniless, maimed, or dead.

One of my jobs as a mental health counselor is to help my clients find connections within the community to aid with any depression or sense of isolation they may be feeling. It really is incumbent upon any therapist to know what resources are available to them. So, besides knowing HRT supervising physicians, surgeons of all types, voice trainers, electrologists, wig stylists and sellers, hair replacement doctors, psychiatrists, other therapists specializing in different modalities, transition socialization guides, HR (human resource) and workplace guidance specialists, welcoming churches of various faiths, the ever-changing laws around name and gender marker changes, school social workers, counsel for one's own practice, and a qualified, gender-specific consultant to run cases past, a therapist must also equip themselves with information on what possible groups, agencies, and advocates a client might turn to for connection and support.

We consider ourselves blessed in the Chicagoland area to have several TGNC service providers of all types: including those that offer legal assistance, social and support networks in the city and suburbs, therapists who work with adults and adolescents, as well as clinics and a children's hospital that specialize in treating the young gender-variant child. We recognize that there are only a handful of such cities in our country that are similar havens for the gender nonconforming. Everyday I receive calls and emails from such persons who live in a state where there are no such supports in place. Their words are full of desperation, fear, and pain. It saddens me that I cannot even deliver my services to them remotely if they are out-of-state because my license through the Illinois Department of Financial and Professional Regulation will not allow me to practice with any client who is not in the state where I reside. And even if the person were within my state, any electronic means of communication must be both HIPAA compliant *and* legal, meaning having a BAA (business associate agreement) contract with me. So, neither Skype nor Zoom would fall into this category, and these are the most commonly requested by clients.

Another aspect I found interesting in the respondents' answers to the second essay question on the survey was how variable they were. Some people wanted gatherings to include spouses, some to include all ages. Some were looking for discussion groups, others support groups, and some strictly social groups or outings such as shopping, movies, dinners, etc.

Others enjoyed attending church services, while other people had bad experiences where they were asked to leave a church. I witnessed this firsthand in my own church with a young client. The head of a committee commented to me after a service that if "that was one of my clients, to tell them to dress more appropriately or don't come back." The church knew I was working with the GNC population, and they assumed I was seeing this young person who was only beginning on the path to self-discovery and expression. I spoke to the pastor who had a conversation with the "righteous one," and no more was said about it. [For the record, it has always confounded me how some religious institutions use their words to excise members of their flock rather than to set the example of warm inclusivity.]

Some might argue this chapter is no place for religious rhetoric, but I would argue it is exactly the place for such an argument because if any group of people have suffered exclusionary behavior at the hands of religionists, surely it is those who present outside the norm of what is deemed acceptable, preferable, and even tolerable in terms of presentation. Think of those 15 pastors I spoke to about hosting our support group, and the only one who was warmly welcoming or welcoming at all was an atheist.

Acknowledgments Chi Chapter Oakbrook, IL
Chicago Gender Society, Chicago, IL
Indiana Transgender Network Online Aggregate Resources
Michigan Transgender Alliance
Mosaic Health Goshen, IN
Over 40 Trans Male Facebook Group
PFLAG Michiana
PFLAG Michigan City
Program in Human Sexuality, University of MN, Minn
SAGE NYC, NY Midtown
SAGE Chicago, IL
T-FEM Chicago, IL
Trans Indy Indianapolis, IN
Trans Lounge LGBT Center, Los Angeles, CA
Transmasculine League of Michiana

Appendix A

Essay question 1. Describe your personal experience with transition and its relevance to shared activities with others during retirement who have or are transitioning.
Responses
"Greater commonality in life experiences related to transition for "baby boomer" population generally than those transitioning younger today. They come into a more informed and welcoming society."
"I get out once a month and that suits me. I enjoy the trans part of my life, but it is just a part of me, and I am okay with that."
"I have enjoyed my years of experience transitioning and the related group activities I have attended."
"Experience with transition has been good. Hostility has been extremely rare. I don't discuss being transgender often, and it is not generally as issue in my activities."
"I went through many purges of clothing. After hearing about Chi Chapter, 20 years later, I attended a meeting. It took time to fully present (en femme) but I did attend Be-All (conference) in 2012. Transition is on hold. (But still attending activities.)"
"Talks and meetings help a lot."
"Transition is a journey, first of discovery, then of progression. I had a close friend, transgender, who was military like me. We talked to each other a couple of times a week, traveled together for weekend adventures, and generally supported each other. She transitioned very late, after her wife died, but my dear friend died last year. She was 80. I Skype with transgender friends that have fully transitioned. It is so helpful to have friends to talk about our lives and activities. We all live full time as women but I'm the only one having completed GCS. Attending Southern Comfort…and transgender organizations in Chicago and Florida were critically important for me in this journey. There are many challenges to overcome. It's so important to have those around you to love and support (you) on this journey."

"Transitioning is tough for me as I am in the closet with family and friends. Knowing no one knows my male self underneath my girl persona was very empowering in that I felt I could express myself. I have met friends who are a lot more active than I am thru (sic) Chi Chapter and social media. They have allowed me to join them in get-togethers in public social settings."

"Transition was a long time coming but joyous since the time came."

"I did not engage in any cross-dressing for over 30 years (1989–2019); worked with a therapist to unblock the repression. I feel supported and accepted at Chi Chapter meetings. They have been very helpful with my self-acceptance."

"I could not imagine transitioning while I was working. I was retired about six months before I started to think about it. I have made a few friends at the T-FEM meeting. Aisha is the only one who is also retired. Being retired, we could drive to the Keystone Conference. During the drive, I learned that we have many things in common, an interest in antiques, woodworking, astronomy, and gardening."

"In my experience, I have no retirees in transition. All of my friends who have or are transitioning are still active in business."

"I have found informal gatherings; i.e., at a bar of people going through the same experiences to be crucial for me. Having the chance to informally and openly talk with others who fully support me has helped me get through the process. I have found meetings to be far less informative and not as open. I have gone to some social events at the Center on Halsted (ice cream social, TG film festival) which I would do more of if closer."

"I have not transitioned. I like trans activities because I can be honest about who I am there."
"Social groups, conventions, support groups have been helpful. Having transgender friends, going out alone, with spouse, with relatives and friends has been very helpful. Coming out to family was the best help along with major help from my HRT doctor, my counselor, my electrologist, my trans friend and her post-op TG dad."

"The first doctor I told asked if I wanted a psychiatric referral. Through other trans men I was able to find a doctor. The cost of hormones and syringes is nominal. I am not involved with other retirees. I am athletic, active and independent. I am concerned about getting older and becoming more vulnerable."

"I tried to come out to a wife of 20 years, but that ended marriage. I went back into closet. Tried coming out to a girlfriend of 4 years, but that ended that relationship. I decided to transition on my own as much as I could. I began attending a Trans focused therapy and a support group where I was (Palm Springs). Great support albeit limited due to small market with limited resources. Much larger gay and lesbian community there. I moved to LA a year ago and have found Trans resources here to be fantastic and very supportive. I go to yoga, occasional (monthly) fitness classes at Trans Lounge where I am the oldest participant, but I love these sessions as I can be healthy …get out of the house presented as I choose. And I see a circle of transwomen and transmen that I am familiar and superficially friendly with. I have also attended a dozen other sessions ranging from the Trans Elder project to social events and skills workshops. All have been good (or most anyway) and I usually leave feeling safe, supported and loving the opportunity to be myself in a social setting with people who share many life experiences. I will not be able to retire although in a way I am due to being very, very underemployed at the moment and for the last few years…having a very difficult time getting hired and I am likely going to need to work way into my senior years."

"I think that I have been very blessed in a couple of ways that many transwomen are not, and so my experiences and answers are heavily influenced by that. I think these advantages make my coming retirement much easier in many ways. First, I have a totally supportive spouse and children. That is a huge advantage that I think makes me much less dependent on specific trans-related activities. But it's not necessarily something that an individual can control. If the support is not there, it's not. We very much have already gradually incorporated a lot of being a cis/trans couple into our pre-retirement life."

"Because of a serious chronic illness, I have had a "homebound transition." Before this transition, I was living as a "sort-of" female at home; but now I see myself as a person who is mostly (roughly 2/3), even when presenting as male with family and some old friends outside my home. As long as I spend most of my time at home presenting as female, the feeling of being female sometimes endures most of the time that I am presenting as male. My homebound transition has been helped immensely by a cisgender female caregiver who accepts me totally as I am and assists me with anything and everything that I need help with- such as laundering my "girl things."
"I retired in 2014, at age 57, in order to address my gender dysphoria. One year after retiring, I fully transitioned. I have used retirement to become an educator regarding gender dysphoria and transgender persons. My blog is eilerspizza.wordpress.com. I have been involved in trans education at Indiana University, had an article featured in Indianapolis Monthly Magazine, and interviewed on three podcasts. Also, I have been active in the trans community in Indianapolis, spoke at the 2015 Trans Day of Remembrance, participated in the drive for civil rights in Indiana, befriended and assisted several trans persons in Indy and have been a regular at Trans Indy group meetings. Because I am older, was a Lutheran minister, am married with children and grandchildren, I am able to be a voice of understanding in the trans community. I have helped them to grasp the difficulties with which their families and others struggle, striving to achieve compassion and unity for all, that all might be accepted, and families love each other. Because I am a blogger, I regularly receive correspondence from those experiencing gender dysphoria, who are trying to sort out all of this, who are facing great marriage, family, faith and work issues. I have used my experience, from every facet of my life to help them think things through." *[I interrupt the flow of responses here because this last response is so carefully articulated and demonstrates so beautifully what Erik Erikson taught us about his psychosocial theory of human development. It is in the seventh of his eight-stage model that he discusses the life crisis of Generativity* vs. *Stagnation. In other words, how do each of us use that time in our life when we are old enough to truly be helpful to younger ones coming up the ropes behind us, to take the time and effort to invest in being a guide and a support while we still have the ability and resources to do so? Clearly, this last response indicates an individual who is using his own life map full of trans-related experiences to assist others attempting to walk that path behind him. He not only holds the map and the lamp, he offers a hand to hold. He offers himself as a model, something each of us has sought since our earliest days. We long to see ourselves in the eyes of another.]*
"My girlfriend (57 years old) and I live far from towns, in south central Oregon. The nearest city has a glbt group but that is an hour drive from here. As far as I know I am trans. I transitioned 44 years ago without a peer or support group."
"There are few transmen in this area and none I have anything in common with besides transition." "I believe there are some folks in my bi-weekly trans group meeting that are retired but the subject hasn't come up while I'm there."
"I THINK I AM THE OLDEST TRANS GUY THAT I KNOW. IT'S AN ISOLATING EXPERIENCE. I'M 67."
Essay Question 2. Explain what kinds of activities you are most likely to attend.
Responses
"Trans group meetings, all ages." "I attend the T-FEM discussion group and the Chicago Gender Society meetings."
"Chi Chapter meetings and Gender Nonconforming occasional dinners with pre-trans friends. Very occasional shopping trips en femme."
"Movies, veterans events, Chi Chapter (as her), Journey Group (as her), Golf."

"I am fully integrated as a woman in all of my activities. I travel the world for a month at a time at least four times a year. In my day-to-day life I am not regarded as transgender, just as a woman. Some might know or suspect but in the past 4 years nobody has ever asked or commented. Next month my wife and I will travel to New Zealand to celebrate our 50th wedding anniversary. While we live separately, we are still married and are together several times a week. Out to dinner; go to a movie, and other social activities."
"Church activities at Holy Trinity Episcopal Church. Experimental Aircraft Association meetings and fly-ins. Local meetings of the National Model Railroad Association."
"Activities where I can socialize with people."
"I like attending scheduled parties at public higher-class lounges where interactions with genetic accepting women are present and dressing in fashionable attire is the norm. That seems to be an important criterion. I also like getting together with friends and go to public shopping malls while in girl mode. The experience is unique in my mind. Being with like-minded friends and sharing mutual interests is also important as going out by yourself is less satisfying."
"Outdoor activities, athletics and photography, spending time with my grandsons."
"Not sure yet. I haven't found any that interest me. Maybe trans and partner events."
"I attend a T-FEM group that meets twice per month. One could say it's a support group, but technically not as it's peer lead. This same group has, on occasion, gone 'out on the town' which was a good time. On other occasions, I've had a quiet dinner in a friend's house who is just starting transition to help answer some of their spouse's questions and to put a face on someone who is well into transition. Being new to the LGBTQ community, I tried to attend as many events of all kinds over the past year. I've been disappointed in the "T" representation at these events. For all I could tell, I was the only visible "T" person there in most cases."
"Same as I currently do but would like to do more events that include more of the LGBTQ rainbow. And would be interested in an arts class or gardening class or hiking, something different. They do a bit of that at that the Center on Halsted but that is hard to get to."
"When I have more time, I plan to attend activities relative to volunteering my time in helping others understand this process who may be struggling. I also hope to work toward educating others who are "NOT" trans to realize the need for understanding and equality."
"I used to be at church weekly, but I was kicked out of several activities, so I don't go anymore. I don't have any social activities I do. I don't play board games available at the Senior Center. I don't like institutional food. I like to work in my kitchen. I like to sew. I like to walk but I can't keep doing that because of broken bone injuries. I ride my bike in warmer weather."
"Mostly lunches and outreach programs and just lots of times with good friends."
"Where I know I can be of help to others."
"I attend a trans men support group. I am getting tickets to a baseball game with friends who are cis-male. I have gone to a couple weekend workshops for trans masculine or trans me anywhere on spectrum. I sing with the Trans Chorus. I've been trying to go on an organized hike, but the activities are in L.A. and I am in Long Beach."
"ACTIVITIES WHERE OTHER TRANSGUYS ARE."
"I am at heart a minister and educator. I have loved the few dozen opportunities I have had to teach students, healthcare professionals and others what it means to be transgender and how we can best live in the world. Though I am an extrovert and outgoing, I tend to be a homebody. I am not interested in social activities, whether or not they are trans-related. Trans Indy helped me tremendously as I (and my wife) started attending as I was beginning my transition. They saw me through it, and now I want to continue attending so that I might help others. This type of setting, peers with peers, appeals greatly to me."
"Fitness and wellness; Social; Skill/transition workshops; Creative projects."

"I like to do some local trans events occasionally, both to support the local community and also to pay back the community by helping others new to the community the way I was helped when I first began getting out. I also enjoy doing some Pride events to show community spirit and support. But what I really love is just getting out in the wider world. I think that trans only events are really helpful as places to start. And in many cases I know that because of all kinds of circumstances some transwomen only feel secure and safe at a trans-related event. But for me it's like a friend of mine once put it, "trans only events all the time are just a bigger closet." As for activities: I love to dance. I mean I really love to dance! I also enjoy museums, concerts, movies and restaurants."
"Online support discussion groups."
"I can't think of any. I connect with other trans guys and allies on Facebook, but I am not interested in socializing face to face. I am an introvert, ha! I garden and spend little time away from home."
"Local symphony and choral events and Community Art Association events."
"I like group meetings or support groups with other people who are trans or also LGBTQIA that are not necessarily social endeavors. Discuss topics of relevance to trans issues or other LGBTQIA issues, how to deal with things, etc. I do also enjoy social outings with similar groups. And also including those outside the LGBTQIA 'family'."

Recommended Reading

1. Hubbard EA, Whitley CT, editors. Trans-kin: a guide for family and friends of transgender people. Boulder: Bolder Press; 2012.
2. Lev A. Transgender emergence: therapeutic guidelines to working with gender-variant people and their families. Binghamton: Haworth Press; 2004.
3. Roughgarden J. Evolution's rainbow. Berkeley: University of California Press; 2004.

Voices: Stories of Resilience 14

Cecilia T. Hardacker, Laura Kelly, Rachael Booth, Johnny Simonello, Estelle Martin, Jesse Harris, Gina Eilers, Jolie Theall, Stefanie Clark, Cornelia Kost, Kelly Ducheny, and Magda Houlberg

14.1 Introduction

Providers and health-care team members who have read this book have been exposed to cutting-edge research and writing designed to support the provision of effective, affirmative care for older transgender and gender nonconforming (TGNC) people. While the previous chapters offered illuminating ideas, research synthesis, and intervention guidance, some were missing the lived experience and direct voice of the TGNC community, especially of TGNC older adults who may have endured decades of healthcare that has not seen them or cared for them in an affirming manner. To intentionally include and amplify these voices, TGNC older adult guest authors were invited to share their experiences in this final chapter. Guest authors were encouraged to speak directly to our

C. T. Hardacker (✉)
Howard Brown Health Center, Chicago, IL, USA
e-mail: ceciliah@howardbrown.org

L. Kelly · J. Simonello · J. Harris · G. Eilers · J. Theall · S. Clark
Chicago, IL, USA

R. Booth
Concord, NH, USA

E. Martin
Cambridge, NH, England

C. Kost
Munich, NH, Germany
e-mail: info@cornelia-kost.de

K. Ducheny
Behavioral Health Services, Howard Brown Health Center, Chicago, IL, USA
e-mail: kellyd@howardbrown.org

M. Houlberg
Medical Services, Howard Brown Health Center, Chicago, IL, USA
e-mail: magdah@howardbrown.org

M. Houlberg et al. (eds.), *Transgender and Gender Nonconforming Health and Aging*,
https://doi.org/10.1007/978-3-319-95031-0_14

audience of health-care providers and offer any guidance they believed health-care providers needed to respectfully and affirmatively care for their community. When we sent out the request, the response was remarkable. We received submissions from around the world and have selected a representative number of guest authors and artists to include. Their ages range from 56 to 73, from all walks of life and three countries.

As said in our first chapter, we celebrate and dedicate this book to the unique set of people, both known and unknown, spanning oceans and time, who have been erased and unwritten throughout history by the patriarchal pen. TGNC people have long stood at the forefront of battles for liberation and equality. With this book, we pay homage to and salute our community's most valuable resource… our TGNC elders.

Our TGNC elders' narratives are uplifting, resilient, generous, and compelling. They are a true representation of lives lived in extraordinary circumstances by extraordinary people. We are grateful for their powerful contribution to this book and to the future of TGNC healthcare providers to come. Here are their stories.

The Editors.

14.2 Laura K. 65

Like most older adults, I have some ongoing medical conditions that require monitoring: because of a brush with malignant melanoma, I see a dermatologist twice a year; because of a history of a vascular event in one eye, a history of narrow-angle glaucoma, and evolving cataracts, I see an ophthalmologist once a year; I see an endocrinologist for my transgender-related hormone therapy; I see a psychologist for an anxiety disorder that stems from years of bullying when I was young; and I must see a general practice person for medication to keep my essential hypertension under control.

I have had the experience of having a provider—it was a clinical psychologist—deny me care because I am transgender. I believe that this was due to the private religious convictions of that provider. I didn't receive the courtesy of an explanation or a referral to someone who would have been willing to see me. I suppose that people like me don't rate courtesy and don't deserve to be treated like fellow human beings. That event sent me into a significant depression that lasted for some time. Many of my peers have had similar experiences.

When I moved to where I now live and was setting up medical care, I spent a good deal of time trying to optimize my chances of not being rejected outright or treated cruelly by a provider. Granted that that is a very low bar in looking for a doctor, but beggars can't be choosers. I immediately crossed out older males. My experience is that men, particularly older men, seem to find transgender women deeply threatening (Page Freud, Sigmund). Medical care associated with a religious group—particularly Christian—got crossed out. Most of the active advocacy for denying transgender people the right to live in peace as ourselves is coming from that quarter.

And I hoped that someone who had themselves experienced prejudice might be at least somewhat sensitive to what it is like to be a member of a marginalized demographic.

What that added up to was looking for female providers, middle-aged or younger, who were persons of color or were members of a non-Christian ethnic group. While not every provider I ended up with ticked all those boxes, they all ticked some of them. All of my initial choices proved to be at least polite and respectful of me as a human being without any noticeable signs of hostility or contempt. None of them misgendered me to my face, nor do I think they did so behind my back. The best of them took pains to address me as "Ms" and to refer to me using feminine pronouns even when they thought I couldn't hear them talking to other medical staff.

I assure you that we are listening. Most of us are terrified of being hurt, yet again.

And I have been. Recently.

I went in for a routine office follow-up for my well-controlled essential hypertension. The nurse practitioner I normally see was on maternity leave, so they scheduled me to see someone else. I expected a drama-free office visit with refills on my prescriptions and a referral for a test I think I need.

I was in the consulting room and heard my chart being taken off the door. After several seconds I heard the provider laugh. I know it says "transgender" on my chart. At that moment, I knew that this was not going to go well.

She came in and was obviously having difficulty not openly laughing at me. She addressed me with a sneer in her voice not as "Ms Kelly," but as "Laura," as if I were a dog or a child and not an elderly woman at least 30 years her senior. Despite the hurt I felt, I tried to be friendly and make conversation, to engage her as another human being, but she was having none of it. She made it clear that she didn't care in the slightest about what I was saying. Obviously someone like me wasn't worth listening to. I decided to do whatever I needed to do to get out of there with my prescription refills. She listened to my chest and said I ought to have a routine metabolic panel done.

She went back out into the hall and told someone, "He will have to come back for labs."

He.

Unless you are transgender yourself, you cannot possibly have any idea of the struggle and heartbreaking sacrifices, the discrimination, the loss of friends, and the realistic fear of deadly violence we live with in order not to wake up every day wishing we were dead. She knew I was trans and called me "he."

I got my prescriptions, went out to my car, and cried.

The test I think I need is a mammogram. (Yes, they're real.) I was not about to give that horrible woman an opportunity for a good belly laugh by raising *that* issue with her. Many of us avoid even necessary medical care because of our all-too-realistic fear of experiences like this. I think I have located another primary care provider who will treat me as a person and not as a joke. Every time one of us walks into the office of a new provider, we are terrified.

Please don't hurt us.

14.3 Rachael B. 66

I am a 66-year-old Vietnam veteran transgender woman who transitioned in 1991 and now describes herself as a woman first and as a transgender woman when I have to. Between that time and now, I have experienced many embarrassing moments in the healthcare field, some that have caused me to become a bit vocal.

Even though I am fortunate enough to "pass" as a genetic female with no problem now, there are a few continuing sources of embarrassment that I've had to endure during the years, most involving my physical history. I asked my doctor once to perform an internal exam on me because I hadn't had one for a while. She knew that I was transgender from previous discussions with me. After my request, she just looked at me and laughed, saying that she didn't think that I really needed one. I have a perfectly functioning vagina, and I am no more or less concerned about the condition of its tissues than any other woman. Yet, she obviously thought that my vagina wasn't "real enough" to warrant being examined. That was the last time I saw this doctor.

Other common sources of embarrassment are any procedures that require me to state when I went through menopause. When I answer that I never had periods, I'm then forced to explain to this complete stranger that I am transgender, so I never had a uterus. Sometimes that elicits a surprised side glance but other times I get silence. I'm not sure which is worse. In any case, it's always annoying to be forced to "out" myself. While I am in no way ashamed to state that I am transgender (I am proud to have had the strength to survive and finally become the person I always knew I was), it is still embarrassing each time I am forced to explain myself.

One of my visits to an emergency room, though, was particularly aggravating. I had been admitted for observation with a high fever and severe headaches and was sitting on a bed in a "room" created by curtains just outside the nurse's station. A nurse came in to ask me the normal preadmission medical questions so they could treat me. One of the questions she asked was when I went through menopause. When I answered that I was transgender and never had periods, she immediately stopped talking and just stared at me. She regained her composure after a few seconds and continued to ask the remaining questions. When she was finished, she walked out of my room and back over to the nurse's station where I could clearly hear her quietly laughing and telling the other nurses about "the thing" she had just talked to. Her scorn was obvious as was the delight she exhibited in telling her coworkers just what she thought of me.

I endured the laughter and ignorance for only a few minutes as my ire rose. I exited my room and walked directly to the nurse's station to confront them all. They suddenly got very quiet. I looked directly at them and said, "I can hear every word you're saying. I'm right there." I pointed over my shoulder to the curtained area. Continuing, I said, "If you're done having fun at my expense and would like to actually learn about the hell I've had to endure throughout my life that caused me to drastically change myself so I wouldn't have to commit suicide, I will be more than happy to explain that to you. All you have to do is come in, sit down, and talk to me. I will answer any and all questions you may have." I turned and walked back into my room. The nurse's station became deathly quiet.

Within a few minutes, the head nurse came in and took my vitals. Looking at me, she said, "Good for you, honey. You handled that well." Then she told me that, if I wanted, she'd have the offending nurse officially reprimanded for her actions. I told her that I didn't want anyone to get in trouble and that I thought what I had said directly to her – and to all of them – was embarrassing enough and hopefully taught her a lesson.

I had no more problems with the nurses after that.

14.4 Artwork by Johnny S. 66

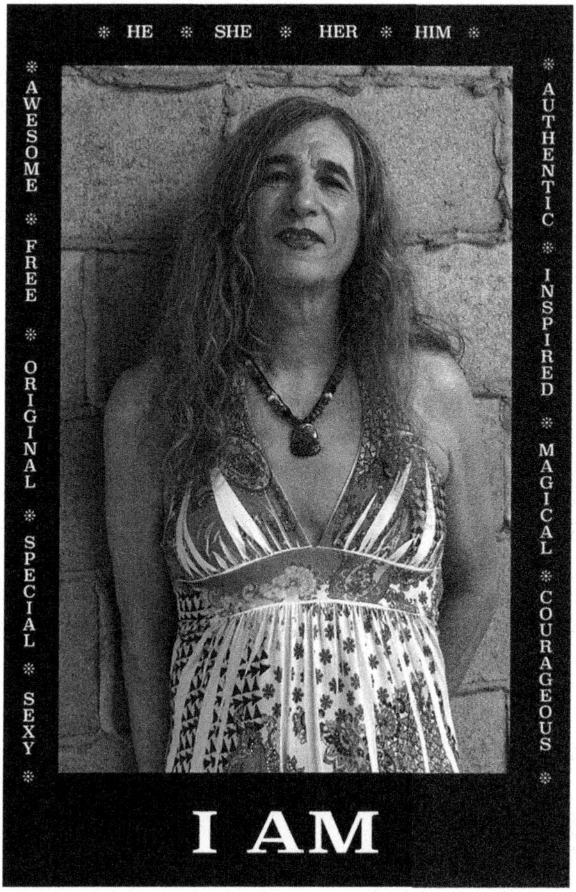

14.5 Estelle M. 66

My name is Estelle M., and I'm trans female and was born in England in 1951. To save you the math, I'm 66.

I was aware of the fact that I was female, even though outwardly I appeared male at the age of 5 years old. I used to secretly pray that I would wake up in the morning as a "normal" girl. By the time I reached 7 or 8, I knew that was not going to happen. It was apparent to me that at this time and place, it would not be healthy for me to tell anyone about how I felt. I went through a decade plus long, "man up" phase. I repressed what I knew and became depressed, developed poor self-esteem, and did poorly school due to learning issues.

Through life I had a number of failed relationship, due largely to what we now know as gender dysphoria.

I first tried to transition in the early to mid-50s. That ended when I met a woman and fell in love and tried to change how I felt with therapy. That did not work and yet again another relationship ended.

My life up until transition was living other people's idea of who I am.

My final attempt to transition started in November 2013 and was on HRT on 22 January 2014. I have had major positive changes to my psychology. I have a more positive outlook, have better mental focus, and have reached a place where I really like who I am.

From my standpoint my gender has not changed; only my presentation has. So in reality the term "transgender" does not work too well for me. I'm not becoming a woman; I am a woman. I'm removing the male facade. I don't have preferred pronouns; I have pronouns she/her. I don't identify as a woman; I'm a woman.

I have changed my name in the courts here in the USA and England. All my legal documents have my correct name and gender. I have been employed as a woman in a male-dominated profession, and my positive attitude has taken me far. This is all due to me living an authentic life. Authenticity should not be denied to anyone.

For me transition is about the truth and mental health. Howard Brown Health has been my health provider through my journey. They provide an informed consent model of healthcare which is excellent.

From my dialog with other trans women in the community, there is an amazing lack of knowledge among the medical fraternity as to the appropriate treatment for trans individuals. As to the dosage, method of ingress into the body, what is an appropriate hormone level. Such things as having older trans women on postmenopausal hormone levels. Some healthcare of trans women seems to border on malpractice.

There is a need for more studies of long-term HRT care. There is a wealth of information out there in the trans community if the research was undertaken.

14.6 Jesse H. 63

The way life is in the 21st century, seniors in just about any community rarely get asked for their venerable thoughts. Everything is youth-centered, and while I know that is important, I also know that when I was in my youth, I wasn't interested in knowing how old age would play out as a senior in the LGBT community.

I came out as **lesbian** in 1976. I spent all of those years politically active and a huge target for homophobes. I had a child and needed housing and employment. The way life was, I was struggling for both and repeatedly denied both, simply for being lesbian. Additionally, there were heterosexuals determined to take my daughter from me. This was based on the archaic belief that homosexuals were the scourge of the earth and harmful to children. I didn't transition because I wanted to be a man—I transitioned to survive. I didn't know how life would play out 32 years later.

I began transitioning in 1986. After the required 1 year minimum for counseling, I was allowed HRT in the form of testosterone and then required to live full time in my gender preference for a minimum of 6 months (1 year. preferred), and I had to get a job as a man. This was all prior to any surgeries. By today's practice, these requirements are considered absurd, but I do not agree. In retrospect, I believe a few of the "gatekeepers" had the right idea.

As a *trans person* in my 30s, I was terrified to go to seek medical attention, even though I have preexisting conditions that needed routine doctor's care. Not only were there no providers safe enough as a lesbian; there were no providers at all for trans medical issues. Transitioning was seriously underground. The computer was new, and the Internet didn't exist; networking by word of mouth was all I had. I've been made the laughingstock in an ER, while being passed around as if I were an exhibit. I recovered from my hysterectomy on a maternity ward. The staff refused to come to my assistance except when vital signs needed charting on each shift.

I began my experiences at the hands of the medical field as a lesbian woman, and I see both as separate topics. I continue my experience today as what the general public would call a trans male and expected to act like a traditional man. I must consider both sides of myself—male and female—while navigating the healthcare system. Generally speaking, it's easier today for many of the younger trans folks—different reasons, different climate. However, it's still not easy for me.

My world view and my political and moral views are still entirely lesbian. I don't identify as man or woman. I'm transgendered, not "transgender." I detest being asked my "pronoun preference" which is current language everywhere. I refuse to use the word "QUEER" to identify myself. I'm very put off by the political correctness of it all. I can't help but see life from a variety of sides and just about every point of view.

In *my* youth I could get in trouble just holding my girlfriend's hand in public. There were no "Hate Law" mandates or anti-discrimination laws. We were afraid to use the word "gay." "Transgender"? What's that? There was no gay pride of any kind.

All of these experiences are what color my perception—and reception—of the medical community as a whole. There are moments when my safety and well-being is completely looked after; the majority of the time is a nightmare in its truest form. Any major medical event (I've had many) is a unique source of stress that very few people can fathom. It's not just another routine clinic visit for me. I may present as irritable, aloof, defensive, and resistant to treatments. I have safety issues regarding body image. You may not want much to do with me because I'm so "crabby." Keep listening. Remember that my aging is your aging and we are all human.

I live the reality every day of being different in every way but one. We all get old, and our society doesn't like it very much. Respect and grace go a very long way.

14.7 Gina E. 61

In April of 2018, I stood before more than one hundred healthcare workers in the IU Health network to speak about my experience as a transgender woman. These doctors, nurses, and others covering every facet of the profession had just heard a presentation—essentially, Trans Ed 101—and I now was putting flesh on the facts.

Days from turning 61, I had recently completed the 5-year trek toward fully transitioning. It began when my wife, Julie, and I lived in rural Michigan. To find a capable therapist meant a drive of almost 2 h, both ways. When I was approved for HRT, a doctor would be equally as far away.

Addressing my gender dysphoria by transitioning meant I had to retire from my calling as a Lutheran minister. I left the world of traditional Christians who lived conservative lives to that of the trans community. E. T. was no more a stranger on this earth than I in my new world. The quality of my healthcare would be foundational to my success in transitioning.

Julie and I moved to Indianapolis. One does not think of Indiana as a bastion of hope for anyone who identifies with LGBTQ+. My first steps were taken with trepidation. Immediately, my concerns were allayed. I needed to engage a local therapist, and I found a woman with a lot of experience with trans clients. Next came an endocrinologist. With IU Health, I found a doctor who has for years treated transgender patients. These two provided me with a good start.

In the meantime, we had to do the usual things—find a dentist, primary care physician, and eye doctor. I was still legally Greg, so I would step directly into each situation and explain whom I was, a male early in transitioning to female. No one blinked. Everyone received me with grace.

As I transitioned, this old body kept falling apart. Our first 3 years in Indy saw me at specialists to have a root canal, a detached retina repaired, a podiatrist to examine my once surgically repaired toe, a cardiologist because I had received two stents when I turned 50, and a different specialist to address a cataract. Mixed in were the scheduling of my transition surgeries, all which I had in 2017, as I turned 60: vocal fold reduction to raise my voice pitch, gender-affirming surgery, and facial feminization and breast implants.

I pretty much have run the gamut of doctors, and I was able to do every bit of transitioning right in Indianapolis. Every experience was almost totally positive. Only one area stands out as a negative. It is a common problem for trans folks: name and pronouns.

I don't pass as a genetic woman. I have found that a person can dress feminine, wear appropriate makeup, and have a big and colorful purse, and if that person still speaks in a manner which is typical of men, even if your name is Gina, you will be gendered male.

When it kept happening, I began asking why. I always received the same answer. "It's your voice." I retorted, "But look how I am dressed, and my name is Gina." And every time the reply came back, "But you sound like a man, so it's natural to think of you as a he." I was learning. I gently corrected, asking them to take care as they referred to me.

I had one other hurdle to jump, the legal changing of my name. Before I achieved that, I had to give my male name. I would ask them to record that I go by Gina. In most cases, they had a way to officially note that, and I was called Gina without fail at those places.

At one place, they were not so up to speed. The woman wrote my preferred name, very largely, at the top of my record. Yet, when sitting among a dozen people in the waiting room, the nurse called for Gregory E. I had to rise and walk to her, all eyes glued on me. I confidently said, "It's Gina."

My trans friends report the same two bugaboos, being wrongly named and incorrect pronouns. Even when everything else about a doctor's appointment goes well, these smart. Ours is a treacherous path to achieving wholeness of being. Our name is as important to us as every person's is.

Ultimately, my experience taught me that we trans folks want nothing more than, or different from, the rest of the population. We long to be addressed with respect, to be taken seriously, and to be treated well.

At that Trans Ed 101 session, my endocrinologist stated that IU Health is behind in formalizing its transgender healthcare. Yet, I was able to stand before that throng of professionals and commend them. At every stop I have made in this city, from the moment I have walked into a doctor's office or hospital, to the reception folks, to the nurses and technicians, and to the doctors, I have been provided their best care and treated with dignity.

No matter our age, we trans persons only want to be treated like everyone else. Because, truly, we are humans in every way as everyone else.

14.8 Artwork by Jolie T.

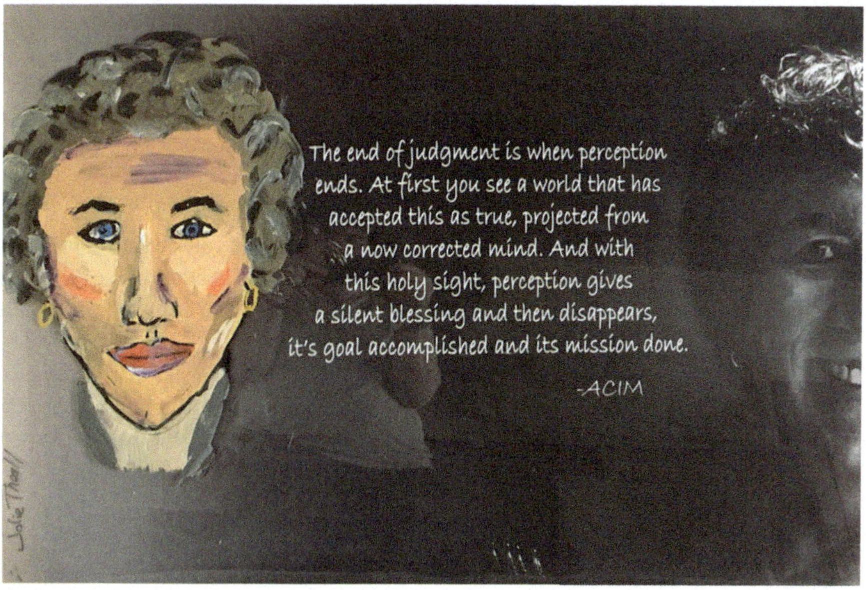
The end of judgment is when perception
ends. At first you see a world that has
accepted this as true, projected from
a now corrected mind. And with
this holy sight, perception gives
a silent blessing and then disappears,
it's goal accomplished and its mission done.
-ACIM
Jolie Thall

14.9 Stefanie C. 73

I was a closeted cross-dressing trans lesbian for 68 years. I knew I was different from age 3 (questioning). When I was 12, I was caught by my mother in her lingerie. In the 1950s, there were only two terms people used: transvestite and transsexual. By the time I went away to college, I knew I was cross-dresser. I dated girls, but liked to "be with" girls. I married a girl in college. We were married for 44 years, have three children and four grandchildren. I told my wife about my cross-dressing urges after we were married. (That is another complete story for another discussion). She did not support the dressing; but we had a good marriage. But I now knew I was a cross-dressing lesbian.

After my wife's death in 2011, I came out and began my journey toward womanhood. I was visible but not out. The first thing I felt I had to do was express myself to my PCP to make sure I was getting the appropriate medical care, so I went to my appointment modestly dressed. No shock! For the next 3 years, I was visible in a very Republican community.

In 2015, after the death of my 102-year-old stepfather, my life's journey changed at an accelerated pace:

I purchased a condo on the Lake in Chicago.
Moved to Chicago.
Became extremely visible in my new community.
Commenced my transition.

Prior to 2015, the regulations concerning transition and legal documents required extensive mental health consultation at a significant cost. Many states required sex reassignment surgery prior to changing a persons' gender marker. Without sex reassignment surgery, you couldn't get a permanent passport so when traveling you were immediately identified as less than a female person. All these requirements presented financial barriers in addition to the medical standards that resulted in time constraints, which emotionally prevent people from obtaining peace of mind and emotional well-being.

This began my journey, thanks to President Obama's Executive Order, the LGBT community became the beneficiary of many more liberalized rules relating to sexuality and marriage. Government forms required for name and gender marker change, passports applications, social security, and the related Medicare applications which feed private health insurance systems; all were rendered obsolete.

The new rules are based upon "informed consent," and a very simple statement, from a Qualified and State Licensed Professional, that the applicant had undergone the "appropriate level of treatment." There was not even a requirement to set forth a treatment plan. Howard Brown was instrumental in helping me understand the concept of "informed consent" and its implementation.

Now, this 73-year-old "closeted" cross-dresser is creating forms that will attempt to change how a person navigates through a morass of bureaucracy. I looked at previous forms to determine past protocol and cut and pasted to fit my perceived needs. With my forms in hand, I set out to achieve and make an "informed consent."

The Center on Halsted helped me to understand the difference between "Gender Presentation and Sexuality." There was extensive consultation which enabled me to understand what it means to be and live as a woman. This process took a total of 5 ½ months. The medical changes, consisting primarily of hormone replacement therapy, commenced in the next month.

The filing process with the State Superior Court is approximately a 5-week process, similar to a married lady wishing to change her name. I had to make an application, publish the name change in an official advertisement, and schedule a court date. The actual time before the Judge was about 10 minutes. After showing proof of who I "was" and an administrative review (just checking the boxes), I received my "Paper Please."

Armed with my new ID and Medicare Card, I began my quest to obtain individual health insurance in Cook County. I have been utilizing Medicare Advantage to obtain my healthcare for 8 years.

Selecting a new PCP presented its own challenge. At a follow-up visit to my newly selected PCP, he, a gay married male doctor, observed that I was one of the most well-adjusted trans woman that he had seen. With pride, I asked: "Why?" "Oh," he said, "Most trans people are dead by the time they are fifty." Suicide, AIDS, murder, 2/3 pay for equal work, and I happily volunteered for this assignment.

Now at 73, I realize I have much to accomplish, with the potential of so little time. People say that I am moving too fast. My response is: "Starting at age 68, I am not moving fast enough"

I began speaking at Chicago City Colleges, universities, and senior centers about the additional challenges relating to LGBT seniors accessing medical care. One year later, I had to modify my presentation from a theoretical basis to actual experience.

Time and finances allowed me to elect to have knee replacement surgery, a procedure I had put off for 50 years. As I was packing my pink nightie, I began to fear for discrimination upon admission to the hospital. Not all hospitals are welcoming to the trans community. Using independent resources, I chose a welcoming institution, which provides semiprivate rooms without a roommate, census allowing. This removed the fear of rejection from a roommate. I still had an unfounded fear from the staff.

The facility didn't just put a "rainbow flag" on their door but demonstrated by their welcoming actions.

Preferred pronouns are very important to the trans community. During the 2-week stay in the hospital and rehab, I was only misgendered one time.

I try to use my life experiences as educational moments. There was one instance when there was an unasked question, centered around a bed pan. My response was that with a trans person, you never know about a trans person, "until you look under the hood."

I love my life. I try to share my experiences. I continue to expand my visibility.

I have traveled alone throughout Europe since transitioning. The acceptance has been gratifying.

"Just remember the light at the end of the tunnel does not have to be a train but God's female smile welcoming you into her new world."

14.10 Cornelia K. 56

Editor's note: Cornelia is German and submitted two versions of her narrative to us, in German and English. Her German narrative is as written; her English translation has had some minor edits for clarity, shown in italics.

14.10.1 Transsexualität und Alter

Mit 56 Jahren arbeite ich seit 24 Jahren als leitende Psychologin in einem Unternehmen der Suchtkrankenhilfe. Wir betreiben mehrere Kliniken und zahlreiche Beratungsstellen. Im Alter von 23 Jahren habe ich meine Transition begonnen und wurde ein Jahr später operiert. Seit 32 Jahren lebe ich in meinem Geschlecht, davon die meiste Zeit stealth.

Während der Transition musste meine Ehe wegen der geltenden Gesetze (TSG) beendet werden. Aus der Ehe habe ich zwei Kinder und mittlerweile 3 Enkelkinder.

Nach einem Zwangsouting durch meine Tochter gegenüber meinem heutigen Ehemann, habe ich im Alter von 54 Jahren wieder geheiratet und wir haben ein Pflegekind aufgenommen.

In den 80er Jahren war die Gruppe der Transsexuellen noch klein und diejenigen, die den ganzen Weg gingen waren noch weniger. Die Szene war geprägt durch die Frauen (amab). Deshalb ist die Gruppe der älteren Transsexuellen klein, deren Transition schon lange zurückliegt. Viele leben stealth und wollen keinen Kontakt zur Szene mehr. Unter den Älteren sind heute vor allem spät transitionierende Menschen öffentlich wahrnehmbar. Diese bringen die gesundheitlichen Themen mit, die für alle Transsexuelle am Anfang ihres Weges stehen.

14.10.2 Körper

Obwohl es heute möglich ist, wird den meisten Transsexuellen viel zu spät geholfen und sie müssen ihre Pubertät beenden. Zu meiner Zeit war eine Hilfe vor der Pubertät undenkbar und zu den lebenslangen Folgen gehören Dysphorien. Sie beziehen sich auf Körpergröße und –proportionen, Gesicht, Haare und Stimme. Da solche Phänomene für Frauen typisch sind, lassen sie sich im Rahmen von Selbstwahrnehmungsgruppen mit anderen (Cis)Frauen gut bearbeiten. Ganz verschwinden werden sie wohl nie. Die genitalangleichende Operation hat mein transsexuelles Wahrnehmen wirkungsvoll und endgültig beendet.

Der Bart wurde mit elektrischer Nadelepilation entfernt. Eine sehr schmerzhafte und langwierige Prozedur. Da ich stealth lebte, konnte ich die Termine nur in größeren Abständen machen, da das Gesicht sehr anschwoll und der Bart eine Mindestlänge brauchte. Die Krankenkasse versagte schließlich die Kostenzusage und ich muss mit den Bartresten bis heute leben.

Mit 22 Jahren bin ich an zwei Ärzte geraten, die mir die Transsexualität wegtherapieren wollten. Dass ich mich zwei Mal versuchte zu Suizidieren, hat seine

Ursache in dem schweren Trauma der Konversionstherapie. Jede Art von nicht-unterstützenden Behandlungsmaßnahmen gehören verboten.

Erst nachdem ich diese Ärzte gewechselt hatte, bekam ich Hilfe und zum ersten Mal Hormone. Für mich ist die lebenslange Hormoneinnahme mit diesem Trauma verbunden. Hormone sind für mich die Erlaubnis zu leben und diese Erlaubnis muss ich mir regelmäßig im Jahr neu holen. Das führt mich fast immer an die Grenze zur Retraumatisierung.

Meine Sexualität habe ich erst im Alter entdeckt. Da ich mit einer Frau Kinder hatte, ging ich davon aus, dass ich nach der Operation weiter mit Frauen Sex haben würde und habe auch zwei längere lesbische Beziehungen gehabt. Mein Körper hatte aber kein Interesse an Sex. Das erklärte ich mit der traumatischen Transition und das mein Interesse an Sex immer eher gering war. Erst mit meinem Mann entdeckte ich zu meinem großen Erstaunen, dass mein Körper heterosexuell war. Ich finde Frauen nach wie vor attraktiv, habe aber gerne Sex mit meinem Mann.

Den Abschnitt Körper möchte ich damit abschließen, dass alt werden mit Transsexualität etwas ganz Normales hat. So habe ich eine Osteokleose von meiner Großmutter geerbt und sie kam unter dem Einfluss von Östrogenen zum Ausbruch. Weil sie nur die Frauen in meiner Familie befällt, wird sie für mich immer ein wunderbarer Beweis für meine biologische, weil genetische, Weiblichkeit jenseits von XY-Chromosomen sein.

14.10.3 Psyche

Transsexualität ist ein Generationenthema, sofern Kinder vorhanden sind. Kinder erleben ähnliche Diskriminierungen, wir ihre transsexuellen Eltern. Sie müssen sich mit dem Thema Outing auseinandersetzen und das setzt sich in die folgende Enkelgeneration fort. Für mich selber habe ich mein ganzes Leben ein und dasselbe Geschlecht, meine Angehörigen haben das als Geschlechtswechsel erlebt. Für mich sind die Begriffe Vater, Mutter, Großvater und Großmutter schwer zu fassen, für meine Kinder und Enkel ebenfalls. Es gibt also weitere Betroffene und andere Perspektiven.

Die Gesetze verlangen die Ehescheidung und die genitalangleichende Operation als Voraussetzung für die Vornamens- und Personenstandsänderung. Deshalb wurde meine Familie von Staats wegen zerstört und die Folgen ziehen sich mittlerweile in die dritte Generation. Vornamens- und Personenstandsänderungen sollten bei allen Institutionen auf Antrag unbürokratisch möglich sein. Allein das kann großes Leid bei Unbeteiligten und völlig unschuldigen Kindern verhindern.

Obwohl das Offenbahrungsverbot für Transsexuelle gilt, bin ich immer wieder zu Outings gezwungen. Vor allem in behördlichen Kontext werden alle Beteiligten in völlig unnötige und peinliche Situationen gezwungen. Für die Ehe war eine Abstammungsurkunde notwendig, die alle Änderungen enthielt. Bei jeder Rentenberatung ist ebenfalls eine Offenlegung meiner Lebensgeschichte notwendig. Menschen wie ich sind häufig in gesellschaftlichen Strukturen nicht vorgesehen.

Mein ganzes Leben lang wollte ich nicht transsexuell sein. Ich habe in meinen jungen Jahren wirklich alles versucht, um ein Mann zu sein. Als ich endlich verstanden habe, wer ich bin, wollte ich den Fehler „Mann“ ungeschehen machen. Ich habe immer mit der Angst des Outings gelebt. Viele meiner Lebensentscheidungen habe ich dieser Frage untergeordnet. Meine politische und berufliche Kariere habe ich bewusst begrenzt, weil ich keinem Menschen aus meiner Vergangenheit begegnen wollte. Die Bedeutung dieser Entscheidung bekam ich zu spüren, als ich trotzdem wegen meiner Transsexualität erpresst wurde. Mich hat das stealth leben von den Menschen in meinem engeren Umfeld entfernt. Am deutlichsten wurde es mit meinem Mann, dem ich 20 Jahre lang nichts über meine Transsexualität sagen konnte. Erst nach meinem Outing konnte ich Nähe zu ihm zulassen. Folglich verstehe ich meine dysphorischen Phasen im Alter als internalisierte Transphobie. Daraus den Umkehrschluss zu ziehen, wenn erst die Transphobie beseitigt ist, hätte ich mit meinem Körper leben können, ist falsch. Für mich ist es ganz einfach, wenn ich nicht als Frau leben kann, bin ich tot.

Dabei ist mein Leben am leichtesten und fühlt sich am richtigsten an, wenn ich einfach nur die Frau sein kann, die ich bin. Dass ich mein Leben der Hilfe anderer Menschen gewidmet habe, hat viel mit der Dankbarkeit zu tun, die ich gegenüber dieser Gesellschaft empfinde, die es mir gestattet hat, als Frau zu leben.

Mit freundlichen Grüßen.

14.10.4 Transsexuality and Age

For 24 years I *have been* working as a leading psychologist for a company which aids addicted people. We have several clinics and many counseling centers. I am now 56 years old and looking back at my transition *which began* when I was just 23. *Only* 1 year later, I had my gender-confirming surgery (GCS). Since then, I am living in my gender as a woman, most of the time stealth. Before my transition I was married, but due to the law effective back then, I had to divorce. From this marriage sprung two children and now three grandchildren. After I *was* outed by my daughter to my current husband, I married again 2 years ago when I was 54. We took in a foster child.

During the 1980s there weren't many transgender people to be found and those who went all the way like me, even fewer. The scene was dominated by women (amab). Thus the group of older transsexuals who transitioned a long time ago is very small. Many want to live stealth and have no more contact to the scene. Among older transgender *people*, *current* society finds mostly those who *have* transitioned *later* in life. They bring along health issues which mark the beginning of transition for all transsexuals.

14.10.5 Body

Even though *it is* possible nowadays, most people with a transgender identity receive medical help far too late and thus have to *transition after they* finish puberty. During my *younger* days, help during prepuberty was unthinkable, and dysphoria *was* part of the lifelong consequences. We are talking body size and proportions, face, hair, and voice. Since those phenomena are typical for women, they can be worked out well with cis-women in self-perception groups. Still, they never disappear completely. Gender confirmation surgery effectively and definitely ended my transsexual perception.

My beard was removed by electric needle epilation which is a very painful and lengthy procedure. Since I lived stealth, I wasn't able to continuously have my appointments but only every once in a while. *The main* reasons were the facial swelling, and the beard hairs had *to be* a certain length. The health insurance didn't want to pay *for* the procedure, and I have to live with the remains of this until today.

When I was 22, I encountered two doctors who wanted to cure my transsexualism. The fact *that* I tried to commit suicide twice was due to the severe trauma of their conversion therapy. Any kind of non-supportive therapy should be prohibited. Only after I changed doctors *was* I finally *able to* receive help and, for the first time, hormones. Personally, lifelong use of hormones is associated with trauma. Hormones are my permission to live. I have to get permission regularly, four times a year. Asking for this permission always leads me to the brink of retraumatization.

Only at my advanced age *did* I discover sexuality. Since I had children with a woman, I thought after surgery I would continue having sex with women. I did have two lesbian *relationships*, but my body wasn't interested in sex. I tried to explain this with my traumatic transition and my generally *low* interest in sex. Only with my husband *did* I discover to my big astonishment that I was heterosexual. I still find women attractive but I enjoy having sex with my husband.

I would like to conclude the section *on the* body with the fact that getting old being transsexual is totally normal. I inherited osteosclerosis from my grandmother, and the outbreak started due to my intake of estrogen. Since it only happens to the women in my family, it is always a wonderful proof of my biological *(because of my genes)* femininity beyond *my* XY chromosomes.

14.10.6 Psyche

Transsexualism involves several generations if children are part of the family. Children experience similar discrimination as their transsexual parents. They too have to deal with outing, and this continues into the next generation of grandchildren. For me personally, I have lived my whole life in the same gender, but for my family, it has been a gender change. It is difficult for me to grasp the terms of father, mother, grandfather, and grandmother, as well as for my children and grandchildren. So there are other sufferers and *other* perspectives.

Laws enforce divorce and gender-conforming surgery for a legal name and gender change. Thus my family *name* was destroyed by the state, and the consequences have now reached the third generation.

Name and gender change should be *as easy as* possible without the use of bureaucracy. That alone could prevent lots of suffering of innocent children and those watching from the sidelines. Even so, prohibition of disclosure includes transsexual persons; I have to out myself continuously. Especially in situations involving public authority, everyone involved *is* forced to go through unnecessary and awkward situations. For my wedding, I had to produce a genealogical certificate which included all changes. Each time I need advice from my pension fund, I have to tell my life history. People like me are seldom included in social structures.

I didn't want to be transsexual at all. When I was young, I tried hard to be a man. Once I understood who I was, I wanted to make the mistake *of "being a man" disappear*. I have always lived with the fear of outing myself. Many of my life decisions I subordinated to this question. I restricted my political and professional career consciously because I didn't want to encounter *anyone from* my past. The significance of this decision I found out when I was blackmailed because of my transsexualism.

Living stealth has detached me from people close to me. *The* most significant example was my husband whom I couldn't tell anything about my transsexuality for 20 years. Only after my forced outing was I able to let closeness happen. Hence I understand my dysphoric phases at this stage as internalized transphobia. To construct a reverse conclusion, *that* if this transphobia would be eliminated, I could have lived with my body, is wrong. For me it is *really* easy, if I can't live as a woman, I am dead.

At the same time, my life is easiest and *right* if I simply can be the woman I am. *The fact* that I devoted my life to help other people has a lot to do with my gratitude *to* the society which permits me to live as a woman.

Index

M. Houlberg et al. (eds.), *Transgender and Gender Nonconforming Health and Aging*,
https://doi.org/10.1007/978-3-319-95031-0

H

I

K